# Updates on Pediatric Health and Diseases

# (*Volume 2*)

# Common Pediatric Diseases: Current Challenges

Edited by

**Nima Rezaei & Noosha Samieefar**
*Network of Interdisciplinarity in Neonates and Infants (NINI)*
*Universal Scientific Education and Research Network*
*(USERN)*
*Tehran, Iran*

# Updates on Pediatric Health and Diseases

*Volume # 2*

*Common Pediatric Diseases: Current Challenges*

Editors: Nima Rezaei & Noosha Samieefar

ISSN (Online): 2972-4449

ISSN (Print): 2972-4430

ISBN (Online): 978-981-5124-18-7

ISBN (Print): 978-981-5124-19-4

ISBN (Paperback): 978-981-5124-20-0

need for a court order if at any point you breach any terms of this License Agreement. In no event will any delay or failure by Bentham Science Publishers in enforcing your compliance with this License Agreement constitute a waiver of any of its rights.

3. You acknowledge that you have read this License Agreement, and agree to be bound by its terms and conditions. To the extent that any other terms and conditions presented on any website of Bentham Science Publishers conflict with, or are inconsistent with, the terms and conditions set out in this License Agreement, you acknowledge that the terms and conditions set out in this License Agreement shall prevail.

**Bentham Science Publishers Pte. Ltd.**
80 Robinson Road #02-00
Singapore 068898
Singapore
Email: subscriptions@benthamscience.net

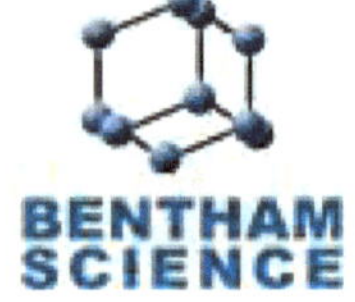

# CONTENTS

# PREFACE

Seeing the world through the eyes of a child/infant sounds inspirational. They are little, lovely and defenseless. Pediatrics is the science of taking care of these cute creations. Pediatrics is a branch of medicine that focuses on the diagnosis and treatment of infants, children and adolescents diseases. As medical sciences are getting more complex with the information explosion, interdisciplinarity is an essential tool to integrate different topics. Therefore, we established an interest group, titled "Network of Interdisciplinarity in Neonates and Infants (NINI)" in the Universal Scientific Education and Research Network (USERN), and invited pediatricians and scientists in the field of pediatrics from all over the world to join this multidisciplinary network: https://usern.tums.ac.ir/Group/Info/NINI

The "Updates on Pediatric Health and Disease" is a comprehensive series of books on infant and adolescent health and diseases. The series features volumes that update readers on the current understanding of basic information and advanced clinical practice in pediatric medicine. Neonatology, as well as different diseases in all subspecialties of pediatrics, including allergy and immunology, cardiology, endocrinology, gastroenterology, hematology, infectious diseases, nephrology, oncology, pulmonology, rheumatology, neurology, psychiatry and dermatology, are represented in each volume.

"Common Pediatric Diseases: Current Challenges" is the second volume of this book series. The first chapter of this book is a rapid introduction to challenges in the field of pediatrics and child health (Chapter 1). The second chapter discusses the positive and negative outcomes of sexting (Chapter 2). Chapter 3 takes a specific view of integrated care of children with neurodevelopmental disorders. The book contains chapters on the influence of non-genetic transgenerational inheritance on children and adolescents' development (Chapter 4) and the approach to pediatric genetic epilepsy (Chapter 5). The medical and social outcomes of cardiac diseases are also discussed (Chapter 6). In addition, the book provides updates on meconium-stained newborns (Chapter 7), transient tachypnea of newborns (Chapter 8) and fetal tumors (Chapter 9). Chapter 10 focuses on Autism Spectrum Disorder during infancy and its early symptoms. Last but not least, medical futility controversies and end-of-life care are discussed in Chapter 11.

The book **"Updates on Pediatric Health and Diseases"** is the result of the valuable contribution of scientists and clinicians from well-known universities/institutes worldwide. I would like to hereby acknowledge the expertise of all contributors, for generously devoting their time and considerable effort in preparing their respective chapters. I would also like to express my gratitude to the Bentham Science publication for providing me with the opportunity to publish the book.

Finally, I hope that this timely book will be comprehensible, cogent, and of special value for researchers and pediatricians who wish to extend their knowledge on pediatric challenges.

**Nima Rezaei & Noosha Samieefar**
Network of Interdisciplinarity in Neonates and Infants (NINI)
Universal Scientific Education and Research Network (USERN)
Tehran, Iran

# ACKNOWLEDGEMENT

I would like to express my gratitude to the Editorial Assistant of this book, Dr. Noosha Samieefar. With no doubt, the book would not have been completed without her contribution.

**Nima Rezaei**
Network of Interdisciplinarity in Neonates and Infants (NINI)
Universal Scientific Education and Research Network (USERN)
Tehran, Iran

# DEDICATION

This book would not have been possible without the continuous encouragement of my family.

I wish to dedicate it to my daughters, Ariana and Arnika, with the hope that we learn enough from today to make a brighter future for the next generation.

**Nima Rezaei**
Network of Interdisciplinarity in Neonates and Infants (NINI)
Universal Scientific Education and Research Network (USERN)
Tehran, Iran

# List of Contributors

| | |
|---|---|
| **Ardeshir Khorsand** | Department of Oral and Maxillofacial Surgery, School of Dentistry, Shahid Beheshti University of Medical Sciences, Tehran, Iran<br>USERN Office, Shahid Beheshti University of Medical Sciences, Tehran, Iran<br>Network of Interdisciplinarity in Neonates and Infants (NINI), Universal Scientific Education and Research Network (USERN), Tehran, Iran |
| **Azar Ghasemi** | USERN Office, Shahid Beheshti University of Medical Sciences, Tehran, Iran<br>USERN Office, Kermanshah University of Medical Sciences, Kermanshah, Iran |
| **Behnaz Moradi** | Department of Radiology, Advanced Diagnostic and Interventional Radiology Research Center (ADIR), Medical Imaging Center, Imam Khomeini Hospital Complex, Tehran University of Medical Sciences, Tehran, Iran<br>Research Center for Immunodeficiencies, Children's Medical Center, Tehran University of Medical Sciences, Tehran, Iran |
| **Cheryl E. Sanders** | Metropolitan State University of Denver, Denver, Colorado 55106, USA |
| **Cornelius Ani** | Division of Psychiatry, Imperial College London, and Consultant Child and Adolescent Psychiatrist, Surrey and Borders Partnership NHS Foundation Trust, Surrey, UK |
| **Delaram J. Ghadimi** | School of Medicine, Shahid Beheshti University of Medical Sciences, Tehran, Iran<br>USERN Office, Shahid Beheshti University of Medical Sciences, Tehran, Iran<br>Network of Interdisciplinarity in Neonates and Infants (NINI), Universal Scientific Education and Research Network (USERN), Tehran, Iran |
| **Elham Pourbakhtyaran** | Department of Pediatric Neurology, Children's Medical Center, Tehran University of Medical Sciences, Tehran, Iran<br>USERN Office, Shahid Beheshti University of Medical Sciences, Tehran, Iran<br>Network of Interdisciplinarity in Neonates and Infants (NINI), Universal Scientific Education and Research Network (USERN), Tehran, Iran |
| **Elizabeth Englander** | Bridgewater State University, Bridgewater, Massachusetts 02325, USA |
| **Fateme Heydari** | School of Medicine, Shahid Beheshti University of Medical Sciences, Tehran, Iran<br>USERN Office, Shahid Beheshti University of Medical Sciences, Tehran, Iran<br>Network of Interdisciplinarity in Neonates and Infants (NINI), Universal Scientific Education and Research Network (USERN), Tehran, Iran |
| **Fahri Ovalı** | Istanbul Medeniyet University, Faculty of Medicine, Department of Pediatrics, Division of Neonatology, Neonatal Intensive Care Unit, Göztepe Education and Traning Hospital, Kadıköy- Istanbul, Turkey |

**Farbod Ghobadinezhad**

USERN Office, Shahid Beheshti University of Medical Sciences, Tehran, Iran
Network of Interdisciplinarity in Neonates and Infants (NINI), Universal Scientific Education and Research Network (USERN), Tehran, Iran
USERN Office, Kermanshah University of Medical Sciences, Kermanshah, Iran

**Fortune A. Ujunwa**

College of Medicine, Department of Pediatrics, University of Nigeria Teaching Hospital (UNTH), Ituku- Ozalla, Enugu State, Nigeria

**Forough Jabbari**

Department of Gynecology, Yas Women's Hospital, Tehran University of Medical Sciences, Tehran, Iran

**Hani F. Ayyash**

Paediatrics Department, Southend University Hospital NHS Foundation Trust, Southend, UK

**Jean Golding**

Centre for Academic Child Health, Population Health Sciences, Bristol Medical School, University of Bristol, Oakfield House, Oakfield Grove, Bristol BS8 2BN, UK

**Josephat M. Chinawa**

College of Medicine, Department of Pediatrics, University of Nigeria Teaching Hospital (UNTH), tuku-Ozalla, Enugu State, Nigeria

**Katalin Parti**

Department of Sociology, Virginia Tech University, Blacksburg, VA 24061, USA

**Kimia Kazemzadeh**

Students' Scientific Research Center, Tehran University of Medical Sciences, Tehran, Iran
Network of Immunity in Infection, Malignancy and Autoimmunity (NIIMA), Universal Scientific Education and Research Network (USERN), Tehran, Iran

**Mario Mastrangelo**

Department of Maternal, Infantile, and Urological Sciences, Sapienza University of Rome, Rome, Italy
Child Neurology and Psychiatry Unit, Department of Neurosciences/Mental Health, Azienda Ospedaliero-Universitaria Policlinico Umberto I, Rome, Italy

**Michael Ogundele**

Consultant Neurodevelopmental Paediatrician, Halton Community Paediatrics Unit, Bridgewater Community Healthcare NHS Foundation, Trust, Runcorn, UK

**Mohammad Moonis Akbar Faridi**

Era's Lucknow Medical College, Era University, Lucknow, India

**Nazanin Taraghikhah**

Network of Immunity in Infection, Malignancy and Autoimmunity (NIIMA), Universal Scientific Education and Research Network (USERN), Tehran, Iran

**Nima Rezaei**

Network of Interdisciplinarity in Neonates and Infants (NINI), Universal Scientific Education and Research Network (USERN), Tehran, Iran
Research Center for Immunodeficiencies, Pediatrics Center of Excellence, Children's Medical Center, Tehran University of Medical Sciences, Tehran, Iran
Department of Immunology, School of Medicine, Tehran University of Medical Sciences, Tehran, Iran

**Noosha Samieefar**  
School of Medicine, Shahid Beheshti University of Medical Sciences, Tehran, Iran  
USERN Office, Shahid Beheshti University of Medical Sciences, Tehran, Iran  
Network of Interdisciplinarity in Neonates and Infants (NINI), Universal Scientific Education and Research Network (USERN), Tehran, Iran

**Parnian Jabbari**  
Network of Immunity in Infection, Malignancy and Autoimmunity (NIIMA), Universal Scientific Education and Research Network (USERN), Tehran, Iran  
Department of Radiology, Yas Women's Hospital, Tehran University of Medical Sciences, Tehran, Iran

**Parnian Shobeiri**  
Network of Immunity in Infection, Malignancy and Autoimmunity (NIIMA), Universal Scientific Education and Research Network (USERN), Tehran, Iran  
School of Medicine, Tehran University of Medical Sciences, Tehran, Iran  
Center for Affective, Stress and Sleep Disorders, Psychiatric Clinics of the University of Basel, Basel, Switzerland

**Sara Zibadi**  
School of Medicine, Shahid Beheshti University of Medical Sciences, Tehran, Iran  
USERN Office, Shahid Beheshti University of Medical Sciences, Tehran, Iran  
Network of Interdisciplinarity in Neonates and Infants (NINI), Universal Scientific Education and Research Network (USERN), Tehran, Iran

**Serge Brand**  
Network of Immunity in Infection, Malignancy and Autoimmunity (NIIMA), Universal Scientific Education and Research Network (USERN), Tehran, Iran  
School of Medicine, Tehran University of Medical Sciences, Tehran, Iran  
Center for Affective, Stress and Sleep Disorders, Psychiatric Clinics of the University of Basel, Basel, Switzerland

**Soroush Khojasteh-Kaffash**  
Student Research Committee, School of Medicine, Birjand University of Medical Sciences, Birjand, Iran  
USERN Office, Shahid Beheshti University of Medical Sciences, Tehran, Iran  
Network of Interdisciplinarity in Neonates and Infants (NINI), Universal Scientific Education and Research Network (USERN), Tehran, Iran

**Sumaiya Shamsi**  
Era's Lucknow Medical College, Era University, Lucknow, India

**Yasmin Iles-Caven**  
Centre for Academic Child Health, Population Health Sciences, Bristol Medical School, University of Bristol, Oakfield House, Oakfield Grove, Bristol BS8 2BN, UK

**Zahra Mohajer**  
USERN Office, Shahid Beheshti University of Medical Sciences, Tehran, Iran  
Network of Interdisciplinarity in Neonates and Infants (NINI), Universal Scientific Education and Research Network (USERN), Tehran, Iran

**Zahra Hosseini Bajestani**  Student Research Committee, Mazandaran University of Medical Sciences, Sari, Iran
USERN Office, Mazandaran University of Medical Sciences, Sari, Iran
Network of Interdisciplinarity in Neonates and Infants (NINI), Universal Scientific Education and Research Network (USERN), Tehran, Iran

CHAPTER 1

# Introduction of Challenges with Pediatric Diseases

**Noosha Samieefar**[1,2,3], **Delaram J. Ghadimi**[1,2,3], **Sara Zibadi**[1,2,3], **Fateme Heydari**[1,2,3], **Elham Pourbakhtyaran**[2,3,4] **and Nima Rezaei**[3,5,6,*]

*[1] School of Medicine, Shahid Beheshti University of Medical Sciences, Tehran, Iran*

*[2] USERN Office, Shahid Beheshti University of Medical Sciences, Tehran, Iran*

*[3] Network of Interdisciplinarity in Neonates and Infants (NINI), Universal Scientific Education and Research Network (USERN), Tehran, Iran*

*[4] Department of Pediatric Neurology, Children's Medical Center, Tehran University of Medical Sciences, Tehran, Iran*

*[5] Department of Immunology, School of Medicine, Tehran University of Medical Sciences, Tehran, Iran*

*[6] Research Center for Immunodeficiencies, Children's Medical Center, Tehran University of Medical Sciences, Tehran, Iran*

**Abstract:** Children and the knowledge of taking care of them, pediatrics, are faced with growing challenges. With the advancement of medical sciences, pediatrics is becoming a group of subspecialties. This could lead to improving the care and management of pediatric disorders, however, transdisciplinary management should not be ignored.

Although the health status of children has improved over the past years, still preventable child deaths are occurring, especially in low-income countries. The increased sexual abuse, discrimination, racism, increased intercountry adoption, malnutrition, environmental hazards like arsenic contamination, pornography, and surrogacy are among the most important current challenges to children's health. Worldwide vaccination coverage has declined from 86% in 2019 to 83% in 2020, and the number of completely unvaccinated children increased by 3.4 million. Approximately, 1 billion children are dealing with multidimensional poverty all around the world among which at least 356 million of them live in extreme poverty, and 100 million more children plunged into poverty as a result of COVID-19.

In this chapter, we will review the most important challenges of children's health and pediatrics with a focus on social and mental health problems.

*Corresponding author Nima Rezaei:* Research Center for Immunodeficiencies, Children's Medical Center Hospital, Dr. Qarib St, Keshavarz Blvd, Tehran 14194, Iran; Tel: +9821-6692-9234; Fax: +9821-6692-9235; E-mail: rezaei_nima@yahoo.com

**Keywords:** Communicable disease, Disease, Epidemiology, Health, Health services, Infectious disease, Integrated medicine, Inter-disciplinary, Pediatrics, Pediatrician, Poverty, Medicine, Mental health, Multi-disciplinary, Non-Communicable disease, Social.

## INTRODUCTION

Children and the knowledge of taking care of them, pediatrics, are faced with growing challenges. Pediatrics is a branch of clinical medicine that deals with the physical, mental, and social health and diseases of infants, children and adolescents.

This specialty of medicine is associated with many challenges. Pediatricians are faced with a child who cannot usually express her/his feelings, needs, and pain. On the other hand, the parents' anxiety and concerns make the situation more challenging [1]. With the advancement of medical sciences, pediatrics is becoming a group of subspecialties. This could lead to improving the care and management of pediatric disorders; however, transdisciplinary management should not be ignored. In fact, the health care team of children should consist of primary care pediatricians, pediatric subspecialists, pediatric surgical specialists, psychiatrists, psychologists, pediatric nurses and social workers.

Children's lives today are at risk of so many challenges. To name a few, increased sexual abuse, discrimination and racism, increased intercountry adoption, malnutrition, and environmental hazards like arsenic contamination, pornography, and surrogacy are among the most important current issues needing planning and investing [2].

Although the health status of children has improved over the past years, still preventable child deaths are occurring, especially in low-income countries. Identifying the cause and challenges could help in reducing the mortality rate, and improving the condition. The most important modifiable factors are as follows: a) delay in accessing health services due to distance, low health literacy or cost, b) social and environmental factors like sanitation or parents' substance abuse, c) primary care inefficiencies like incorrect recommendations by primary health care workers due to ignorance or the lack of a referral system to transport critically ill patients to high facility centers, and d) hospital inefficiencies like lack of triage, misdiagnosis and maltreatment, nosocomial infections, ineffective monitoring and malnutrition [3].

In this chapter, we will review the most important challenges of children's health and pediatrics.

## ACCESS TO HEALTH SERVICES

Although immunization is one of the most important health achievements in the last century, global immunization rates remain below expectations. Worldwide coverage has declined from 86% in 2019 to 83% in 2020, and the number of completely unvaccinated children increased by 3.4 million. Approximately 23 million children under the age of one year have not received basic vaccines. More than 60% of these children live in Angola, Brazil, the Democratic Republic of the Congo, Ethiopia, India, Indonesia, Mexico, Nigeria, Pakistan and the Philippines [4].

Factors that decrease the rate of pediatric immunization can be classified into three groups: 1) system barriers including persistent and equivocal changes in the guidelines, the complexity of vaccine schedules and poverty or low socioeconomic status leading to missed immunization opportunities, 2) healthcare provider barriers such as their lack of information about contraindications and involvement of multiple healthcare providers in any child's immunization process and parent, and 3) patient barriers including misperception of uneducated parents about vaccination and possible side effects, having a child too ill to vaccinate and religious objections [5 - 7].

More than 50% of the world's population does not have access to essential health services. Efficient healthcare services in Sub-Saharan Africa and Southern Asia are harder to access, and even in more affluent regions such as Eastern Asia, Latin America and Europe, it is a challenge to spend a noticeable fraction of household budget on health expenses. National averages can conceal low levels of health service coverage in deprived population groups; for example, only 17 percent of mothers and children in the poorest fifth of households in low- and lower-middl--income countries obtained at least six of seven basic maternal and child health interventions, compared to 74 percent for the wealthiest fifth of households [2]. Every six-second, a child younger than 5 years old dies in the world, mostly by preventable causes, and 40% of them occur in countries involving humanitarian crises.

Despite all the endless challenges, United Nations International Children's Emergency Fund (UNICEF) tries to enhance the rate of maternal, newborn and child survival by establishing efficient healthcare services, immunization programs and preventive promotive curative systems for pediatric diseases such as pneumonia, diarrhea and malaria all around the world. UNICEF also focuses on child and adolescent health and well-being by supporting national health plans and helping countries combat non-communicable diseases. Moreover, UNICEF works on strengthening health systems focusing on health, nutrition, early childhood development, water, sanitation and hygiene; and also tries to improve access to healthcare services in emergencies and humanitarian crises [8].

## POVERTY AND SOCIAL PROBLEMS

Poverty is the state of not having enough income to provide basic needs including food, clothing and shelter. Approximately 1 billion children are dealing with multidimensional poverty all around the world among which at least 356 million of them live in extreme poverty, and 100 million more children plugged into poverty as the result of Coronavirus disease (COVID-19) [9]. Poverty can affect many aspects of children's well-being [10]; First, it may affect their physical health; poor children are likely to be twice in fair health compared to non-poor children. Low birth weight and increased neonatal mortality rate are some of the serious consequences of poverty [11, 12]. It also has been proved that there is a meaningful relationship between poverty and pediatric malnutrition which leads to failure to thrive [13]. Moreover, lead poisoning is more common among poor children living in older houses, which can cause hearing loss, vitamin D deficiency, anemia, nephrotoxicity, and growth stunting [14]. Poverty can also affect children's cognitive abilities; children below the poverty threshold are 1.3 times more susceptible to experience learning disabilities and developmental delays compared to non-poor children [10, 15]. Poverty is also linked to lower IQ and verbal abilities among children. The effect of long-term poverty is more significant than-short term poverty [10]. Furthermore, poverty can come up with emotional and behavioral outcomes, and can be a strong predictor of pediatric behavioral and emotional problems. Long-term poverty is associated with internalizing behaviors such as dependence, anxiety and unhappiness, whereas short-term poverty is more associated with externalizing problems such as hyperactivity [16].

On the other hand, social problems such as war, natural disasters and other emergencies are big threats to children's health. Approximately 50% of newborn mortality happens in humanitarian crises and children who survive, often fail to thrive, and suffer from maltreatment [17]. Between 2005 and 2020, more than 104100 children were verified as armed conflict victims, and more than 93000 children were verified as hired or forced to conflict. In the same years, at least 14200 children were raped, sexually exploited, forcibly married, and experienced other forms of sexual violence which affected predominantly girls [18]. Terrorism can affect children in different ways; first, it can make a stressful environment for both mother and fetus which elevates cortisol levels for both of them, and leads to birth adverse events [19]. Second, attacks may damage local markets or prevent children from having proper food which causes malnutrition and stunting [20, 21].

Third, terrorism can cause economic problems and interfere with getting efficient healthcare [21].

## ADOLESCENTS PREGNANCY AND ABORTION

Another challenge we are facing is adolescents' pregnancy and abortion. Although the global adolescent-specific fertility rate has declined by 11.6% over the past 20 years, still nearly 21 million girls aged 15-19 years become pregnant annually, and at least 12 million of them give birth. In developing countries, more than 777000 girls under 15 give birth each year. Moreover, 3.9 million unsafe abortions occur among girls aged 15-19 annually. Adolescents' pregnancy rate is different from one place to another, but it is more often in developing countries, especially Eastern Asia (951,353) and Western Africa (70,423). Socio-economic factors such as poverty, lack of education, being forced by families to marry early and low employment opportunities are contributed to adolescents' pregnancy and giving birth. This often leads to serious health consequences for both mother and child, as the leading cause of death among girls aged 15-19 years in developing countries is pregnancy and labor complications which are responsible for 99% of universal maternal deaths of women aged 15-49 years. Teenage mothers are facing higher risks of eclampsia, puerperal endometritis and systemic infections than 20–24-year-old women, while their babies are at higher risks of low birth weight, preterm delivery and severe neonatal conditions. In addition to serious health conditions, unmarried adolescent mothers tend to experience social problems including slur, rejection and violence by their partners or parents. Pregnancy and giving birth may also cause educational and occupational deprivation [22].

## ETHNICITY

Ethnicity may also affect children's health, regardless of family income, parents' educational level, age and sex. Native American, black and Hispanic children ascendingly have lower rates of health compared to Asian/Pacific Islander and white children. Asian/Pacific Islander children spend the fewest mean days in a year in bed for health conditions followed by black and Hispanic children, while Native American and white children spend more than 3 days [23].

## MENTAL DISORDERS

According to DSM-5, "a mental disorder is a syndrome characterized by clinically significant disturbance in an individual's cognition, emotion regulation or behavior that reflects a dysfunction in the psychological, biological or developmental processes underlying mental functioning" [24].

In the past two decades, mental disorders have been among the five top causes of lost life due to disability and death (Disability-Adjusted Life Year (DALY)) in children worldwide with a constant increase in its proportional impact, have been recognized as the main reason for disability in childhood. The most prevalent mental disorders were conduct disorder, anxiety disorder, major depressive disorder and autistic spectrum disorders [25 - 27].

Early life experiences and environment affect brain development in children and, consequently, their mental health throughout their life [28]. There is no surprise that in many cases, mental disorders early in life lead to adulthood derangements, as well [29 - 31]. Disruption in education and social development, interpersonal relationships, higher risk of substance abuse and poor reproductive health, and suicide are some of the consequences of mental disorders in children and adolescents [29, 32, 33]. Unfortunately, there are disparities in resources for childhood mental disorders around the globe even in developed western counties [34 - 36], along with a rise in the rate of mental disorder diagnosis in children and adolescents [37]. There is a need to make mental health care more accessible by providing it in pediatric and primary care clinics [38, 39].

## DEPRESSION

Depressive mood disorders consist of defined clinical conditions exhibiting the following symptoms: sadness, anhedonia, irritability, cognitive and somatic alterations, and reduced functionality in patients. Recently, a new diagnosis was added to DSM-V named disruptive mood dysregulation disorder in pediatric patients younger than 12 years-old, and it was defined as constant irritable mood and repeated temper outbursts and the usual development of depressive or anxiety disorders later in life [24]. Depressive presentations in children and adults are different, even symptoms are various before and after puberty, and its diagnosis may be challenging [40 - 42].

Roughly 1% of children and about 10% of teenagers meet the criteria for depressive disorders [41, 43]. It is essential to bear in mind that the prevalence of depression increases throughout life, and reaches its adulthood rates in late adolescence [40]. In a cohort study, 40% of participants developed at least one episode of depressive and anxiety disorder before adulthood [44].

Antidepressants and cognitive behavior therapy are the most successful and widely used treatments in depressed pediatric patients [45, 46]. Many studies have demonstrated earlier diagnosis and treatment of depression leads to better prognosis and lower recurrence rates [44, 47]. Given that many patients with psychiatric conditions remain untreated, and have low accessibility to mental health care providers [41, 48], advancing pediatricians with evidence-based knowledge of diagnosis and treatment of depressive disorders can lower the risk of treatment resistance and episodes of depression in adulthood [40, 49, 50].

## SUICIDE

Suicide in children and adolescents is not common, but it is the second cause of death in young adults [51]. In the past decades, scarce data showed a minor global increase in suicide rates in the pediatric population. However, the overall trend was decreasing in North America and Europe [52, 53]. Age and gender differences and racial variation are present in suicidal rates as adolescents and male youths are at higher risk of committing suicide; along with the fact that discriminated racial groups are at a higher risk. For example, despite the reduction in pediatric suicide rates in the USA, the prevalence of African-American boys committing suicide has been rising in the past years [53 - 57]. It is important to be aware that many children older than ten comprehend taking one's own life, but they seldom talk about it, and children as young as 11 years old commit suicide [55, 58].

Pediatricians play a pivotal role in suicide prevention and management. The American Academy of Pediatrics recommends pediatricians to screen suicidal ideation in adolescents during their visits by identifying patients with risk factors and cultivating pediatric patients and their parents. For example, educating parents to identify "warning signs" or to reduce access to suicide methods [51, 59 - 61]. Suicide risk factors include a history of self-harm and prior suicidal attempts, mental disorders, chronic diseases, bullying, abuse and academic or emotional difficulties [54, 59]. Every chronic illness imposes a different suicide risk, for example, patients with cancer, severe asthma and epilepsy are at higher risk, and pediatricians can support their patients through timely identification and intervention [60, 61].

## BULLYING

Bullying is defined as repeated and consistent exposure to peers' negative actions (intentional attempts to inflict injury or discomfort) [62]. Bullying can be direct (physical or verbal), indirect (for example, gossip or social exclusion, *etc.),* or cyberbullying Note: Please remove (define and give an example) [63]. Across Europe and North America, 10 to 50% of school-aged children are exposed to bullying, with an overall prevalence of 30% [64]. Although verbal bullying is the most prevalent type, physical bullying can lead to serious injuries [63, 65]. Cyberbullying, on the other hand, allows anonymous perpetuation without being identified, and can occur anytime, anywhere [66].

Studies have demonstrated both the bully and the victim are affected in their social and academic lives, and are prone to mental disorders and even suicide [67 - 69].

## SOCIAL MEDIA

Social media are platforms where social interaction is available [70]. Smartphones are available for 10-year-old children who use the internet for 8 hours a day on average. About 80% of adolescents aged 13 to 16 use social media [71, 72].

Every day, more children and adolescents –and at a younger age- use social media to connect to their peers [70, 71], which is a double-edged sword. It brings benefits such as strengthened friendships and more opportunities for learning and collaboration. However, it also brings mental health problems like anxiety and depression, or exposes children to cyberbullying or explicit content. Social media may trigger low self-esteem and isolation [70, 73, 74]. Lack of knowledge may lead to disrupting privacy of the young population and has deleterious effects even years later [75].

Pediatricians should guide families about the risks and benefits of social media, encourage them to talk about it, and screen children for social media overuse or other unfavorable consequences [70, 75].

## CHILD ABUSE

It is estimated that 4.2 homicides occur per 100,000 under the age of 15 years old worldwide, primarily due to child abuse [76]. The World Health Organization (WHO) defines child abuse as physical, emotional or sexual abuse, neglect or exploitation, resulting in actual or potential harm to the child's health, survival, development or dignity. Estimates show a 30% prevalence of any type of child abuse worldwide with equal distribution for girls and boys, except for sexual abuse that women are far more prone to it [77]. The more abuse is imposed upon victims, the more consequences and adverse effects would be. However, the rate of child abuse is declining, fortunately [78 - 80].

History of trauma in childhood is related to subsequent mental disorders, learning deficits, substance abuse, cerebrovascular and cardiac diseases, diabetes, and malignancies [78, 81].

Pediatricians play a crucial role in preventing and identifying risk factors for child abuse and its victims. For example, a survey showed 90% of the parents charged with child maltreatment with head trauma had asked a clinician to help with their infants crying [82, 83].

## SUBSTANCE ABUSE

Alcohol and tobacco are the most misused drugs worldwide [84], and are among the greatest risk factors for DALYs throughout the lifetime [85]. The trend of substance abuse among adolescents varies in different countries; as the USA is going through a decline (except for cannabis), the drift in the UK is increasing [84, 86, 87].

Alcohol consumption in adolescents can disrupt structural and functional brain development, unsafe driving and sex, alcohol use disorder and death [88, 89]. Data from the USA shows that alcohol consumption is among the major causes of death in adolescents (car crashes, homicide and suicide). The alcohol or marijuana use rate among them is about 30% and 20%, respectively [88, 90, 91]. While substance abuse rarely starts as early as childhood, it peaks in late adolescence [89, 92], many studies have demonstrated the link between early substance abuse and a greater risk of dependence later in life, and the link between mental disorders and substance abuse [86, 88, 93, 94]. American Academy of Pediatrics recommends screening for substance abuse or its risk factors in visits, and screening tools have been developed to help clinicians [88, 95]. Early detection and referral to more specialized care providers can defer the harmful consequences [90, 92].

## ADOPTION AND FOSTER CARE

The foster care system started in 1987 to protect children in Spain. About 143 million children don't live with their birth parents, and about 95% of these children are in family foster care support. About 2.4% of the United States children (about 2.1 million) are adopted.

These children are faced with emotional crises, and may feel lonely at the beginning of being in a foster family [96, 97].

When these children grow up they want to know more about their birth family, and they may reunite with them. We must prepare them about the possibility of birth parents rejection before the reunion. The most common rationale causing a child entering in foster care system include neglect (62%), substance abuse by parents (36%), poor child coping skills (14%) physical abuse and child behavioral problems [98].

Psychological and early foster care support might reduce the risk of subsequent problems. Adopting these children in families after this deprivation may lead to better adaptive functioning in adolescence.

Children often don't want to speak about foster care as they prefer to keep it private [99 - 101].

Foster and adoptive families need help and support to manage the challenges of the relationship between children and new parents. These children often are afraid of forming a secure relationship because of adverse life experiences [102].

## ENVIRONMENTAL TOXINS

Children take in proportionally more water, food and air than adults, and are experiencing fundamental nervous system developments. Therefore, they are more prone to the detrimental effects of environmental toxins. Environmental toxins are found in the tap or well water, food, furniture, toys, dust and surroundings. The most well-known toxins are lead, mercury, insecticides, polychlorinated biphenyls, nitrogen dioxide, and so forth. They increase the risk of low birth weight, developmental delay, and a wide range of neurological deficits. Pediatricians can provide families with information about protecting children from exposure [103 - 105].

## NATURAL DISASTERS

Children are more vulnerable to the turmoil natural disasters bring. Even small-scale ones will negatively impact their mental and physical health or education. Direct injuries, infectious diseases, disturbed health care and vaccination, malnutrition, mental disorders, and child abuse are all aftermaths of natural disasters. Exposure to disasters before or after birth significantly impacts children's growth indices [106 - 112].

## CHILD INJURY

Traffic accidents, drowning, thermal injuries, poisoning and falls cause trauma in the pediatric population. WHO estimated that unintentional injuries cause about a million deaths under the age of 20 every year, and they cause more deaths in countries with lower incomes. Trauma kills more children in the USA in comparison with any other causes [113, 114]. Mortality rates and causes vary among different age groups [115 - 117]. For example, adolescents tend to suffer from road accidents more frequently, while accidents commonly occur in houses of younger children [114 - 117].

The morbidity and its impact on families of child injury survivors are a public health crisis. It is important to remember that child injury is preventable, and its consequences can be reduced by proper management when healthcare workers are trained to care for pediatric trauma patients, and primary healthcare providers can upskill families to prevent child injury [118, 119].

## BREASTFEEDING

Breast milk is the natural and best way to feed all infants and is recommended for the first 6 months of life, and then breastfeeding should be continued with complementary solids for up to 2 years and beyond.

Nowadays inappropriate advertisements and marketing of breast milk substitutes have led to the failure of our efforts to increase the duration of breastfeeding.

Breastfeeding can protect against infectious diseases like respiratory tract disease, urinary tract diseases, Otitis media, and Gastrointestinal illness. Furthermore, it protects against childhood obesity [120, 121].

Breastfeeding can reduce the risk of childhood leukemia. When it lasts longer than 6 months, it can reduce the risk of asthma by 30% compared to infants with less than 6 months of breastfeeding. When it lasts equal to or longer than 3 or 4 months, it can lead to lower total behavior and conduct disorders in childhood [122 - 124].

Breastfeeding has an inverse effect on weight gain velocity, and its effect is dose-dependent.

Direct feeding with breast appears to have a more beneficial effect than feeding expressed breast milk, and expressed milk has a more beneficial effect than formula [125].

There is also an inverse association between very early breastfeeding initiation and neonatal mortality. Infants who initiate breastfeeding equal to or lower than 1 hour after birth, have a 33% lower risk of mortality compared to those who initiate breastfeeding 2-23 hours after birth, and infants who initiate breastfeeding equal to or more than 24 hours after birth have twice the likelihood for mortality rate [126].

## CHRONIC ILLNESSES AND NON-COMMUNICABLE DISEASES

The prevalence of pediatric chronic illnesses has increased over time, especially, in developing countries, and approximately 13-27% of children are dealing with Non-Communicable Diseases (NCDs [127]. In 2019, half of the Disability-Affected Life Years (DALYs) were caused by NCDs, and they were responsible for 20 percent of deaths among those aged 10-19 [128]. Children and adolescents with NCDs often face more challenges as they have to handle their illness, treatment and self-management skills, in addition, to accommodating its possible obstacles [129]. NCDs may affect their school performance and also cause low self-esteem, negative body image and decreased social contact which can lead to psychiatric disorders [130]. Furthermore, these children are disposed to have lower rates of graduation, employment, salary and marriage in adulthood [131].

Mental health disorders are the most common NCDs among adolescents [132]. The currency of asthma is related to socioeconomic status as, according to studies, about 18% of poor children are affected by asthma while only 7.3-9.5% of all children are involved [133, 134]. Food allergies have become the most common reason for anaphylaxis, and nearly 4% of children and adolescents are involved [135]. Epilepsy is one of the most important neurological problems that can lead to psychosocial problems, and affects about 0.7% of children and adolescents [136]. Pediatric hypertension is also an important risk factor for cardiovascular and kidney problems which affects 1-5% of children, and has a higher contingency with obesity [137]. Moreover, the annual prevalence of diabetes increased from 1.86 to 2.82 per 1,000 during 2002–2013: 1.48 to 2.32 per 1,000 for type 1 diabetes, and 0.38 to 0.67 per 1,000 for type 2 diabetes in 2002–2006 [138]. Obesity is an important risk factor of developing diabetes, as more than 25% of obese adolescents have signs of diabetes by age 15 [139]. 1 million children are born each year with congenital heart disease, and more than 90% of them live in deprived areas. Chronic illnesses not only affect children's concentration and academic performance, but can also be very disruptive to families [140, 141].

Prematurity and low birth weight in neonates are predisposing factors to NCDs in early life [142]. Generally, harmful behaviors such as smoking, sedentary lifestyle, poor diet, alcohol and drug abuse are known to be risk factors for NCDs [132]. Nowadays, sedentary behaviors (such as watching TV, using laptops and cell phones) are becoming more common among children all around the world [143]. Moreover, adolescents' alcohol consumption becomes more prevalent which increases the possibility of dependence, neurological problems, nonintentional injury and violence [144, 145]. Overweight and obesity are increasing in developed countries which can cause higher incidence of diabetes and cardiovascular diseases [146, 147].

## EARLY GENETIC AND PRENATAL DIAGNOSIS

Although advances have been made in screening and early diagnosis of prenatal problems and genetic anomalies, there is a long way to achieve the goal. Genetic tests could help us in determining the recurrence risk of diseases for parents to inform reproductive decision-making. Pediatricians should consider genetic etiologies and screening when they clinically suspect an underlying genetic problem, after taking medical and family developmental history and pedigree. To confirm this diagnosis, genetic testing could be used [148]. The first genetic screening was performed in the 1960s to detect the high level of phenylalanine.

Non-invasive screening tests include ultrasound, biochemical screening, non-invasive prenatal testing (using cell-free fetal DNA) and so on. Invasive tests are Amniocentesis, Fetoscopy, Chorionic villus sampling and percutaneous umbilical blood sampling.

Now the focus is on decreasing the use of prenatal invasive procedures, as they are operator-dependent.

Genetic assessment techniques are case dependent and may include karyotype, molecular DNA testing, fluorescence *in situ* hybridization, comparative genomic hybridization, microarray analysis and next-generation sequencing [149 - 151].

## PREMATURITY AND LOW BIRTH WEIGHT

Prematurity and low birth weight are the most important risk factors for neonatal mortality.

Low birth weight is defined when weight at birth is lower than 2500 grams, this is a cause of morbidity and mortality in childhood. It may cause chronic disease and cognitive developmental problems.

Children with small gestational age have higher insulin resistance, and consequently have higher risks of developing type 2 diabetes in adolescence. Preterm children are exposed to more psychiatric disorders and neurodevelopmental problems [152 - 154].

## CONGENITAL ANOMALIES

About 3.2 million children in the world are born with congenital anomalies, and about 300,000 children with birth defect anomalies die during the first 28 days of their life. Congenital anomalies are responsible for 25% of infant mortality. Therefore, prevention strategies are essential for the health care systems [155].

Congenital anomalies are divided into 2 categories: minor anomalies are associated with structural abnormalities that have little effect on function, and major congenital anomalies can cause protracted illness, often affect life expectancy, and could be lethal.

Some of the congenital anomalies are preventable, such as spina bifida and anencephaly by folate supplementation during pregnancy. Therefore, early detection of anomalies might help in reducing newborn, infant and child morbidity and mortality rate [156, 157].

## MALIGNANCY

Cancer is the leading cause of death in the population under age 20 [158]. Estimates have shown an incidence of 400,000 childhood cancers in 2015, and almost half remained undiagnosed [159].

In the last few decades, the overall incidence rate of cancer has increased, while the mortality for all types of cancer has declined [160 - 162]. Although the 5-year survival is about 80% in high-income countries, the statistics are not as fortunate in the rest of the world, where most of the young population lives [163, 164]. Cancer survivors are more likely to have another malignancy or chronic disease (cognitive dysfunction, mental disorders, cardiac and pulmonary problems and chronic pain) later in life. Also, their all-cause mortality after 30 years remains higher than the normal population. The prevalence of chronic health conditions increases as there are more cancer survivors, and they grow older [165, 166].

Unfortunately, childhood cancers are not preventable -except for the well-known carcinogenicity due to radiation in early years- nor can they be screened, because most symptoms are similar to more common and less detrimental diseases of their age [160].

The most common types of cancer in children are acute lymphoid leukemia, Central Nervous System (CNS) tumors and neuroblastomas, while in adolescents, they are Hodgkin lymphoma, thyroid cancers, and CNS tumors [160].

## MEDICAL FUTILITY AND END-OF-LIFE-CARE

Although there has been considerable progress in child survival since 1990 (61% improvement), however, in 2020, 5 million children under 5 years old died; therefore, physicians are involved with 13800 children's deaths every day [167]. Approximately, two-third of infant deaths happen in the first month of life often as a result of congenital abnormalities, while 20% of deaths during the first year of life are because of unexpected events including such as trauma. The leading cause of school-aged children and adolescents' death respectively are trauma and accidents (*e.g.* homicide, suicide, *etc.*).

Extensive variety of children mortality causes can come up with some challenges of End-Of-Life (EOL) care. One of the pediatric EOL challenges is infrequency; it is estimated that each physician in North America cares for less than 3 children's deaths which leads to a lack of experience and discomfort while dealing with a child's death. They may also feel guilty and have severe emotional response as they couldn't cure them. Moreover, many neonatal deaths happen as a result of congenital abnormalities, which may be rare, and makes the prognosis unclear or hard to estimate due to limited data. Also, differentiating a fatal disease from a life-lasting condition is another challenge we are facing, especially, in cases of congenital diseases. As it may prevent the child from getting palliative or proper EOL care if the physician only emphasizes increasing the duration of life. Furthermore, children may not be able to understand the conception of death or ask questions about the meaning of their life which can be so difficult for the caregiver to explain [168].

While Pediatric Palliative Care (PPC) has a critical role in children with life-threatening conditions, it also can come up with several challenges [169]: First of all, there have been some disagreements over the definition of PPC. WHO has defined it as embracing the needs of children with life-threatening diseases. The main argument or question is whether we should use the term "life-threatening" which is curable or "life-limiting" which is fatal; however, it seems that "life-threatening" seems to be more relevant. Second, there are so many barriers in the way of getting proper PPC that can be classified into four groups including; general barriers (such as lack of healthcare coverage and data), community barriers (such as geographic diversity and lack of experienced staff), hospital barriers (such as frequent changes of clinicians) and developing nations barriers (such as limited access to proper drugs and pain killers). To overcome these barriers and offer proper end-of-life health care, we need a better comprehension of PPC settings. Third, there might be some cultural and religious differences among children that should be merged with PPC; so, children and their parents should be involved with the EOL care process, and should be asked about their preferences. Fourth, children's feelings and suffering are often neglected; also, the way of giving hope to them and their parents is negotiable so attempts should be made in order to reduce children's suffering and improve hope. Finally, caring for a child with an end-stage disease or condition may be too distressing for healthcare personnel so, the proper support and coping strategies to manage their stress can be useful [169]. Nevertheless, questions like how to minimize pain or bereavement still remain unanswerable.

Euthanasia is another option for end-stage children approved in Netherlands and Belgium. Although there is no age restriction given, the child should be in a situation that understands the condition and the explanations given by pediatrician; also, the decision should be supported by the child's parent or legal guardian [170]. Some opponents claim that even competent children and adolescents lack the capacity of making the right decision between choosing palliative care and euthanasia [171]. Furthermore, it has been proven that dealing with chronic illnesses can impact children's making decisions especially when it concerns health problems [172].

A child's death can have several consequences for families, marriage and siblings [173]. Parents who have lost a child tend to feel lonely, desperate, sad, vulnerable, panic, stressed and wishing for death [173, 174]. They also may develop physical symptoms including anorexia, confusion, distraction, insomnia and overthinking [175]. Furthermore, child's death can come up with marriage issues such as feeling anger towards spouse, low intimacy, avoidance of communication and in some cases divorce [173, 176 - 178]. In addition to parents, siblings are affected as well, and they tend to feel isolation, depression, and guilt or reveal physical symptoms such as anxiety, Post-Traumatic Stress Disorder (PTSD), nightmares and trouble sleeping [179 - 182].

## HOW TO INTERACT WITH A SICK CHILD

In the management of pediatric illnesses, families are also inadvertently involved. Dealing with a sick child can be distressful and carry lots of psychological pressure on families. Families with a sick child can demonstrate overprotectiveness and rigidity towards their child; they may feel desperate, and overwhelmed and neglect their duties as family members. Therefore, considering family concerns is important while managing the disease. Cooperation with families can reduce the psychological burden of the disease, and maximize the efficiency of treatment. In cases of surgery, parents often expect the physician to explain to them the duration of the procedure, the location of incision and intravenous lines, the amount of hair to be removed and the child's appearance after surgery [183]. Parents want information about their children's condition, treatment process and their future prospects [184]; they also want advice about their child's attitude, Inheritance of the disease and a long-term care plan [185, 186]. Therefore, it is important for the pediatrician to explain a clear definition of the disease, treatment process and prognosis to families, and necessarily recommend them a psychotherapist [187].

Effective interaction with a sick child is necessary during history taking, examination and treatment process; thus, pediatricians should be able to overcome barriers and learn communication skills despite children's young age or their lack of information and find a way to explain the condition to them. Between 35-70% of medico-legal actions are the result of some factors, including poor transmission of information, failure to understand the patient's and family's opinions, failure to request and include patient's values into the medical strategy and perceptions of desertion [188]. Interaction with families from a different language or culture also can be challenging that using a translator and asking families about their preferences can be helpful [189]. Moreover, many pediatricians are uncomfortable giving bad news.

To overcome communication problems, time management skills and using closed interview conversation techniques by asking yes or no questions are helpful [188].

## CONCLUSION

"Every child has the right to survive and thrive"

UNICEF

Pediatric health, as one of the measures of society's values and productivity, depends on the interaction of many factors like social and physical environment, children's family, genes and behaviors. Although tremendous progress has been made in the diagnosis and treatment of childhood disorders, health problems are on the rise.

To improve the health status of children, we are faced with many challenges and barriers. To overcome them, a greater emphasis should be on prevention measures, and collaboration of health care providers and policymakers is needed.

Pediatricians and those who work in the field of children's health should be aware of the most important challenges. Working in the field of pediatrics is challenging but rewarding!

## ACKNOWLEDGEMENT

Declared none.

## REFERENCES

[1]    Corno AF. Great challenges in pediatrics. Front Pediatr 2013; 1: 5.
       [http://dx.doi.org/10.3389/fped.2013.00005] [PMID: 24400252]

[2]    World Bank and WHO: Half the world lacks access to essential health services, 100 million still pushed into extreme poverty because of health expenses. Available From: https://www.who.int/news/item/13-12-2017-world-bank-and-who-half--he-world-lacks-access-to-essential-health-services-100-million-still-pushed-into-extreme-poverty-because-of-health-expenses

[3]    World Health Organization. Improving the quality of paediatric care: An operational guide for facility-based audit and review of paediatric mortality. 2018.

[4]    World Health Organization. Immunization coverage. Available From: https://www.who.int/news-room/fact-sheets/detail/immunization-coverage

[5]    Whyte MD, Whyte J IV, Cormier E, Eccles DW. Factors influencing parental decision making when

parents choose to deviate from the standard pediatric immunization schedule. J Community Health Nurs 2011; 28(4): 204-14.
[http://dx.doi.org/10.1080/07370016.2011.615178] [PMID: 22053765]

[6]     Anderson EL. Recommended solutions to the barriers to immunization in children and adults. Mo Med 2014; 111(4): 344-8.
[PMID: 25211867]

[7]     Kimmel SR, Burns IT, Wolfe RM, Zimmerman RK. Addressing immunization barriers, benefits, and risks. Journal of Family Practice 2007; 56(2): S61-9.

[8]     https://www.unicef.org/health

[9]     https://www.unicef.org/social-policy/child-poverty

[10]    Brooks-Gunn J, Duncan GJ. The effects of poverty on children. Future Child 1997; 7(2): 55-71.
[http://dx.doi.org/10.2307/1602387] [PMID: 9299837]

[11]    Corman H, Grossman M. Determinants of neonatal mortality rates in the U.S. J Health Econ 1985; 4(3): 213-36.
[http://dx.doi.org/10.1016/0167-6296(85)90030-X] [PMID: 10300553]

[12]    Frank RG, Strobino D, Salkever DS, Jackson CA. Updated estimates of the impact of prenatal care on birthweight outcomes by race. National Bureau of Economic Research 1991. Report No.: 0898-2937.
[http://dx.doi.org/10.3386/w3624]

[13]    Miller JE, Korenman S. Poverty and children's nutritional status in the United States. Am J Epidemiol 1994; 140(3): 233-43.
[http://dx.doi.org/10.1093/oxfordjournals.aje.a117242] [PMID: 8030626]

[14]    Mushak P, Crocetti A. Nature and extent of lead poisoning in children in the United States: A report to Congress Final report. Atlanta, GA (USA): Agency for Toxic Substances and Disease Registry 1988.

[15]    Duncan GJ, Brooks-Gunn J, Klebanov PK. Economic deprivation and early childhood development. Child Dev 1994; 65(2): 296-318.
[http://dx.doi.org/10.2307/1131385] [PMID: 7516849]

[16]    McLeod JD, Shanahan MJ. Poverty, parenting, and children's mental health. Am Sociol Rev 1993; 58(3): 351-66.
[http://dx.doi.org/10.2307/2095905]

[17]    https://www.who.int/teams/maternal-newborn-child-adolescent-health-and-ageing/child-health

[18]    https://www.unicef.org/protection/protecting-children-in-humanitarian-action

[19]    Talge NM, Neal C, Glover V, Early Stress TR, Fetal PSN. Antenatal maternal stress and long-term effects on child neurodevelopment: how and why? J Child Psychol Psychiatry 2007; 48(3-4): 245-61.
[http://dx.doi.org/10.1111/j.1469-7610.2006.01714.x] [PMID: 17355398]

[20]    Bozzoli C, Quintana-Domeque C. The weight of the crisis: Evidence from newborns in Argentina. Rev Econ Stat 2014; 96(3): 550-62.
[http://dx.doi.org/10.1162/REST_a_00398]

[21]    Grossman D, Khalil U, Ray A. Terrorism and early childhood health outcomes: Evidence from Pakistan. Soc Sci Med 2019; 237: 112453.
[http://dx.doi.org/10.1016/j.socscimed.2019.112453] [PMID: 31442823]

[22]    World    Health    Organization.    Available    From:    https://www.who.int/news-room/fac-sheets/detail/adolescent-pregnancy

[23]    Flores G, Bauchner H, Feinstein AR, Nguyen US. The impact of ethnicity, family income, and parental education on children's health and use of health services. Am J Public Health 1999; 89(7): 1066-71.
[http://dx.doi.org/10.2105/AJPH.89.7.1066] [PMID: 10394317]

[24]     Edition F. Diagnostic and statistical manual of mental disorders 5: A quick glance. Indian J Psychiatry 2013; 55(3): 220-3.

[25]     Baranne ML, Falissard B. Global burden of mental disorders among children aged 5–14 years. Child Adolesc Psychiatry Ment Health 2018; 12(1): 19.
[http://dx.doi.org/10.1186/s13034-018-0225-4] [PMID: 29682005]

[26]     Collaborators GMD. Global, regional, and national burden of 12 mental disorders in 204 countries and territories, 1990–2019: a systematic analysis for the Global Burden of Disease Study 2019. Lancet Psychiatry 2022; 9(2): 137-50.
[http://dx.doi.org/10.1016/S2215-0366(21)00395-3] [PMID: 35026139]

[27]     Erskine HE, Moffitt TE, Copeland WE, *et al.* A heavy burden on young minds: the global burden of mental and substance use disorders in children and youth. Psychol Med 2015; 45(7): 1551-63.
[http://dx.doi.org/10.1017/S0033291714002888] [PMID: 25534496]

[28]     Räikkönen K, Pesonen AK. Early life origins of psychological development and mental health. Scand J Psychol 2009; 50(6): 583-91.
[http://dx.doi.org/10.1111/j.1467-9450.2009.00786.x] [PMID: 19930257]

[29]     Patel V, Flisher AJ, Hetrick S, McGorry P. Mental health of young people: a global public-health challenge. Lancet 2007; 369(9569): 1302-13.
[http://dx.doi.org/10.1016/S0140-6736(07)60368-7] [PMID: 17434406]

[30]     Kessler RC, Berglund P, Demler O, Jin R, Merikangas KR, Walters EE. Lifetime prevalence and age-of-onset distributions of DSM-IV disorders in the National Comorbidity Survey Replication. Arch Gen Psychiatry 2005; 62(6): 593-602.
[http://dx.doi.org/10.1001/archpsyc.62.6.593] [PMID: 15939837]

[31]     Copeland WE, Adair CE, Smetanin P, *et al.* Diagnostic transitions from childhood to adolescence to early adulthood. J Child Psychol Psychiatry 2013; 54(7): 791-9.
[http://dx.doi.org/10.1111/jcpp.12062] [PMID: 23451804]

[32]     Brännlund A, Strandh M, Nilsson K. Mental-health and educational achievement: the link between poor mental-health and upper secondary school completion and grades. J Ment Health 2017; 26(4): 318-25.
[http://dx.doi.org/10.1080/09638237.2017.1294739] [PMID: 28266232]

[33]     Carvajal L, Requejo JH, Irwin CE. The measurement of mental health problems among adolescents and young adults throughout the world. J Adolesc Health 2021; 69(3): 361-2.
[http://dx.doi.org/10.1016/j.jadohealth.2021.06.009] [PMID: 34452726]

[34]     Larson S, Chapman S, Spetz J, Brindis CD. Chronic childhood trauma, mental health, academic achievement, and school□based health center mental health services. J Sch Health 2017; 87(9): 675-86.
[http://dx.doi.org/10.1111/josh.12541] [PMID: 28766317]

[35]     McEnany FB, Ojugbele O, Doherty JR, McLaren JL, Leyenaar JK. Pediatric mental health boarding. Pediatrics 2020; 146(4): e20201174.
[http://dx.doi.org/10.1542/peds.2020-1174] [PMID: 32963020]

[36]     Belfer ML. Child and adolescent mental disorders: the magnitude of the problem across the globe. J Child Psychol Psychiatry 2008; 49(3): 226-36.
[http://dx.doi.org/10.1111/j.1469-7610.2007.01855.x] [PMID: 18221350]

[37]     Olfson M, Blanco C, Wang S, Laje G, Correll CU. National trends in the mental health care of children, adolescents, and adults by office-based physicians. JAMA Psychiatry 2014; 71(1): 81-90.
[http://dx.doi.org/10.1001/jamapsychiatry.2013.3074] [PMID: 24285382]

[38]     Foy JM. Enhancing pediatric mental health care: algorithms for primary care. Pediatrics 2010; 125 (Suppl. 3): S109-25.
[http://dx.doi.org/10.1542/peds.2010-0788F] [PMID: 20519563]

[39]    Patel V, Kieling C, Maulik PK, Divan G. Improving access to care for children with mental disorders: a global perspective. Arch Dis Child 2013; 98(5): 323-7.
[http://dx.doi.org/10.1136/archdischild-2012-302079] [PMID: 23476001]

[40]    Williams SB, O'Connor EA, Eder M, Whitlock EP. Screening for child and adolescent depression in primary care settings: a systematic evidence review for the US Preventive Services Task Force. Pediatrics 2009; 123(4): e716-35.
[http://dx.doi.org/10.1542/peds.2008-2415] [PMID: 19336361]

[41]    Garber J, Gallerani CM, Frankel SA. Depression in children. In: Gotlib IH, Hammen CL (Eds.) Handbook of depression. The Guilford Press 2009: pp. 405-43.

[42]    Rice F. Genetics of childhood and adolescent depression: insights into etiological heterogeneity and challenges for future genomic research. Genome Med 2010; 2(9): 68.
[http://dx.doi.org/10.1186/gm189] [PMID: 20860851]

[43]    Ghandour RM, Sherman LJ, Vladutiu CJ, Ali MM, Lynch SE, Bitsko RH, *et al.* Prevalence and treatment of depression, anxiety, and conduct problems in US children. The Journal of pediatrics 2019; 206(1): 256-67.
[http://dx.doi.org/10.1016/j.jpeds.2018.09.021]

[44]    Patton GC, Coffey C, Romaniuk H, *et al.* The prognosis of common mental disorders in adolescents: a 14-year prospective cohort study. Lancet 2014; 383(9926): 1404-11.
[http://dx.doi.org/10.1016/S0140-6736(13)62116-9] [PMID: 24439298]

[45]    Forti-Buratti MA, Saikia R, Wilkinson EL, Ramchandani PG. Psychological treatments for depression in pre-adolescent children (12 years and younger): systematic review and meta-analysis of randomised controlled trials. Eur Child Adolesc Psychiatry 2016; 25(10): 1045-54.
[http://dx.doi.org/10.1007/s00787-016-0834-5] [PMID: 26969618]

[46]    Lawton A, Moghraby OS. Depression in children and young people: identification and management in primary, community and secondary care (NICE guideline CG28): Table 1. Arch Dis Child Educ Pract Ed 2016; 101(4): 206-9.
[http://dx.doi.org/10.1136/archdischild-2015-308680] [PMID: 26459492]

[47]    Curry J, Rohde P, Simons A, *et al.* Predictors and moderators of acute outcome in the Treatment for Adolescents with Depression Study (TADS). J Am Acad Child Adolesc Psychiatry 2006; 45(12): 1427-39.
[http://dx.doi.org/10.1097/01.chi.0000240838.78984.e2] [PMID: 17135988]

[48]    Collins KA, Westra HA, Dozois DJA, Burns DD. Gaps in accessing treatment for anxiety and depression: Challenges for the delivery of care. Clin Psychol Rev 2004; 24(5): 583-616.
[http://dx.doi.org/10.1016/j.cpr.2004.06.001] [PMID: 15325746]

[49]    Hopkins K, Crosland P, Elliott N, Bewley S. Diagnosis and management of depression in children and young people: summary of updated NICE guidance. BMJ 2015; 350(mar04 9): h824.
[http://dx.doi.org/10.1136/bmj.h824] [PMID: 25739880]

[50]    DeFilippis M, Wagner KD. Management of treatment-resistant depression in children and adolescents. Paediatr Drugs 2014; 16(5): 353-61.
[http://dx.doi.org/10.1007/s40272-014-0088-y] [PMID: 25200567]

[51]    World Health Organization. Preventing suicide: A global imperative. World Health Organization 2014.

[52]    Skinner R, McFaull S. Suicide among children and adolescents in Canada: trends and sex differences, 1980–2008. CMAJ 2012; 184(9): 1029-34.
[http://dx.doi.org/10.1503/cmaj.111867] [PMID: 22470172]

[53]    Kõlves K, De Leo D. Suicide rates in children aged 10–14 years worldwide: changes in the past two decades. Br J Psychiatry 2014; 205(4): 283-5.
[http://dx.doi.org/10.1192/bjp.bp.114.144402] [PMID: 25104833]

[54]   Rodway C, Tham SG, Ibrahim S, Turnbull P, Kapur N, Appleby L. Children and young people who die by suicide: childhood-related antecedents, gender differences and service contact. BJPsych Open 2020; 6(3): e49.
[http://dx.doi.org/10.1192/bjo.2020.33] [PMID: 32390589]

[55]   Bridge JA, Asti L, Horowitz LM, *et al.* Suicide trends among elementary school–aged children in the United States from 1993 to 2012. JAMA Pediatr 2015; 169(7): 673-7.
[http://dx.doi.org/10.1001/jamapediatrics.2015.0465] [PMID: 25984947]

[56]   Kõlves K, de Leo D. Suicide methods in children and adolescents. Eur Child Adolesc Psychiatry 2017; 26(2): 155-64.
[http://dx.doi.org/10.1007/s00787-016-0865-y] [PMID: 27194156]

[57]   Hepp U, Stulz N, Unger-Köppel J, Ajdacic-Gross V. Methods of suicide used by children and adolescents. Eur Child Adolesc Psychiatry 2012; 21(2): 67-73.
[http://dx.doi.org/10.1007/s00787-011-0232-y] [PMID: 22130898]

[58]   Mishara BL. Conceptions of death and suicide in children ages 6-12 and their implications for suicide prevention. Suicide Life Threat Behav 1999; 29(2): 105-18.
[PMID: 10407964]

[59]   Dilillo D, Mauri S, Mantegazza C, Fabiano V, Mameli C, Zuccotti GV. Suicide in pediatrics: epidemiology, risk factors, warning signs and the role of the pediatrician in detecting them. Ital J Pediatr 2015; 41(1): 49.
[http://dx.doi.org/10.1186/s13052-015-0153-3] [PMID: 26149466]

[60]   Iannucci J, Nierenberg B. Suicide and suicidality in children and adolescents with chronic illness: A systematic review. Aggress Violent Behav 2021; 64(2): 101581.

[61]   Shain BN. Suicide and suicide attempts in adolescents. Pediatrics 2007; 120(3): 669-76.
[http://dx.doi.org/10.1542/peds.2007-1908] [PMID: 17766542]

[62]   Olweus D. Bullying at school: basic facts and effects of a school based intervention program. J Child Psychol Psychiatry 1994; 35(7): 1171-90.
[http://dx.doi.org/10.1111/j.1469-7610.1994.tb01229.x] [PMID: 7806605]

[63]   Waseem M, Ryan M, Foster CB, Peterson J. Assessment and management of bullied children in the emergency department. Pediatr Emerg Care 2013; 29(3): 389-98.
[http://dx.doi.org/10.1097/PEC.0b013e31828575d7] [PMID: 23462401]

[64]   Adamson P. Child well-being in rich countries: A comparative overview. 2013.

[65]   Vieno A, Gini G, Santinello M. Different forms of bullying and their association to smoking and drinking behavior in Italian adolescents. J Sch Health 2011; 81(7): 393-9.
[http://dx.doi.org/10.1111/j.1746-1561.2011.00607.x] [PMID: 21668879]

[66]   Vaillancourt T, Faris R, Mishna F. Cyberbullying in children and youth: Implications for health and clinical practice. Can J Psychiatry 2017; 62(6): 368-73.
[http://dx.doi.org/10.1177/0706743716684791] [PMID: 28562091]

[67]   Rigby K. Consequences of bullying in schools. Can J Psychiatry 2003; 48(9): 583-90.
[http://dx.doi.org/10.1177/070674370304800904] [PMID: 14631878]

[68]   Smith PK. Bullying: Definition, types, causes, consequences and intervention. Soc Personal Psychol Compass 2016; 10(9): 519-32.
[http://dx.doi.org/10.1111/spc3.12266]

[69]   Kaltiala-Heino R, Fröjd S. Correlation between bullying and clinical depression in adolescent patients. Adolesc Health Med Ther 2011; 2: 37-44.
[http://dx.doi.org/10.2147/AHMT.S11554] [PMID: 24600274]

[70]   Hadjipanayis A, Efstathiou E, Altorjai P, *et al.* Social media and children: what is the paediatrician's role? Eur J Pediatr 2019; 178(10): 1605-12.

[http://dx.doi.org/10.1007/s00431-019-03458-w] [PMID: 31468108]

[71]   Dyer T. The effects of social media on children. Dalhousie Journal of Interdisciplinary Management 2018; 14.

[72]   McCrae N, Gettings S, Purssell E. Social media and depressive symptoms in childhood and adolescence: A systematic review. Adolesc Res Rev 2017; 2(4): 315-30.
[http://dx.doi.org/10.1007/s40894-017-0053-4]

[73]   Hamm MP, Newton AS, Chisholm A, *et al.* Prevalence and effect of cyberbullying on children and young people: A scoping review of social media studies. JAMA Pediatr 2015; 169(8): 770-7.
[http://dx.doi.org/10.1001/jamapediatrics.2015.0944] [PMID: 26098362]

[74]   Richards D, Caldwell PHY, Go H. Impact of social media on the health of children and young people. J Paediatr Child Health 2015; 51(12): 1152-7.
[http://dx.doi.org/10.1111/jpc.13023] [PMID: 26607861]

[75]   O'Keeffe GS, Clarke-Pearson K. The impact of social media on children, adolescents, and families. Pediatrics 2011; 127(4): 800-4.
[http://dx.doi.org/10.1542/peds.2011-0054] [PMID: 21444588]

[76]   World Health Organization. Global status report on violence prevention 2014. World Health Organization 2014.

[77]   Zeanah CH, Humphreys KL. Child abuse and neglect. J Am Acad Child Adolesc Psychiatry 2018; 57(9): 637-44.
[http://dx.doi.org/10.1016/j.jaac.2018.06.007] [PMID: 30196867]

[78]   Afifi TO, MacMillan HL, Boyle M, Taillieu T, Cheung K, Sareen J. Child abuse and mental disorders in Canada. CMAJ 2014; 186(9): E324-32.
[http://dx.doi.org/10.1503/cmaj.131792] [PMID: 24756625]

[79]   Radford L, Corral S, Bradley C, *et al.* Child abuse and neglect in the UK today. 2011.

[80]   Giardino AP, Hanson N, Hill KS, Leventhal JM. Child abuse pediatrics: new specialty, renewed mission. Pediatrics 2011; 128(1): 156-9.
[http://dx.doi.org/10.1542/peds.2011-0363] [PMID: 21646255]

[81]   Yang BZ, Zhang H, Ge W, *et al.* Child abuse and epigenetic mechanisms of disease risk. Am J Prev Med 2013; 44(2): 101-7.
[http://dx.doi.org/10.1016/j.amepre.2012.10.012] [PMID: 23332324]

[82]   Flaherty EG, Stirling J Jr. Clinical report—the pediatrician's role in child maltreatment prevention. Pediatrics 2010; 126(4): 833-41.
[http://dx.doi.org/10.1542/peds.2010-2087] [PMID: 20945525]

[83]   Talvik I, Alexander RC, Talvik T. Shaken baby syndrome and a baby's cry. Acta Paediatr 2008; 97(6): 782-5.
[http://dx.doi.org/10.1111/j.1651-2227.2008.00778.x] [PMID: 18397351]

[84]   Degenhardt L, Charlson F, Ferrari A, *et al.* The global burden of disease attributable to alcohol and drug use in 195 countries and territories, 1990–2016: a systematic analysis for the Global Burden of Disease Study 2016. Lancet Psychiatry 2018; 5(12): 987-1012.
[http://dx.doi.org/10.1016/S2215-0366(18)30337-7] [PMID: 30392731]

[85]   Griswold MG, Fullman N, Hawley C, *et al.* Alcohol use and burden for 195 countries and territories, 1990–2016: a systematic analysis for the Global Burden of Disease Study 2016. Lancet 2018; 392(10152): 1015-35.
[http://dx.doi.org/10.1016/S0140-6736(18)31310-2] [PMID: 30146330]

[86]   McArdle P. Alcohol abuse in adolescents. Arch Dis Child 2008; 93(6): 524-7.
[http://dx.doi.org/10.1136/adc.2007.115840] [PMID: 18305075]

[87]   Miech R, Johnston L, O'Malley P, Bachman J, Schulenberg J, Patrick M. Monitoring the Future

national survey results on drug use. 1975-2018: Volume I, Secondary school students. 2019.

[88]   Ryan SA, Kokotailo P, Camenga DR, *et al.* Alcohol use by youth. Pediatrics 2019; 144(1): e20191357.
[http://dx.doi.org/10.1542/peds.2019-1357] [PMID: 31235608]

[89]   Das JK, Salam RA, Arshad A, Finkelstein Y, Bhutta ZA. Interventions for adolescent substance abuse: An overview of systematic reviews. J Adolesc Health 2016; 59(4): S61-75.
[http://dx.doi.org/10.1016/j.jadohealth.2016.06.021] [PMID: 27664597]

[90]   Pompili M, Serafini G, Innamorati M, *et al.* Substance abuse and suicide risk among adolescents. Eur Arch Psychiatry Clin Neurosci 2012; 262(6): 469-85.
[http://dx.doi.org/10.1007/s00406-012-0292-0] [PMID: 23304731]

[91]   Kann L, McManus T, Harris WA, *et al.* Youth risk behavior surveillance—United States, 2017. MMWR Surveill Summ 2018; 67(8): 1-114.
[http://dx.doi.org/10.15585/mmwr.ss6708a1] [PMID: 29902162]

[92]   Degenhardt L, Stockings E, Patton G, Hall WD, Lynskey M. The increasing global health priority of substance use in young people. Lancet Psychiatry 2016; 3(3): 251-64.
[http://dx.doi.org/10.1016/S2215-0366(15)00508-8] [PMID: 26905480]

[93]   Hadland SE, Knight JR, Harris SK. Alcohol use disorder: a pediatric-onset condition needing early detection and intervention. Pediatrics 2019; 143(3): e20183654.
[http://dx.doi.org/10.1542/peds.2018-3654] [PMID: 30783023]

[94]   Strasburger VC. Policy statement--children, adolescents, substance abuse, and the media. Pediatrics 2010; 126(4): 791-9.
[http://dx.doi.org/10.1542/peds.2010-1635] [PMID: 20876181]

[95]   Kulig JW. Tobacco, alcohol, and other drugs: the role of the pediatrician in prevention, identification, and management of substance abuse. Pediatrics 2005; 115(3): 816-21.
[http://dx.doi.org/10.1542/peds.2004-2841] [PMID: 15741395]

[96]   Navarro-Soria I, Servera M, Burns GL. Association of foster care and its duration with clinical symptoms and impairment: Foster care versus non-foster care comparisons with Spanish children. J Child Fam Stud 2020; 29(2): 526-33.
[http://dx.doi.org/10.1007/s10826-019-01596-1]

[97]   Steenbakkers A, Van Der Steen S, Grietens H. The needs of foster children and how to satisfy them: A systematic review of the literature. Clin Child Fam Psychol Rev 2018; 21(1): 1-12.
[http://dx.doi.org/10.1007/s10567-017-0246-1] [PMID: 29075894]

[98]   Jones VF, Schulte EE, Waite D, *et al.* Pediatrician Guidance in Supporting Families of Children Who Are Adopted, Fostered, or in Kinship Care. Pediatrics 2020; 146(6): e2020034629.
[http://dx.doi.org/10.1542/peds.2020-034629] [PMID: 33229466]

[99]   Humphreys KL, Miron D, McLaughlin KA, *et al.* Foster care promotes adaptive functioning in early adolescence among children who experienced severe, early deprivation. J Child Psychol Psychiatry 2018; 59(7): 811-21.
[http://dx.doi.org/10.1111/jcpp.12865] [PMID: 29389015]

[100]  Wade M, Fox NA, Zeanah CH, Nelson CA. Effect of foster care intervention on trajectories of general and specific psychopathology among children with histories of institutional rearing: a randomized clinical trial. JAMA Psychiatry 2018; 75(11): 1137-45.
[http://dx.doi.org/10.1001/jamapsychiatry.2018.2556] [PMID: 30267045]

[101]  Dansey D, Shbero D, John M. Keeping secrets: how children in foster care manage stigma. Adopt Foster 2019; 43(1): 35-45.
[http://dx.doi.org/10.1177/0308575918823436]

[102]  Schoemaker NK, Wentholt WGM, Goemans A, Vermeer HJ, Juffer F, Alink LRA. A meta-analytic review of parenting interventions in foster care and adoption. Dev Psychopathol 2020; 32(3): 1149-72.

[http://dx.doi.org/10.1017/S0954579419000798] [PMID: 31366418]

[103]   Hauptman M, Woolf AD. Childhood ingestions of environmental toxins: what are the risks? Pediatr Ann 2017; 46(12): e466-71.
[http://dx.doi.org/10.3928/19382359-20171116-01] [PMID: 29227523]

[104]   Liu J, Lewis G. Environmental toxicity and poor cognitive outcomes in children and adults. J Environ Health 2014; 76(6): 130-8.
[PMID: 24645424]

[105]   Lanphear BP, Vorhees CV, Bellinger DC. Protecting children from environmental toxins. PLoS Med 2005; 2(3): e61.
[http://dx.doi.org/10.1371/journal.pmed.0020061] [PMID: 15783252]

[106]   Seddighi H, Salmani I, Javadi MH, Seddighi S. Child abuse in natural disasters and conflicts: a systematic review. Trauma Violence Abuse 2021; 22(1): 176-85.
[http://dx.doi.org/10.1177/1524838019835973] [PMID: 30866745]

[107]   Dyregrov A, Yule W, Olff M. Children and natural disasters. Taylor & Francis 2018; p. 1500823.

[108]   Cerna-Turoff I, Fischer HT, Mansourian H, Mayhew S. The pathways between natural disasters and violence against children: a systematic review. BMC Public Health 2021; 21(1): 1249.
[http://dx.doi.org/10.1186/s12889-021-11252-3] [PMID: 34247619]

[109]   Kousky C. Impacts of natural disasters on children. Future Child 2016; 26(1): 73-92.
[http://dx.doi.org/10.1353/foc.2016.0004]

[110]   Watson JT, Gayer M, Connolly MA. Epidemics after natural disasters. Emerg Infect Dis 2007; 13(1): 1-5.
[http://dx.doi.org/10.3201/eid1301.060779] [PMID: 17370508]

[111]   Datar A, Liu J, Linnemayr S, Stecher C. The impact of natural disasters on child health and investments in rural India. Soc Sci Med 2013; 76(1): 83-91.
[http://dx.doi.org/10.1016/j.socscimed.2012.10.008] [PMID: 23159307]

[112]   Ahsanuzzaman , Islam MQ. Children's vulnerability to natural disasters: Evidence from natural experiments in Bangladesh. World Development Perspectives 2020; 19: 100228.
[http://dx.doi.org/10.1016/j.wdp.2020.100228]

[113]   Peden M, Oyegbite K, Ozanne-Smith J, Hyder AA, Branche C, Rahman F, Rivara AKMF, Bartolomeos K. World report on child injury prevention. World Health Organization United Nations Children's Fund (Global Headquarters, New York) 2008: p. 228.

[114]   Sengoelge M, Hasselberg M, Laflamme L. Child home injury mortality in Europe: A 16-country analysis. Eur J Public Health 2011; 21(2): 166-70.
[http://dx.doi.org/10.1093/eurpub/ckq047] [PMID: 20430805]

[115]   Akhavan Rezayat A, Zarifian A, Maamouri G, *et al.* Child injury mortality in Iran: A systematic review and meta-analysis. J Transp Health 2020; 16: 100816.
[http://dx.doi.org/10.1016/j.jth.2019.100816]

[116]   Meddings D. Child injury prevention and child survival. BMJ Publishing Group Ltd 2011; pp. 145-6.

[117]   Aoki M, Abe T, Saitoh D, Oshima K. Epidemiology, patterns of treatment, and mortality of pediatric trauma patients in Japan. Sci Rep 2019; 9(1): 917.
[http://dx.doi.org/10.1038/s41598-018-37579-3] [PMID: 30696939]

[118]   Shook JE, Chun TH, Conners GP, *et al.* Management of pediatric trauma. Pediatrics 2016; 138(2): e20161569.
[http://dx.doi.org/10.1542/peds.2016-1569] [PMID: 27456509]

[119]   Falcone RA Jr, Daugherty M, Schweer L, Patterson M, Brown RL, Garcia VF. Multidisciplinary pediatric trauma team training using high-fidelity trauma simulation. J Pediatr Surg 2008; 43(6): 1065-71.

[http://dx.doi.org/10.1016/j.jpedsurg.2008.02.033] [PMID: 18558184]

[120]   Meek J, Abrams S, Hoppin A. Infant benefits of breastfeeding. UpToDate Waltham: UpToDate Accesed. 2020; 25.

[121]   World Health Organization. Breastfeeding. Available From: https://www.who.int/health-topics/breastfeeding#tab=tab_2

[122]   Su Q, Sun X, Zhu L, *et al.* Breastfeeding and the risk of childhood cancer: a systematic review and dose-response meta-analysis. BMC Med 2021; 19(1): 90.
[http://dx.doi.org/10.1186/s12916-021-01950-5] [PMID: 33845843]

[123]   Xue M, Dehaas E, Chaudhary N, O'Byrne P, Satia I, Kurmi OP. Breastfeeding and risk of childhood asthma: a systematic review and meta-analysis. ERJ Open Res 2021; 7(4): 00504-2021.
[http://dx.doi.org/10.1183/23120541.00504-2021] [PMID: 34912884]

[124]   Poton WL, Soares ALG. Oliveira ERAd, Gonçalves H. Breastfeeding and behavior disorders among children and adolescents: a systematic review. Rev Saude Publica 2018; 52: 9.

[125]   Azad MB, Vehling L, Chan D, *et al.* Infant Feeding and Weight Gain: Separating Breast Milk From Breastfeeding and Formula From Food. Pediatrics 2018; 142(4): e20181092.
[http://dx.doi.org/10.1542/peds.2018-1092] [PMID: 30249624]

[126]   Smith ER, Hurt L, Chowdhury R, Sinha B, Fawzi W, Edmond KM. Delayed breastfeeding initiation and infant survival: A systematic review and meta-analysis. PLoS One 2017; 12(7): e0180722.
[http://dx.doi.org/10.1371/journal.pone.0180722] [PMID: 28746353]

[127]   Van Cleave J, Gortmaker SL, Perrin JM. Dynamics of obesity and chronic health conditions among children and youth. JAMA 2010; 303(7): 623-30.
[http://dx.doi.org/10.1001/jama.2010.104] [PMID: 20159870]

[128]   https://data.unicef.org/topic/child-health/noncommunicable-diseases/

[129]   Nylander C, Seidel C, Tindberg Y. The triply troubled teenager - chronic conditions associated with fewer protective factors and clustered risk behaviours. Acta Paediatr 2014; 103(2): 194-200.
[http://dx.doi.org/10.1111/apa.12461] [PMID: 24117768]

[130]   Shorey S, Ng ED. The lived experiences of children and adolescents with non-communicable disease: A systematic review of qualitative studies. J Pediatr Nurs 2020; 51: 75-84.
[http://dx.doi.org/10.1016/j.pedn.2019.12.013] [PMID: 31926405]

[131]   Pinquart M. Achievement of developmental milestones in emerging and young adults with and without pediatric chronic illness--a meta-analysis. J Pediatr Psychol 2014; 39(6): 577-87.
[http://dx.doi.org/10.1093/jpepsy/jsu017] [PMID: 24727750]

[132]   Akseer N, Mehta S, Wigle J, *et al.* Non-communicable diseases among adolescents: current status, determinants, interventions and policies. BMC Public Health 2020; 20(1): 1908.
[http://dx.doi.org/10.1186/s12889-020-09988-5] [PMID: 33317507]

[133]   Akinbami OJ. Trends in asthma prevalence, health care use, and mortality in the United States, 2001-2010: US Department of Health and Human Services. Centers for Disease Control and 2012.

[134]   Barnett SBL, Nurmagambetov TA. Costs of asthma in the United States: 2002-2007. J Allergy Clin Immunol 2011; 127(1): 145-52.
[http://dx.doi.org/10.1016/j.jaci.2010.10.020] [PMID: 21211649]

[135]   Liu AH, Jaramillo R, Sicherer SH, *et al.* National prevalence and risk factors for food allergy and relationship to asthma: results from the National Health and Nutrition Examination Survey 2005-2006. Journal of Allergy and Clinical Immunology 2010; 126(4): 798-806.

[136]   Russ SA, Larson K, Halfon N. A national profile of childhood epilepsy and seizure disorder. Pediatrics 2012; 129(2): 256-64.
[http://dx.doi.org/10.1542/peds.2010-1371] [PMID: 22271699]

[137]  Bassareo PP, Mercuro G. Pediatric hypertension: An update on a burning problem. World J Cardiol 2014; 6(5): 253-9.
[http://dx.doi.org/10.4330/wjc.v6.i5.253] [PMID: 24944755]

[138]  Li L, Jick S, Breitenstein S, Michel A. Prevalence of diabetes and diabetic nephropathy in a large US commercially insured pediatric population, 2002–2013. Diabetes Care 2016; 39(2): 278-84.
[http://dx.doi.org/10.2337/dc15-1710] [PMID: 26681728]

[139]  Goran MI, Ball GDC, Cruz ML. Obesity and risk of type 2 diabetes and cardiovascular disease in children and adolescents. J Clin Endocrinol Metab 2003; 88(4): 1417-27.
[http://dx.doi.org/10.1210/jc.2002-021442] [PMID: 12679416]

[140]  Tchervenkov CI, Jacobs JP, Bernier PL, et al. The improvement of care for paediatric and congenital cardiac disease across the World: a challenge for the World Society for Pediatric and Congenital Heart Surgery. Cardiol Young 2008; 18(S2) (Suppl. 2): 63-9.
[http://dx.doi.org/10.1017/S1047951108002801] [PMID: 19063776]

[141]  Forrest CB, Bevans KB, Riley AW, Crespo R, Louis TA. School outcomes of children with special health care needs. Pediatrics 2011; 128(2): 303-12.
[http://dx.doi.org/10.1542/peds.2010-3347] [PMID: 21788226]

[142]  Gillman MW. Developmental origins of health and disease. N Engl J Med 2005; 353(17): 1848-50.
[http://dx.doi.org/10.1056/NEJMe058187] [PMID: 16251542]

[143]  Rideout VJ, Foehr UG, Roberts DF. Generation m 2: Media in the lives of 8-to 18-year-olds. Henry J Kaiser Family Foundation 2010.

[144]  DeWit DJ, Adlaf EM, Offord DR, Ogborne AC. Age at first alcohol use: a risk factor for the development of alcohol disorders. Am J Psychiatry 2000; 157(5): 745-50.
[http://dx.doi.org/10.1176/appi.ajp.157.5.745] [PMID: 10784467]

[145]  Bonomo YA, Bowes G, Coffey C, Carlin JB, Patton GC. Teenage drinking and the onset of alcohol dependence: a cohort study over seven years. Addiction 2004; 99(12): 1520-8.
[http://dx.doi.org/10.1111/j.1360-0443.2004.00846.x] [PMID: 15585043]

[146]  Wang Y, Lobstein T. Worldwide trends in childhood overweight and obesity. Int J Pediatr Obes 2006; 1(1): 11-25.
[http://dx.doi.org/10.1080/17477160600586747] [PMID: 17902211]

[147]  Must A, Strauss RS. Risks and consequences of childhood and adolescent obesity. Int J Obes 1999; 23(S2) (Suppl. 2): S2-S11.
[http://dx.doi.org/10.1038/sj.ijo.0800852] [PMID: 10340798]

[148]  Savatt JM, Myers SM. Genetic testing in neurodevelopmental disorders. Front Pediatr 2021; 9: 526779.
[http://dx.doi.org/10.3389/fped.2021.526779] [PMID: 33681094]

[149]  Tabor A, Alfirevic Z. Update on procedure-related risks for prenatal diagnosis techniques. Fetal Diagn Ther 2010; 27(1): 1-7.
[http://dx.doi.org/10.1159/000271995] [PMID: 20051662]

[150]  Couce M, Ed. Cincuenta años de cribado neonatal de enfermedades congénitas en España. Anales de Pediatría 2019; 90(4): 205-6.
[http://dx.doi.org/10.1016/j.anpedi.2018.11.013]

[151]  Levy B, Stosic M. Traditional prenatal diagnosis: past to present. Methods Mol Biol 2019; 1885: 3-22.
[http://dx.doi.org/10.1007/978-1-4939-8889-1_1] [PMID: 30506187]

[152]  Josiane SF. Role of Maternal Education and Prenatal Care on Child Health in Cameroon. 2020.

[153]  Martín-Calvo N, Goni L, Tur JA, Martínez JA. Low birth weight and small for gestational age are associated with complications of childhood and adolescence obesity: Systematic review and meta□analysis. Obes Rev 2022; 23(S1) (Suppl. 1): e13380.

[http://dx.doi.org/10.1111/obr.13380] [PMID: 34786817]

[154]   Linsell L, Johnson S, Wolke D, Morris J, Kurinczuk JJ, Marlow N. Trajectories of behavior, attention, social and emotional problems from childhood to early adulthood following extremely preterm birth: a prospective cohort study. Eur Child Adolesc Psychiatry 2019; 28(4): 531-42.
[http://dx.doi.org/10.1007/s00787-018-1219-8] [PMID: 30191335]

[155]   Baldacci S, Gorini F, Santoro M, Pierini A, Minichilli F, Bianchi F. Environmental and individual exposure and the risk of congenital anomalies: A review of recent epidemiological evidence. Epidemiol Prev 2018; 42(3-4 Suppl 1): 1-34.

[156]   Ogbole GI, Akinmoladun JA, O Oluwasola TA. Pattern and outcome of prenatally diagnosed major congenital anomalies at a Nigerian Tertiary Hospital. Niger J Clin Pract 2018; 21(5): 560-5.
[http://dx.doi.org/10.4103/njcp.njcp_210_17] [PMID: 29735854]

[157]   Bhide P, Kar A. A national estimate of the birth prevalence of congenital anomalies in India: systematic review and meta-analysis. BMC Pediatr 2018; 18(1): 175.
[http://dx.doi.org/10.1186/s12887-018-1149-0] [PMID: 29801440]

[158]   World Health Organization. CureAll framework: WHO global initiative for childhood cancer: increasing access, advancing quality, saving lives. Geneva: World Health Organization 2021.

[159]   Ward ZJ, Yeh JM, Bhakta N, Frazier AL, Atun R. Estimating the total incidence of global childhood cancer: a simulation-based analysis. Lancet Oncol 2019; 20(4): 483-93.
[http://dx.doi.org/10.1016/S1470-2045(18)30909-4] [PMID: 30824204]

[160]   Ward E, DeSantis C, Robbins A, Kohler B, Jemal A. Childhood and adolescent cancer statistics, 2014. CA Cancer J Clin 2014; 64(2): 83-103.
[http://dx.doi.org/10.3322/caac.21219] [PMID: 24488779]

[161]   Smith MA, Seibel NL, Altekruse SF, *et al.* Outcomes for children and adolescents with cancer: challenges for the twenty-first century. J Clin Oncol 2010; 28(15): 2625-34.
[http://dx.doi.org/10.1200/JCO.2009.27.0421] [PMID: 20404250]

[162]   Hubbard AK, Spector LG, Fortuna G, Marcotte EL, Poynter JN. Trends in international incidence of pediatric cancers in children under 5 years of age: 1988–2012. JNCI Cancer Spectr 2019; 3(1): pkz007.
[http://dx.doi.org/10.1093/jncics/pkz007] [PMID: 30984908]

[163]   Force LM, Abdollahpour I, Advani SM, *et al.* The global burden of childhood and adolescent cancer in 2017: an analysis of the Global Burden of Disease Study 2017. Lancet Oncol 2019; 20(9): 1211-25.
[http://dx.doi.org/10.1016/S1470-2045(19)30339-0] [PMID: 31371206]

[164]   Israels T, Challinor J, Howard S, Arora RH. Treating children with cancer worldwide—challenges and interventions. Pediatrics 2015; 136(4): 607-10.
[http://dx.doi.org/10.1542/peds.2015-0300] [PMID: 26371201]

[165]   Phillips SM, Padgett LS, Leisenring WM, *et al.* Survivors of childhood cancer in the United States: prevalence and burden of morbidity. Cancer Epidemiol Biomarkers Prev 2015; 24(4): 653-63.
[http://dx.doi.org/10.1158/1055-9965.EPI-14-1418] [PMID: 25834148]

[166]   Armstrong GT, Liu Q, Yasui Y, *et al.* Late mortality among 5-year survivors of childhood cancer: a summary from the Childhood Cancer Survivor Study. J Clin Oncol 2009; 27(14): 2328-38.
[http://dx.doi.org/10.1200/JCO.2008.21.1425] [PMID: 19332714]

[167]   https://data.unicef.org/topic/child-survival/under-five-mortality/

[168]   Guyer B, Martin JA, MacDorman MF, Anderson RN, Strobino DM. Annual summary of vital statistics--1996. Pediatrics 1997; 100(6): 905-18.
[http://dx.doi.org/10.1542/peds.100.6.905] [PMID: 9374556]

[169]   Liben S, Papadatou D, Wolfe J. Paediatric palliative care: challenges and emerging ideas. Lancet 2008; 371(9615): 852-64.

[http://dx.doi.org/10.1016/S0140-6736(07)61203-3] [PMID: 17707080]

[170]   Samanta J. Children and euthanasia: Belgium's controversial new law. Divers Equal Health Care 2015; 12(1): 4-5.

[171]   Siegel AM, Sisti DA, Caplan AL. Pediatric Euthanasia in Belgium. JAMA 2014; 311(19): 1963-4.
[http://dx.doi.org/10.1001/jama.2014.4257] [PMID: 24743867]

[172]   Fielding D, Duff A. Compliance with treatment protocols: interventions for children with chronic illness. Arch Dis Child 1999; 80(2): 196-200.
[http://dx.doi.org/10.1136/adc.80.2.196] [PMID: 10325743]

[173]   Christ GH, Bonanno GA, Malkinson R, Rubin S. Bereavement Experiences after the Death of a Child. In: Field MJ, Behrman RE (Eds.) When Children Die: Improving Palliative and End-of-Life for Children and Their Families. Washington DC: National Academy Press; 2003: pp. 553-79.

[174]   Sanders CM. Grief: The mourning after: Dealing with adult bereavement. John Wiley & Sons. 1989.

[175]   Bowlby J. Attachment and loss: Loss, sadness and depression. New York: Basic Books 1980; Vol. 3.

[176]   Schwab R. Effects of a child's death on the marital relationship: A preliminary study. Death Stud 1992; 16(2): 141-54.
[http://dx.doi.org/10.1080/07481189208252564]

[177]   Lang A, Gottlieb L. Marital intimacy in bereaved and nonbereaved couples: A comparative study Children and death. Taylor & Francis 2013; pp. 291-300.

[178]   DeFrain J. Learning about grief from normal families: SIDS, stillbirth, and miscarriage. J Marital Fam Ther 1991; 17(3): 215-32.
[http://dx.doi.org/10.1111/j.1752-0606.1991.tb00890.x]

[179]   Rosen H. Prohibitions against mourning in childhood sibling loss. Omega (Westport) 1985; 15(4): 307-16.
[http://dx.doi.org/10.2190/DPFA-URA4-CH2K-UMQ5]

[180]   Fanos JH, Nickerson BG. Long-term effects of sibling death during adolescence. J Adolesc Res 1991; 6(1): 70-82.
[http://dx.doi.org/10.1177/074355489161006]

[181]   Applebaum DR, Burns GL. Unexpected childhood death: Posttraumatic stress disorder in surviving siblings and parents. J Clin Child Psychol 1991; 20(2): 114-20.
[http://dx.doi.org/10.1207/s15374424jccp2002_1]

[182]   Powell M. The Psychosocial Impact of Sudden Infant Death Syndrome on Siblings. Ir J Psychol 1991; 12(2): 235-47.
[http://dx.doi.org/10.1080/03033910.1991.10557840]

[183]   Lashley M, Talley W, Lands LC, Keyserlingk EW. Informed proxy consent: communication between pediatric surgeons and surrogates about surgery. Pediatrics 2000; 105(3): 591-7.
[http://dx.doi.org/10.1542/peds.105.3.591] [PMID: 10699114]

[184]   Perrin EC, Lewkowicz C, Young MH. Shared vision: concordance among fathers, mothers, and pediatricians about unmet needs of children with chronic health conditions. Pediatrics 2000; 105(1 Pt 3) (Suppl. 2): 277-85.
[http://dx.doi.org/10.1542/peds.105.S2.277] [PMID: 10617736]

[185]   Walker DK, Epstein SG, Taylor AB, Crocker AC, Tuttle GA. Perceived needs of families with children who have chronic health conditions. Child Health Care 1989; 18(4): 196-201.
[http://dx.doi.org/10.1207/s15326888chc1804_1] [PMID: 10296095]

[186]   Wharton RH, Levine KR, Buka S, Emanuel L. Advance care planning for children with special health care needs: a survey of parental attitudes. Pediatrics 1996; 97(5): 682-7.
[http://dx.doi.org/10.1542/peds.97.5.682] [PMID: 8628607]

[187]  Sargent J. The sick child: family complications. J Dev Behav Pediatr 1983; 4(1): 131.
       [http://dx.doi.org/10.1097/00004703-198303000-00010] [PMID: 6833505]

[188]  Mărginean CO, Meliţ LE, Chinceşan M, *et al.* Communication skills in pediatrics – the relationship
       between pediatrician and child. Medicine (Baltimore) 2017; 96(43): e8399.
       [http://dx.doi.org/10.1097/MD.0000000000008399] [PMID: 29069036]

[189]  Levetown M. Communicating with children and families: from everyday interactions to skill in
       conveying distressing information. Pediatrics 2008; 121(5): e1441-60.
       [http://dx.doi.org/10.1542/peds.2008-0565] [PMID: 18450887]

CHAPTER 2

# Positive and Negative Outcomes of Sexting

**Elizabeth Englander**[1,*], **Cheryl E. Sanders**[2] and **Katalin Parti**[3]

[1] *Bridgewater State University, Bridgewater, Massachusetts 02325, USA*

[2] *Metropolitan State University of Denver, Denver, Colorado 55106, USA*

[3] *Department of Sociology, Virginia Tech University, Blacksburg, Virginia 24061, USA*

**Abstract:** Historically, the concept of "sexting" (the sending of nude pictures or videos between teenage youth) has been associated with extremely negative outcomes, including legal vulnerabilities, lost future opportunities, and depression and suicide. These negative outcomes have been widely promoted in the news media and in research on the phenomena. Yet despite diligent efforts by adults to warn youth of these negative outcomes, sexting persists and may even be more common than was first thought. Almost a decade ago, the first research began to emerge that suggested that these risks may be less common than first thought. More recent research has filled out our knowledge about sexting by outlining positive outcomes of sexting that may help explain why underage youth persist in these behaviors despite draconian warnings. This paper outlines some of these positive outcomes, such as improved feelings of self-confidence and attractiveness; strengthening of existing relationships; and the view that sexting is a safe way to explore emerging sexuality. Given this mix of both potential positive and negative feelings about sexting, I propose here that sexting education should follow the best practices long established for sex education, namely, ensuring that youth understand risks, consider relationships and feelings, and do not engage in sexting because of pressure or coercion.

**Keywords:** Cellphone, Computer, Cyberbullying, Digital Behaviors, Digital sexual harassment, Internet sex, Nude, Nudity, Online sex, Photos, Pictures, Sex, Sext, Sexting, Sexual content, Sexual harassment, Videos, Virtual, Virtual behavior, Virtual nudes.

## INTRODUCTION

The concept of sexting was brought to the public's attention in 2005. That year, the Los Angeles Times published a news story about a phenomenon they referred

* **Corresponding author Elizabeth Englander:** Bridgewater State University, Bridgewater, Massachusetts 02325, USA: Tel: (508) 531-1784, Fax: (508) 531-5784, Email: eenglander@bridgew.edu

Nima Rezaei and Noosha Samieefar (Eds.)<br>

to as "sext-messaging." Within a few years, the National Campaign to Prevent Teen and Unplanned Pregnancy, in partnership with Cosmogirl.com, released the results of a survey of 1,280 teens and young adults about that topic. In that survey, 22% of teenage girls and 18% of teenage boys reported that they had sent or posted a nude or semi-nude photo of themselves [1].

This was the emerging phase in knowledge and research about sexting. Sexting was, without a doubt, a shocking and disturbing phenomenon for most adults. In this first phase, adults understood that such pictures could be fascinating and stimulating for youth, but they also viewed sexting as an activity that could have dangerous and potentially life-changing consequences. Early cases of sexting reported in the media tended to reinforce this viewpoint. Young girls, in particular, were viewed as hapless victims who commonly found their pictures were widely distributed; one girl interviewed in the NCPTUP study described how a topless photo was sent around and, within hours, "the whole county had it" [2]. Tragic cases made headlines; all too often sexting and the chronic sexual harassment that seemed to inevitably follow led to tragic cases of suicide. Sexting seemed, at least at times, to be a life-or-death issue. Parental anxiety increased steadily, fed, no doubt, by discomfort with adolescent sexuality, combined with a sense that sexting was a new and scary digital behavior. National Public Radio's headline in 2009 reflected the public mood: "Sexting: A Disturbing New Teen Trend?" [3]. The article focused on a high school in Seattle, Washington, where adults discovered that football players were distributing nude photos of two female students. One parent told NPR that she feared the incident would permanently scar her daughter's life. Meanwhile, legal prosecutions of sexting cases began in earnest, and states often used felony child pornography laws. In all the cacophony, few attempted to understand why sexting was occurring, how risky it was in reality, and how sexting might be engaged in for different reasons.

## SEXTING: POSITIVE AND NEGATIVE OUTCOMES

Around 2012, in what might be viewed as the second phase of this understanding of sexting behaviors, researchers began to introduce studies that explored the possibility that sexting was a more complicated and nuanced behavior. The first author of this article published just such a report in 2012, titled "Low Risk Associated with Most Teenage Sexting." In that report, I reported on a study of 617 18-year-olds that found that most sexting did not, in fact, lead to draconian consequences, such as peer harassment or detection and punishment by adults [4]. Other studies showed similar findings, pointing out that sexting was not strongly related to other high-risk variables such as high risk sexual behavior or poor self-image [5, 6]. Contrary to media depictions, it was not found to be reliably associated with sexual harassment [7]. Victimization online, such as through cyberbullying, was related to suicidal ideation, but sexting didn't appear to follow the same pattern [8]. At the same time, professionals in law enforcement, such as District Attorneys, were beginning to seek out alternatives to using felony child pornography laws in sexting cases. Generally the sense was that such laws were inappropriate, especially when cases involved voluntary sexting between two minors [9].

On the other hand, researchers began to perceive that sexting was not always a fun and fully consensual activity, and that at times youth were pressured or coerced into sexting [10, 11]. The consequences of pressure or coercion were noted, in studies at MARC, to be an increase in negative outcomes [4]. Other researchers have framed coercive sexting as part of the larger issue of sexual coercion [10]. Increased partner aggression and physical coercion have also been associated with coerced sexting [7].

A recent survey of 742 youth aged 18 and 19 studied as part of research at the Social and Emotional Research Consortium (SERC) examined sexting behaviors. Youth were surveyed online between October 2019 and May 2020, at universities in Massachusetts and Colorado.

The results of this study reflect the most current knowledge about sexting. Currently, while research on sexting is significantly more advanced than even a few years ago, the state of knowledge has not always filtered down to the general public. For example, we know that sexting is not, as was first assumed, a deviant behavior engaged in by a small slice of youth. In reality, it often happens between dating couples, especially for females [11]. The current study found that more than half of the sample had engaged in sexting by age 18, and 64% of all sexting occurred within a romantic relationship.

Further, while early attempts at sexting education often emphasized the legal troubles that, were suggested, engulfed youth; in contrast, this study found that very few cases of sexting were ever actually detected by adults. That in turn suggests that legal consequences are almost certainly the exception, rather than the rule.

Perhaps most interestingly, the current study found that while sexting has often been depicted in the media as an overwhelmingly negative experience for youth, it leads to positive outcomes. As with adolescent in-person sexual behaviors, some experiences with sexting are negative but, importantly, not all. The positive outcomes that were most commonly reported were increased self-confidence, a more positive self-image, the strengthening of a romantic relationship, and viewing sexting as a positive way to explore sexuality. These positive outcomes were actually reported by subjects at higher rates, compared to negative outcomes such as legal prosecution or problems, opportunity losses, or bullying or harassment by peers [12]. Another recent study reported on similar findings, noting that approximately one half of subjects reported experiencing positive outcomes after sexting, and only 10% reported experiencing negative outcomes [11].

This is not to suggest that negative outcomes do not exist or are unimportant. However, they may be substantially different than those first conceptualized. For example, legal prosecution was hardly the most likely problem. In fact, the most common negative outcomes in the SERC study were emotional consequences, such as anxiety or concern about the picture. These emotional outcomes are important and should not be minimized, especially among some more vulnerable groups of sexters (such as very young teenagers or those who 'sext' as the result of coercion or negative pressure). Among those vulnerable subjects, negative outcomes were noted significantly more frequently.

Researchers have established that sexting is significantly less common among younger teens, but it still occurs. Several studies have established this, including one of more than a thousand middle school students in Los Angeles. That study found that 20% of middle school students had received a sext, and 5% had sent one [13]. Previous studies at the Massachusetts Aggression Reduction Center (MARC) have also found that slightly higher percentages (10%) of middle school students (under age 15) have sent a nude photo of themselves to a peer [4]. In the current study, 38% of youth reported having sent their first sext prior to age 18. Among this sample, sexting prior to age 18 was more common than first sexting at age 18 or 19.

Pressure to sext also seems to be more nuanced than at first glance. Overwhelmingly, research has only focused on pressure as a negative influence. While such negative pressure is noted in this study to be much more common among younger sexters, some pressure was experienced as neutral or even positive. For example, teens involved in a romantic and sexual relationship reported finding some pressure from their partners flattering or, at least, understandable.

## CONCLUSION

Education about sexting seems to rely primarily on fear-based messaging, that is, trying to frighten youth by describing draconian consequences to sexting and suggesting that such consequences are in fact common. In this study, these messages were not highly effective. They had more of an impact upon females, but even among the girls who these fear-based messages as impactful, 40% still admitted sending a sext, suggesting that this approach is at best only minimally effective in reducing sexting behaviors [12].

Almost two-thirds of youth in the SERC study reported that they knew of friends who sexted, but who had no negative consequences, contrary to what adults emphasized; this led them to disregard adult advice. Happily, fear-based messaging is not the only option to ensure that youth are aware of risks associated with sexting. Other strategies involve the use of social norming approaches, which emphasize that not all teens sext, that there are risks, and that each person should feel free to decide against it instead of submitting to social pressure to comply (a similar approach is often used in adolescent sex education). Social norms education has been effective with other risk behaviors, such as texting while driving [14, 15].

Adults often ask what can be told to youth to completely stop them from sexting. Similar to sexual behaviors, there is probably nothing that adults can do to entirely eliminate these behaviors. However, if adults reframe our approach to sexting, for example, by viewing it as a type of sexual behavior, we may be able to help youth make wise personal choices. The data suggests that with the right partner, sexting is not always a negative experience. However, with the wrong partner, it can a traumatic or damaging experience. Because sexting occurs in the context of relationships (even when it happens with people who don't know each other well), discussions can and should focus on how to build healthy relationships. For adolescents, choosing or rejecting sexual activity, including sexting, is part of any relationship. While it may not always be possible to definitely halt adolescent sexting or sexual activity, adult responsibility probably lies with our ability to connect with youth and teach them how to make thoughtful choices about their sexual behaviors, including reminding all teens that no one knows the long-term outcomes of sexting.

## CONSENT FOR PUBLICATION

Not applicable.

## CONFLICT OF INTEREST

The authors declare no conflict of interest, financial or otherwise.

## ACKNOWLEDGEMENT

Declared none.

# REFERENCES

[1]     National Campaign to Prevent Teen & Unplanned Pregnancy. Sex and Tech: Results from a survey of teens and young adults. 2008. Washington, DC; 2008. (Cosmogirl.com).

[2]     Garfinkle S. Sex + Texting = Sexting - On Parenting. 2008. Available From: http://voices.washingtonpost.com/parenting/2008/12/sexting.html

[3]     Joffe-Walt C. "Sexting": A Disturbing New Teen Trend? 2009. Available From: https://www.npr.org/templates/story/story.php?storyId=101735230

[4]     Englander E. Low Risk Associated With Most Teenage Sexting: A Study Of 617 18-Year-Olds. 2012. Available From: http://webhost.bridgew.edu/marc/SEXTING%20AND%20COERCION%20report.pdf

[5]     Brown D, Sarah K, Stern S. Sex, Sexuality, Sexting, and SexEd: Adolescents and the Media. The prevention researcher 2009; 16(4): 12-6.

[6]     Temple JR, Choi H. Longitudinal association between teen sexting and sexual behavior. Pediatrics 2014; 134(5): e1287-92.
[http://dx.doi.org/10.1542/peds.2014-1974] [PMID: 25287459]

[7]     Ross JM, Drouin M, Coupe A. Sexting Coercion as a Component of Intimate Partner Polyvictimization. J Interpers Violence 2019; 34(11): 2269-91.
[http://dx.doi.org/10.1177/0886260516660300] [PMID: 27443412]

[8]     John A, Glendenning AC, Marchant A, *et al.* Self-Harm, Suicidal Behaviours, and Cyberbullying in Children and Young People: Systematic Review. J Med Internet Res 2018; 20(4): e129.
[http://dx.doi.org/10.2196/jmir.9044] [PMID: 29674305]

[9]     Wolak J, Finkelhor D, Mitchell KJ. How often are teens arrested for sexting? Data from a national sample of police cases. Pediatrics 2012; 129(1): 4-12.
[http://dx.doi.org/10.1542/peds.2011-2242] [PMID: 22144707]

[10]    Van Ouytsel J, Lu Y, Shin Y, Avalos BL, Pettigrew J. Sexting, pressured sexting and associations with dating violence among early adolescents. Comput Human Behav 2021; 125: 106969.
[http://dx.doi.org/10.1016/j.chb.2021.106969]

[11]    Wachs S, Wright MF, Gámez-Guadix M, Döring N. How Are Consensual, Non-Consensual, and Pressured Sexting Linked to Depression and Self-Harm? The Moderating Effects of Demographic Variables. Int J Environ Res Public Health 2021; 18(5): 2597.
[http://dx.doi.org/10.3390/ijerph18052597] [PMID: 33807667]

[12]    Choi H, Van Ouytsel J, Temple JR. Association between sexting and sexual coercion among female adolescents. J Adolesc 2016; 53(1): 164-8.
[http://dx.doi.org/10.1016/j.adolescence.2016.10.005] [PMID: 27814493]

[13]    Drouin M, Coupe M, Temple JR. Is sexting good for your relationship? It depends …. Comput Human Behav 2017; 75: 749-56.
[http://dx.doi.org/10.1016/j.chb.2017.06.018]

[14]    Englander E, Milosevic T, Staksrud E. Sexting: Healthy or Harmful? Comparative Analyses of Teens in Colorado, Massachusetts, Norway, and Serbia. In Dublin, Ireland; 2019.

[15]    Rice E, Gibbs J, Winetrobe H, *et al.* Sexting and sexual behavior among middle school students. Pediatrics 2014; 134(1): e21-8.
[http://dx.doi.org/10.1542/peds.2013-2991] [PMID: 24982103]

CHAPTER 3

# The Role of Integrated Services in the Care of Children and Young People with Neurodevelopmental Disorders and Co-Morbid Mental Health Difficulties: An International Perspective

**Hani F. Ayyash**[1,*], **Cornelius Ani**[2] and **Michael Ogundele**[3]

*[1] Paediatrics Department, Southend University Hospital NHS Foundation Trust, Southend, UK*

*[2] Division of Psychiatry, Imperial College London, and Consultant Child and Adolescent Psychiatrist, Surrey and Borders Partnership NHS Foundation Trust, Surrey, UK*

*[3] Consultant Neurodevelopmental Paediatrician, Halton Community Paediatrics Unit, Bridgewater Community Healthcare NHS Foundation Trust, Runcorn, UK*

**Abstract:** Children and Young People (CYP) affected by Neurodevelopmental, Emotional, Behavioural and Intellectual Disorders (NDEBIDs) such as Attention Deficit and Hyperactive Disorder (ADHD) and Autism Spectrum Disorder (ASD) are at increased risk of other Mental Health (MH) difficulties such as anxiety and depression. Therefore, they require comprehensive and holistic services to meet their complex needs. However, many countries still offer them disjointed services involving different healthcare providers and professionals each looking at only one aspect of the CYP's needs. To address this problem, the framework of "Integrated Care" is recommended as a template for providing comprehensive and joined-up care to meet the complex needs of these CYP with NDEBIDs and MH difficulties. This chapter aims to explore integrated care. It outlines the adverse impacts of disjointed care including: unnecessary multiple referrals, inefficient multiple assessments, delays in accessing required assessment and treatment, frustration and distress for affected CYP and their families and conflicts among professionals. Identified barriers to integrated care include problems with health planning, limited evidence-base, inter-professional difficulties related to different training and professional cultures and mental health stigma. The chapter highlights the benefits of integrated care including user satisfaction, the shortened path to point of care, systemic efficiencies and improved professional relationships. Finally, the chapter discusses the following desirable characteristics of integrated care: joint care commissioning, adequate ring-fenced funding, strategic leadership and planning, cross-training for professionals and good

---

* **Corresponding author Hani F. Ayyash:** Paediatrics Department, Southend University Hospital NHS Foundation Trust, Southend, UK; Tel: 0044 1702 435555; E-mail: hfayyash15@gmail.com

**Nima Rezaei and Noosha Samieefar (Eds.)**
**All rights reserved-© 2023 Bentham Science Publishers**

adherence to evidence-based protocols. Perspectives from Low and Middle-Income Countries (LMICs) were also discussed to acknowledge the international nature of the problem.

**Keywords:** Adolescent, Children, child-health services, Co-morbidities, Holistic services, Integrated care, Mental-health difficulties, mental-health services, Neurodevelopmental disorders, Paediatric services, young people.

## INTRODUCTION

Millions of Children and Young People (CYP) worldwide are affected by Neurodevelopmental, Emotional, Behavioural and Intellectual Disorders (NDEBIDs) such as Attention Deficit and Hyperactive Disorder (ADHD), Autism Spectrum Disorder (ASD), tics and Tourette Syndrome (TS), motor coordination disorder, dyspraxia, sensory processing disorders, developmental delay and learning disabilities [1 - 7]. Prevalence rates of up to 15% have been reported for NDEBID in High-Income Countries (HIC), including up to 10% prevalence for developmental delay [8, 9]. The co-existence of a number of NDEBIDs within the same CYP and sharing of symptoms across other disorders (co-morbidity) is the rule rather than the exception [10, 11]. CYP with NDEBIDs are typically managed by a wide range of professionals including health visitors, nurses, social workers, education specialists, paediatricians, General Practitioners (GP), Speech and Language Therapists (SALT), child neurologists, child psychiatrists, psychologists, neurophysiologists, dentists, clinical geneticists, Occupational Therapists (OT) and Physiotherapists [10, 12].

Studies show that CYP with NDEBIDs are at increased risk of developing sleep disorders [13] and secondary Mental Health (MH) difficulties such as anxiety, depression, Obsessive Compulsive Disorder (OCD), self-harming, suicidal behaviours and conduct disorder in up to 50% of those affected [9, 14] (Table **1**). For example, CYP with ASD have elevated rates of anxiety and depression compared with typically developing children. A recent large scale comprehensive systematic review examining a total of 2755 records, revealed a high burden of co-morbid psychiatric disorders including anxiety disorders, depressive disorders, bipolar and mood disorders, schizophrenia spectrum, suicidal behaviour disorders, attention deficit/hyperactivity disorder, disruptive, impulse-control and conduct disorders amongst diverse age groups with ASD. These findings provide high-quality evidence for the integration of MH services for people with ASD at both clinical and policy-level decision-making from a global viewpoint [15, 16].

Co-morbidities such as conduct disorders (45%), emotional difficulties (14%), learning difficulties (17%), autism (7%), motor coordination difficulties (7%),

Tourette syndrome (3%) and specific scholastic difficulties (3%) were also found among young people with ADHD who recently transitioned to adult services [17]. Furthermore, CYP with ADHD are known to be at higher risk of suicidal behaviour compared to their peers [18]. Thus, many CYP with NDEBIDs experience additional MH difficulties which can lead to further personal suffering, extra functional and education impairment, and in some cases, elevated risk of death from suicide. There is also increasing evidence that these additional MH risks can be long-term and extend into adulthood [19].

**Table 1. Prevalence of anxiety and depressive disorder among CYP with three common NNDs.**

| Neurodevelopmental Disorder | Prevalence of Anxiety Disorders (Source) | Prevalence of Depressive Disorder (Source) | Prevalence of Conduct Disorder (Source) |
|---|---|---|---|
| ADHD | 23% [117] | 9% [118] | 25-50% [119] |
| ASD | 55.3% [120] | 12.5% [121] | 12% [122] |
| Tourette Syndrome | 36.1% [123] | 29.8% [123] | 29.7% (DBD) [123] |
| FASD | 21% [124] | 7% [124] | 7% [125] |
| DCD | Emotional problems 70% [126] | - | 43% [126] |
| Developmental delay | 13.7% [127] | 3.2% [127] | 43.2% (ODD) [127] |
| Intellectual disabilities | 8.7% [128] | 1.5% [128] | 25% [128] |

The bio-psycho-social and ecological origins [20] of NDEBIDs and associated MH difficulties make it imperative that the assessment and treatment of affected CYP should be multimodal, comprehensive and holistic. Such comprehensive assessments are required to capture the full range of CYP's needs in order to produce a full formulation and profile to inform their care plans. Unfortunately, clinical practice in many countries does not reflect this self-evident rationale for holistic assessment and treatment for affected CYP [21]. Services that are designed to support these CYP often tend to be fragmented and disjointed such that the CYP have to attend multiple clinic appointments with different healthcare providers and professional groups each looking at only one aspect of their complex need often without any coordination [22, 23]. In some countries, one or more of the NDEBIDs would be assessed and treated by Paediatric and Child Health Services (PCHS) while others and any associated MH difficulties may be addressed by Child and Adolescent Mental Health Services (CAMHS) [22]. The split between these services can be even more complex such that for the same NDEBIDs such as ASD, some younger children may be seen by PCHS while older young people are seen by CAMHS [23]. The rationale for these service-splits is often opaque and seems arbitrary. Some of the splits may have arisen from historical structures that have persisted without evidence-base. Unsurprisingly, these fragmented and disjointed approaches to assessment and treatment of CYP with NDEBIDs, and additional MH difficulties tend to result in adverse outcomes for affected CYP and their families including multiple ineffectual referrals, delayed assessments, repetitive inefficient assessments and sub-optimal care plans informed by incomplete profiles [23, 24].

The concept of "Integrated Care" was introduced to address difficulties such as disjointed care for CYP with complex needs. The World Health Organization (WHO) defines "Integrated care" as *"Health services organized and managed so that people get the care they need, when they need it, in ways that are user-friendly, achieve the desired results and provide value for money"* [25]. Integrated care provides a framework for comprehensive, holistic and joined-up assessment and treatment in a manner that is more compatible with the complex needs of CYP with NDEBIDs and MH difficulties [22]. Integrated care often involves overcoming the breakdown in communication and collaboration that can arise between different parts of the system and different groups of professionals. An important feature of integrated care is moving beyond pathways for specific diseases [26, 27]. Two dimensions of integrated care relevant to the management of CYP with NDEBIDs and additional MH problems include: (a) at the horizontal level, linking health and education and social care for a whole approach to child care, and (b) at the longitudinal level, linking services across the life course stages for smooth transitions [28].

The need for integrated care for CYP with NDEBIDs and MH mental health difficulties has been recognized for many years, and is a priority goal for the World Health Organization [29]. However, this recognition has not translated into widespread positive changes in practice, often because many countries still have care systems that focus on acute care [30]. This lack of change in focus toward integrated care has resulted in the fact that many countries are still providing fragmented services for this vulnerable group of children with NDEBIDs and MH difficulties.

This chapter explores the core issues related to integrated care for CYP with NDEBIDs and additional MH difficulties. After exploring the scale and impact of the problem, the chapter discusses barriers to integrated care and the benefits of overcoming these obstacles. Given the international nature of the problems associated with disjointed care for CYP with NDEBIDs and MH difficulties, the chapter also explores integrated care from the perspective of Low and Middle-Income Countries (LMICs). Finally, the desirable characteristics of integrated services are explored. The chapter is not intended to provide an exhaustive exploration of the wider subject of integrated care. Rather it specifically focused on CYP with NDEBIDs and additional MH difficulties whose complex needs occur at the interface between PCHS and CAMHS.

## EVIDENCE-BASED DIAGNOSIS OF NDEBID

Diagnosis of NDEBIDs is traditionally based on the assessment of behaviour by clinicians and carers in different settings, however, this approach is prone to biases. Recent advances in computerized Continuous Performance Task (CPT) tests and Quantified Behaviour (Qb) Test [31] have greatly improved their clinical utility in the assessment of some NDEBIDs [32]. As there is no single laboratory test or set of physiological features that have been identified as an unequivocal "Gold Standard", the "reference standard" is often the clinician's judgment. For this reason, in an integrated neurodevelopmental service, the use of an objective representation of the symptoms of NDEBIDs visually presented with the aid of diagrams and graphs, would enable parents, and often patients, to gain a better understanding of the condition and to better appreciate and adhere to the medical management proposed by the physician, whether this includes medications or not. Conversely, visual presentation of a normal CPT test of Qb test, for example, may help to convince a parent that their child's difficulties are not due to ADHD [32]. The Qb Test and other computerized testing systems may be helpful as a part of a comprehensive neurodevelopmental assessment, especially in High-Income Countries where local studies have supported their reliability and usefulness.

## ANALYSIS OF INTEGRATED CARE

### The Negative Impact of Disjointed Services for CYP With NDEBIDs and Co-Morbid Mh Disorders

The most serious and immediate impact of non-integration of services for CYP with NDEBIDs and additional MH difficulties is on the affected CYP and their families. In addition, care providers and the wider health economy are also adversely affected.

### *Inefficient Multiple Assessments*

In relation to CYP with NDEBIDs and additional MH difficulties and their families, the adverse experiences of non-integrated services include distress from going through multiple assessments whereby they repeatedly give the same or similar information to different professionals with no additional benefit to the CYP concerned [24, 33]. For example, the assessment of each NDEBIDs and or MH difficulties involves inquiries into the CYP's developmental, family, social and medical histories. However, when services are not integrated, this information gets repeated at each different assessment, even though most of this information is stable and not likely to have changed. Thus, diagnostic pathway modelling has shown that by avoiding unnecessary repetition, it takes an integrated service 785 minutes to complete assessment of NNDs while it takes 1245 minutes to complete the same assessment in a disjointed service [24]. Integrated service also achieved a 40% reduction in cost and a 75% reduction in time from referral to completion of the assessment [24].

Our clinical experience shows that background histories make up about 40% of a typical new assessment for a CYP with suspected NDEBIDs or MH difficulty. Therefore, for a CYP with three possible NDEBIDs (*e.g.,* ADHD, ASD, and Tourette syndrome) and an additional MH difficulty (*e.g.,* depression) who is assessed by four disparate non-integrated services, the family would end up repeating this background information on four separate occasions. This is likely to be not only annoying and distressing to the family but is also wasteful of time and effort for each of the four different professionals who must assess the CYP. Each of these professionals could easily have saved 40% of the time taken up in their interview and report writing if they did not have to repeat this background information unnecessarily. The aforementioned modelling [24] demonstrates how huge cumulative inefficiency occurs in non-integrated services. The frustration engendered by the confusing referral pathways in disjointed services can result in families making complaints, which is understandable. However, the time taken up in each service to deal with these multiple complaints leads to even more ineffectual service delivery.

### Confusing Multiple Referral Pathways

Another source of distress for CYP with NDEBIDs and additional MH difficulties who have to access disjointed services is the need for multiple referrals for their different NDEBIDs and or MH difficulties [33, 34]. Due to the fact that these separate and multiple referrals do not get pooled to a single point of access, there is an increased risk of confusion as the referrals get redirected back and forth between different services and the original referrer. Some referrals may get lost or mislaid in the process. Where healthcare providers operate "waiting lists" due to demand-capacity imbalance, the initial confusion about which service is responsible for each of the multiple referrals can lead to a significant delay before the CYP joins the "right" waiting list. In some cases, the need for a further assessment for another NDEBID or MH difficulty only becomes known during the assessment for the first NDEBID the CYP was referred for. If the CYP is subsequently referred elsewhere for the newly recognized NDEBID or MH difficulty, they may be placed on a waiting list by the next service provider as a "new referral" not considering that the CYP may have already waited for several months to be assessed by the first service. It is therefore not surprising that these confusions and delays cause considerable frustration and distress for affected CYP and their families, as well as for referrers.

### *Delays in Accessing the Required Assessment and Treatment*

Non-integrated services for CYP with multiple NDEBIDs and MH difficulties can lead to prolonged wait before the young person's full needs, and profile can be understood and used to inform their care and educational planning [24]. This wait arises because even when a healthcare provider can be identified that accepts responsibility for assessing each suspected NDEBIDs or MH difficulty (which is not always the case), the timescales for each assessment may vary widely, and the CYP's needs may have evolved further in the meantime.

The disjointed nature of non-integrated services also means that while each healthcare provider can come to a narrow formulation based on their specialty assessment of the CYP's separate NDEBIDs and or MH difficulties, there may be no overarching formulation that links the separate narrow formulations into the single cohesive and coherent profile that is required for planning the CYP's care and education. The resulting incomplete or incoherent profile could mean that some but not all the CYP's needs are met which can lead to persisting challenges in settings such as education. The consequences of disjointed service provision often led to CYP bouncing between services, with subsequent long delays and patients 'falling through the gaps' [24].

### *Conflicts Among Professionals*

Disjointed services for CYP with NDEBIDs and additional MH difficulties also have adverse effects on professionals providing care for the affected CYP [35]. Non-integrated services engender a sense of territoriality among professionals which may be subconscious or overt. The resulting territorial approach to service delivery can lead to mistrust between staff in the different organizations that are meant to be working together to support an affected CYP [36]. Unhealthy competition [37] and "bunker mentality" can emerge among professionals in separate organizations within the local health system. This unhelpful atmosphere can lead to professionals in one organization making unfounded assumptions about the demand-capacity or efficiency of service delivery in other organizations. Professionals in each organization may start having unrealistic expectations from each other, which can lead to healthcare providers blaming each other unfairly for unmet needs of the CYP, whose needs overlap between the organizations. Professionals may also inadvertently undermine one another by offering conflicting messages at various clinical encounters with the patients and their carers [22]. Overall, the sense of cooperation and collaboration which is essential for good clinical outcomes for the CYP with NDEBIDs and MH difficulties can become unwittingly undermined by the negative undercurrents caused by non-integration of the services designed to support them.

## Barriers to Integrated Care for CYP with NDEBIDs and Additional MH Difficulties

Given the huge negative impact of disjointed services for CYP with NDEBIDs and additional MH difficulties, it is self-evident that services for this vulnerable group of CYP should be integrated [22]. This begs the question of why such service integration has not become the norm in most countries. This section of the chapter explores some of the barriers holding back the integration of services for CYP with NDEBIDs and MH difficulties. These barriers apply in many High-Income Countries (HICs) as well as in Low and Middle-Income Countries (LMICs) all over the world [30].

### *Strategic Difficulties in Service Commissioning, Funding and Planning*

Systematic reviews have tended to identify more proximal barriers to service integration such as poor interagency communication, lack of valuing across agencies, poor understanding across agencies and confidentiality issues [21]. However, while these factors matter, others have argued that the more overarching barriers are strategic macro factors related to the fact that health systems in many countries are organized with a focus on the needs of people with acute episodic care based on one condition rather than on people with long-term conditions such as CYP with NDEBIDs and MH difficulties [30]. This historical focus on acute care has for example contributed to the structuring of services for CYP into separate PCHS and CAMHS [28]. The manner in which these historical structures are currently commissioned and funded appears to have perpetuated the focus on acute care and continuing separation of services for CYP where integration should be the goal [24].

Many countries operate health services in a commissioner (or funders) vs provider split [38]. Within this arrangement, the commissioners specify the remit of health services that they would fund. If the healthcare provider accepts the commission, they will deliver services within the remit and funding limits set by the commissioning / funding body. In some countries such as the United States of America, the commissioners / funders may be insurance companies [38]. However, in other countries such as the United Kingdom where healthcare is state-funded, the commissioners may be another agency of the government (*e.g.,* integrated care systems (ICS). A multidisciplinary team of professionals including paediatricians, child psychiatrists and allied medical and mental health workers has identified the need to engage service development, commissioning and service managers for addressing primary care involvement and definition of service models for effective management of people with NDEBIDs such as ADHD [39]. In either case, the outcome is that commissioning remits and the linked funding, and outcome measures may constrain providers on how they organize and provide services at a lower meso level which can compound the more overarching barriers created at the macro level by the national health system focus on acute care. For example, healthcare providers may have limited incentive to provide integrated care where local commissioning remits specify separate clinical pathways instead of a more holistic care system. Some services are commissioned based on a particular NDEBID or age grouping rather than aiming at holistic/multidisciplinary assessment/intervention for each CYP [24, 40]. This tendency against integrated care may be irrespective of favourable higher macro policies by national governments or the World Health Organization [30].

Health commissioners and funders seek financial accountability and "value for money" from healthcare providers, which is understandable. However, the way healthcare providers organize and deliver services may be positively or adversely influenced depending on how the accountability and expected outcomes are operationalized [41]. For example, where commissioners set simplistic short-term outcome measures because they are easier to "count" (*e.g.,* time to diagnosis), the healthcare providers may become incentivized to focus narrowly on the pursuit of assessment of one NDEBID because the "time to reach a diagnosis" would be quicker and more easily defined than for multiple NDEBIDs with additional MH difficulties. Such provider organizations may also become less favourably disposed towards cooperation with other organizations in the local health system to provide more comprehensive services that would better meet the needs of CYP with multiple NDEBIDs and MH difficulties. This is because while their contribution could be of crucial benefit to affected CYP, it may be more difficult to evidence it (*i.e.,* count) based on the simple narrow outcomes set for their organization by the service commissioners. Thus, commissioning criteria and expectations can be powerful barriers that can hamstring well-meaning healthcare providers, and stop them from delivering integrated care where they may otherwise wish to do so [42].

Another strategic barrier to service integration for CYP with NDEBIDs and MH difficulties relates to how the services designed to meet their needs are set up. Traditionally, many countries set up services along "Clinical Pathways". The reasons given for this approach include greater consistency of care and cost reduction [43]. This type of service design has resulted in PCHS and CAMHS often being set up separately, despite the obvious close interface between these two services in meeting the needs of CYP with NDEBIDs and additional MH difficulties [24, 40]. Thus, the mere fact that PCHS and CAMHS are seen by Commissioners, professionals and the wider public as "different" immediately creates artificial boundaries, and potential barriers for CYP who must use these otherwise complementary services. As already noted, the presence of actual or perceived boundaries by professionals working within PCHS and CAMHS could lead to unhelpful competition, and mistrust such that some professionals in both services could start going against their instinctive clinical sense of cooperation for the common good of the patient. At a practical level, these services often have different health information systems that are not shared either due to patient confidentiality or technological barriers [30].

Insufficient funding of services for CYP with NDEBIDs and MH difficulties is another factor that militates against service integration. Innovative integrated services often face significant challenges both to obtain initial funding to cover the costs of change, and then to secure sustainable funding for the longer term [21, 22]. Poorly funded services may be more likely to focus on narrow objectives to meet what managers often refer to as their "core goals". The obvious difficulty is that disparate services working narrowly to meet their core goals miss the point that for CYP with NDEBIDs, the so-called core goals are of limited value if not coordinated to produce an overarching joined up profile for the CYP. This tendency for services to focus on narrower goals can become accentuated during times of economic downturn which results in governments instituting austerity measures. At such times, health funders and commissioners sometimes place additional pressures on provider organizations to adopt "lean" practices as a means to financial savings. While lean policies have shown demonstrable benefits in some business environments such as manufacturing, they do not necessarily apply well to the complex environment of healthcare delivery [44]. Thus, unsophisticated application of lean methods to health care delivery for CYP with NDEBIDs and mental health difficulties can result in the narrowing of clinical assessments and treatments where a more comprehensive and holistic approach should be the goal.

### Limited Evidence-Base

Good evidence-base is essential to persuade health funders, commissioners and planners to commit effort and additional resources to redesigning services for CYP with NDEBIDs and MH difficulties in order to make them more integrated. Although the benefits of integrated services are self-evident, and have a good face value, policy makers still need robust research evidence to support their decision making if they are to change the status quo. However, assessment of the effects of service integration has largely been limited to HICs and mainly at the patient level and less at the meso or macro levels [22, 30]. Furthermore, the quality of the evidence is hampered by challenges in assessing complex interventions in "real-world" settings [30]. The need for evidence base is particularly important where redesigning services will require extra funding and significant initial disruption for existing users and staff delivering services in the current configuration. In these circumstances, overcoming the inertia of existing patterns of service delivery becomes harder, and so requires even more robust evidence of likely benefit to convince professionals to change their practice.

Systematic reviews indicate that the research evidence to support service integration is mixed [21, 22]. While some studies suggest that both users and professionals find integrated services helpful, others suggest negative outcomes in terms of quality [21]. One of the limitations of the current evidence base is the fact that evaluations of some services are based on soft data such as anecdotes [45]. Even where services are already integrated, lack of robust evidence can make it difficult to convince funders to maintain ongoing support [45].

### *Difficulties Related to Professionals*

Several factors related to the professionals involved in service delivery can become barriers to integrating services for CYPs with NDEBIDs and MH difficulties. Historically, the training of specialists in paediatric and child health has limited overlap with the training of child and adolescent mental health professionals [46]. This reduced cross-over in the formative years of these core professional groups who work with CYPs with NDEBIDs and MH difficulties can result in clinicians having a narrow focus on the needs of CYP related to the professional's core area of training. For example, Community Child Health (CCH) clinicians in the UK are not usually trained to assess and treat MH and behavioural difficulties [22].

Once qualified and in the frontline of care provision, if opportunities are not offered for further cross-over of experience between the professional groups, the narrow focus could become entrenched, and may in time create barriers to join-up working. This gap in cross-over training has been acknowledged by some educators across the world with the result that new curricula are being implemented to foster closer inter-professional exposure both in training and during the working life of professionals. For example, in the UK, the Royal College of Pediatrics and Child Health (RCPCH) created an opportunity in 2018 for pediatric trainees to gain additional training in child mental health (https://www.rcpch.ac.uk/resources/child-mental-health-sub-specialty).     The American Academy of Paediatrics has also introduced similar mental health competencies for paediatric primary care clinicians [47].

Stigma among professionals is another potential barrier to the integration of services for CYPs with NDEBIDs and co-morbid MH difficulties. The subject of stigma is sensitive to discuss especially when it relates to stigma by professionals toward mental illness. There is nonetheless research evidence to suggest that some health professionals have negative attitudes toward CYP affected by mental illness [48, 49]. The stigmatizing attitude towards CYP with MH could extend to stigmatization of professionals who work in CAMHS [50] through a process known as "courtesy stigma" [51]. The implication is that if professionals working in PCHS have negative stigmatizing attitudes towards CYP with MH difficulties and or towards professionals working in CAMHS, such child health professionals may be less likely to think favourably about integrating services for CYPs with NDEBIDs and additional MH difficulties [52].

## Benefits of Integrated Care for CYP with NDEBIDs and Co-Morbid MH Difficulties (Box 1)

Overcoming the challenges discussed in the previous section has obvious advantages for CYP with NDEBIDs and additional MH difficulties and their families. There are also clear benefits for professionals and the wider health system [22].

### *User Preference and Satisfaction*

Studies indicate that users and their families prefer integrated services for several reasons, including less exposure to stigma and receipt of continuity of care from familiar providers [22, 30]. Other reasons include the fact that integrated services provide streamlined "one-stop" and joined up access that meets the multiple needs of CYP with multiple NDEBIDs and co-morbid MH difficulties. The benefit of this joined up approach by integrated services starts from having a single point of access for referrals. This removes the need for multiple referrals that are known to cause frustration to families. Furthermore, the holistic approach to assessment within integrated services means that essential background information such as developmental, family and medical histories are collected once only and not repeated unnecessarily. Also, if the family had to wait initially for an assessment, this wait time may be more bearable as they know that all the suspected NDEBIDs and or MH difficulties will be assessed concurrently without the likelihood of going to the back on another waiting list. The joined up assessment is more likely to produce a more complete profile of the CYP's needs which aids adequate planning for their education and care. Better and comprehensive planning is particularly important in reducing the risk of multiple disruptive changes to the affected CYP's educational placements.

### *Improved Equity of Access and Reduced Time to Point-of-Care*

Joined up services operating single point of access can handle the referral process more quickly and equitably [53]. Referrers only have to know one address or point of contact. The joined-up service is then able to internally match the referred child's assessment needs to the most appropriate clinician within the integrated service. This reduces potential inequity in access that might otherwise arise depending on how well-informed the referrer might be about the local services. For example, given that many referrals for CYP with NDEBIDs and or MH difficulties come from primary care or General Practitioners (GPs), a newly qualified GP who is new to an area might struggle to get referrals correctly channeled through disjointed services whereas a well-established GP who has taken time to map the local services may not have the same difficulty. However, both GPs would have a similar ease of making referrals to integrated services that operate at a single point of access.

## Improved Care Efficiency

Children have the right to the highest standard of healthcare, and to a standard of living and social security that facilitates full physical, mental, spiritual, moral and social development [54]. The UN Convention on the Rights of the Child provides a basis for health professionals to promote optimal health and development of infants, children and young people. A comprehensive strategy to improve UK child health should therefore include action across all the domains and determinants of health. Integrated care provides a comprehensive strategy to meet children's health needs in ways that make sense to children and families [28].

Integrated services for CYP with NDEBIDs and or MH difficulties have the necessary ingredients to bring huge benefits to the wider health system [22]. The efficiencies gained through integrated services often result in wider advantages to the local health system including shorter waiting times, better quality of care, improved client satisfaction and fewer complaints and, ultimately reduction in healthcare spending. These benefits arise from the fact that integrated services are more naturally aligned toward meeting the complex needs of CYP with multiple NDEBIDs and MH difficulties compared with disjointed services that create artificial boundaries and "pigeon holes" in a way that is unnatural [24].

## Improved Protection for More Vulnerable Children

Integrated services are particularly likely to benefit CYP with additional vulnerabilities such as those "Looked After" by the state or who are refugees or seeking asylum [22, 55]. These groups of CYP often have an increased prevalence of multiple health needs including several NDEBIDs and MH difficulties such as Post Traumatic Stress Disorder (PTSD) [56]. These CYP are also more likely to experience instability in placements. For example, if a child "Looked After" by the State is referred to disparate non-integrated services due to having multiple NDEBIDs, they may need multiple new referrals each time they move to a new placement if they have not had all their required assessments while in the previous placement. While pending referrals and assessments are meant to be transferred to the child's new placement, this may not happen promptly, especially where services are disjointed. This scenario increases the potential risk of the CYP's needs not being met which can result in poorer outcomes. On the contrary, if the CYP was accessing an integrated service prior to change of placement, the handover of ongoing assessment and treatment of the CYP's NDEBIDs and MH problems would be more streamlined and more likely to be successful [57].

### *Improved Transitional Care Services for Young People?*

It is important to remember that service integration is both horizontal and vertical. An example of horizontal integration is the focus on meeting the current needs of CYP with NDEBIDs and co-morbid MH difficulties [22, 28]. However, the vertical dimension of service integration is also important. The latter focuses on the longitudinal picture such as transition from the child-focused to adult-oriented support of the CYP. Verity and his colleagues [17] addressed the need for developing a transitional comprehensive evidence based service for young people with NDEBIDs requiring adult mental health services in accordance with the national service framework. This led to the establishment of a transitional adolescent NDEBID clinic and stimulus for an adult ADHD service [58]. Establishing a formal transitional process early from the age of 13 years among patients with chronic NDEBID may help minimize the high rate of attrition and poor treatment adherence among adolescents. For example, a study of care transitions in the North West of England [59] demonstrated that only 12.5% of the adolescents who were eligible for transition to adult NDEBID services were receiving follow-up services. Among those that were successfully transferred to adult services, 19% of them were already discharged within two years. Multi-disciplinary team approach providing holistic care encompassing the medical, psychosocial and educational/vocational needs of adolescents and young adults will greatly facilitate the successful move from paediatric to adult services [60]. Adult NDEBID services across the UK should be developed as a matter of urgency to avoid patients dropping out of treatment during the transitional period after paediatric care stops at age 16 or 18 if in full education [39, 61]. Thus, integrated services are not only beneficial to CYP with NDEBIDs and MH difficulties in the present but they should also benefit them as they transition to adulthood [62]. Having a long-term view of integrated service into adulthood would help to prevent "cliff-edge" transitions for CYP with NDEBIDs when they become adults and continue to need assessment and treatment [63].

### Improved Understanding and Cooperation Among Professionals

Integrated services for CYP with multiple NDEBIDs and co-morbid MH difficulties also bring benefits to professionals [21]. For example, there is considerable overlap between the clinical practice of Paediatricians and Child and Adolescent Psychiatrists (CAP) that is less obvious in services that are not joined up [22]. On the contrary, when services are integrated, the close working between Paediatricians and CAPs enhances this overlap, and produces synergy [55] in the quality of care provided to CYP.

As there is a complex relationship between NDEBIDs and mental health disorders as well as significant overlap between the roles and skills of PCHS and CAMHS teams, more and more children presenting with internalizing and externalizing disorders are first presenting to the PCHS teams who are increasingly expected to assess and manage these conditions. For this reason, it is essential that the paediatric and psychiatric teams are integrated and co-located to provide holistic diagnosis and management of children with NDEBID and mental health problems [64].

Integrated services also enhance the opportunity for each professional group to learn from the others in an informal naturalistic process that complements formal training. In the UK, a multidisciplinary group of professionals involved in the management of NDEBID met in August 2010 with the objective of defining themes and statements for service development. One of the consensuses and recommendations agreed upon by the majority of the multidisciplinary team was that wider education is needed to ensure that policymakers at national and local levels are fully aware of the impacts of untreated NDEBID, particularly those with ADHD, on the individual patients and the entire society [39, 61]. The symbiotic learning among professional groups in integrated services helps to extend individual clinicians' skills in a helpful lateral manner that improves task-sharing [30]. For example, child and adolescent psychiatrists may become more conversant with recognizing medical needs or medication side effects or requirements for medical investigations such as ECG. On the other hand, paediatricians may become more familiar with psychosocial interventions and recommend them to CYP and families who may otherwise have missed out on such interventions. These benefits for professional groups working in integrated services can improve their job satisfaction and retention [21].

### Reduced Impact of Mental Health Stigma

Integrated services could help mitigate the negative impact of mental health stigma on help-seeking behaviour. Evidence from many countries and cultures shows that fear of mental health stigma can prevent CYP from seeking help for NDEBIDs and or MH difficulties [65]. The negative impact of stigma on help-seeking may be more noticeable among minority ethnic groups living in Western Europe and North America [66, 67]. For example, fear of stigma has been hypothesized as a possible reason for relatively lower mental health service utilization among children of Asian background in the United Kingdom [68]. Stigma related to mental illness in CYP is also well documented in LMICs as one of the factors militating against access to MH services [49]. Therefore, where mental health stigma is a concern for a family, they may be more willing to attend an integrated service to seek help for their CYP with NDEBIDs and co-morbid MH difficulties because the service does not have an obvious "Mental Health" label compared with a provision that is explicitly described as "Mental Health Service" [69 - 71].

## *Alignment with Emerging Government Policy*

Integrated health care services are increasingly being recognized by governments and health policymakers as the desirable service models for the future, in the face of rising healthcare costs and limited financial and human resources [22]. For example, the UK Government has used its recent major health policy document (NHS Long-term plan) to promise greater funding for breaking down traditional barriers between care institutions so as to support the increasing number of people with long-term health conditions, rather than viewing each encounter with the health service as a single, unconnected 'episode' of care (https://www.longterm plan.nhs.uk/wp-content/uploads/2019/08/nhs-long-term-plan-version-1.2.pdf).

## Integrated Services in the Context of Low and Middle Income Countries

## *Significant Needs*

While integrated services for CYP with NDEBIDs and co-morbid MH difficulties are desirable all over the world, such services are particularly relevant to the situation in LMICs. About 90% of the CYP in the world live in LMICs where they make up more than 50% of the population [72]. This also means that proportionately, the vast majority of CYP with NDEBIDs and co-morbid MH difficulties live in LMICs. Also, CYP in LMICS are exposed to more risk factors for developing NDEBIDs, such as Low Birth Weight (LBW), obstetric complications and malnutrition [73, 74]. The magnitude of the specific risk associated with LBW is illustrated by the fact that 91% of LBW babies are born in LMICs [75]. CYP in LMICs are also more likely to experience environmental risk factors for mental health difficulties such as extreme poverty, lack of access to education and societal dislocation due to wars and famine [76]. Overall, the burden of NDEBIDs and MH difficulties among CYP in LMICs is projected to continue to grow due to two factors [77]. The first factor relates to persisting biological and environmental risks. The second reason is due to the projected increase in the overall population of CYP living in LMICs resulting from a combination of persisting high fertility rates and reduction in mortality rates.

## Resource Gaps

Unfortunately, the high and rising burden of CYP with NDEBIDs and MH difficulties in LMICs is not matched by the availability of services. Studies continue to document huge treatment gaps for mental illnesses among all ages in LMICs, more so for CYP [78]. For example, many LMICs have only one psychiatrist per million population [79]. The very few psychiatrists in these settings often have no specific expertise in Child and Adolescent Mental Health (CAMH). Furthermore, the few available psychiatrists are often based in major cities whereas majority of the population of CYP in LMICs live in rural areas [80]. Although the availability of paediatric and child health professionals in LMICs is also limited, they are much more widely available compared to child and adolescent mental health professionals.

Thus, the situation in LMICs means that services to meet the needs of CYP with NDEBIDs and MH difficulties would need to be integrated because it may not be viable to rely on the extremely limited or non-existent CAMH professionals to run stand-alone MH services. In these settings, the limited number of professionals with expertise in CAMH may be better used for training and supervision of other professionals. For example, the CAMH professionals could help to extend the expertise of paediatric and child health professionals to enable the latter group to deliver services for CYP with NDEBIDs and associated MH difficulties. This process of inter-professional skill extension which is termed "task shifting" is being advocated in LMICs as an important mechanism for bridging treatment gaps [70, 81].

Some CAMH training programs in LMICs, such as Nigeria are starting to recognize the important need for integrated services for CYP with NDEBIDs and MH difficulties [76]. For example, the training programme run by the centre for child and adolescent mental health at the University of Ibadan in Nigeria encourages professionals with backgrounds in paediatrics and child health to apply for training in CAMH. Also, the training curriculum is designed to overlap significantly between paediatrics and child health and CAMH. This overlap is illustrated by the fact that the clinical component of the training requires students to have a mandatory experience of participating in clinics run jointly by paediatricians and child and adolescent mental health professionals [76].

### *Limited Evidence-Base*

Presently, the evidence for integrated services is mainly available from HICs, and there is limited information from LMICs. While some of the information from HICs may be relevant to LMICs, direct relevance between the two settings cannot be assumed due to huge cultural and socio-economic differences. For example, it has been suggested that the concept of task-shifting may be more applicable in LMICs due to more severe shortage of highly trained professionals. Similarly, the impact of out-of-pocket payment for health services by families of CYP with NDEBIDs and MH difficulties may be more relevant to LMICs. This is because many LMICs have limited or no public funding for healthcare. Overall, the limited evidence from LMICs suggests that the region has a low level of preparedness for service integration due to factors such as insufficient multidisciplinary personnel, limited training opportunities, insufficient or fragmented health information systems and implementation that is not contextualized to take into account local health and religious belief systems [82].

### DESIRABLE FEATURES OF INTEGRATED SERVICES FOR CYP WITH NDEBID AND CO-MORBID MENTAL HEALTH DIFFICULTIES

Research has shown that services that already offer integrated assessment and treatment of CYP with NDEBIDs and MH difficulties vary in the extent to which their practices are integrated [45]. While some services offer joint assessment and or treatment for one or more NDEBIDs without provision for meeting additional MH needs, others include multiple NDEBIDs with support for additional MH needs. Some services provide only assessments while others offer both assessments and treatments. The services also differ in how they are funded, with some based on "block" funding, while others are funded for specific patients. Despite these variations, the integrated services are working toward similar goals albeit to varying degrees. Systematic reviews and other primary studies have identified factors that can help to improve the commissioning, design, and implementation of integrated services for CYP with NDEBIDs and co-morbid MH difficulties. Overall, systemic changes are required in health systems to support service integration [22, 30]. This starts at the macro level with national policy formulation that supports service integration.

Introducing service integration may not require new structures or staff. Instead, the required change may be to repurpose existing infrastructure and staff, while changing the culture and expectations in the system towards one of cooperation and collaboration between professionals with the shared goal of providing a holistic care package for affected CYP. These changes in thinking and culture need to involve several aspects as discussed next.

## Joint Service Commissioning

A previous section of this chapter highlighted the crucial role of commissioners and funders in relation to service development and integration. Therefore, it follows that one of the main desirable strategic factors to support the development of integrated services at the meso level is gaining the support of local commissioners and health funders. Service integration is more likely to be initiated and sustained if the funders make integration an explicit goal for the service being commissioned [22]. Such a goal for joined-up service delivery tends to be easier where PCHS and CAMHS are commissioned by the same funders.

Even when overarching central government policy is favourable towards service integration, the buy-in of local funders remains crucial, especially where service specifications (and hence funding streams) are decentralized and locally determined. Funders who wish to support service integration for CYP with NDEBIDs and MH difficulties need to specify clear goals and outcome measures for service providers that explicitly support service integration [22]. In this situation, unambiguous goals that include measures of demonstrable aspects of service integration are more useful than "buzz words" that can be differently interpreted [83].

Given that service integration for CYP with NDEBIDs and MH difficulties interface mainly between PCH and CAMHS, the funding and commissioning specification needs to capture components that are typically associated with both professional groups. The unambiguous expectation for joined up working is more likely to unite the clinicians from these and other related professional groups towards achieving the common goals of providing a comprehensive and holistic service for CYP with NDEBIDs and MH difficulties. Both groups then know and own both the success and failure of the joined up service delivery. The resulting service environment is likely going to reduce the potential for unwitting interdisciplinary competition, territoriality and mistrust that can all undermine the primary goal of meeting the complex needs of CYP with NDEBIDs and MH difficulties.

A team of commissioners and funders spread across a wide conjoint area or specializing in different aspects of healthcare provision for the CYP would need to come together, and constitute a "joint team" with an identified "fund manager" to coordinate the alignment of all resources towards the implementation of the integrated service. Close collaboration among all the local stakeholders should be prioritized right from the onset through all the stages of planning, implementation and evaluation of the integrated services. In the UK, a set of forty consensus statements covering ten topics that would define the ideal structure and direction of integrated multidisciplinary services for CYP with NDEBIDs have been presented by a multidisciplinary group of paediatricians and child psychiatrists, including joint commissioning and optimization of the relevant care pathways [61].

## Adequate and Ring-Fenced Funding

Adequate funding is crucial for integrated services to avoid them being "set up to fail". The specification should provide for sufficient funding to meet the projected demand for holistic and comprehensive assessment of the needs of CYP with NDEBIDs and co-morbid MH difficulties as well as treatment [22]. Even when the goal is for the integrated service to become more cost-effective over time, they may require additional initial "set-up" funding to get it running. It is also possible, and may even be desirable for the new joined up service to require more funding than was available for the disparate services that preceded it. The important point is that insufficient funding and resources would result in predictable demand-capacity imbalance in the new integrated service. Unfortunately, such an imbalance could not only exacerbate unmet needs for affected children but may restart internal boundaries whereby professional groups may start pulling back to defensive positions in the same way as might have been the case before integration. It is also important that funders do not use the process of service integration as a "Trojan horse" for "cost-cutting" which would effectively reduce the funding and resources available to the joined-up service. Such a move would be predictably counterproductive.

## Effective Service Planning and Implementation

An integrated service requires realignment of procedures and practices in such a way as to reduce duplication and gain efficiency [24, 53]. This usually involves having a single point of access so that referrers and users only need to know one point of access. From this point, the referral can be internally triaged to ensure that the CYP is seen by the right clinicians for assessment and treatment in a seamless process that minimizes repetition and duplication [84]. Joined up administrative and record keeping systems would further reduce repetition and improve efficiency [22, 24]. It could also lead to some cost savings for some office equipment and recurring expenses. For example, common database for all CYP with NDEBIDs and co-morbid MH disorders could be utilized across a range of specialist services [85, 86].

One of the important goals for integrated services for CYP with NDEBIDs is multidisciplinary assessment to determine the needs of CYP referred to the service. This often includes making a determination about whether the CYP meets the criteria for a formal diagnosis of one or more NDEBIDs. Accurate and reliable diagnostic assessments can hugely improve the profiling of a CYP's needs in a way that can inform their educational and other care plans. However, it is important to remember that diagnostic assessments are designed to categorize symptoms and behaviours that are, in reality, dimensionally distributed in the population. This means that even when a CYP does not meet the specific criteria for diagnosis of a particular NDEBID such as ASD, the child may still have sufficient traits of ASD that can be almost as impairing as for other CYP with a diagnosis. Therefore, CYP assessed within integrated services but who do not meet diagnostic criteria for any specific NDEBID can benefit from a more dimensional profiling of their needs that can still usefully inform their support in education and at home [45]. A successful and efficient NDEBID service should implement Integrated Care Pathways (ICPs) to ensure appropriate assessment, diagnosis and management of each case. ICPs will also offer the chance for improved outcomes and resource optimization [61].

The multiple and complex needs of CYP with NDEBIDs and co-morbid MH problems mean that they and their families need to be working with multiple members of the team simultaneously. Therefore, in order to make these care plans coherent for the family, it is essential that each CYP is allocated a care coordinator who remains responsible for the family as other clinicians make their input and exit from the plan [61]. The care coordinator provides a constant point of focus for the family in their care journey which can help to avoid confusion for the families and ensure that access to services and local agencies is optimized. The care coordinator could either be a member of the PCHS or CAMHS, depending on whether the NDEBID or MH disorder is the predominant presentation of the CYP, but with scope for flexibility.

**Evidence-Based Practice**

The evidence base for service integration is continuing to develop, and better evidence is required to guide modelling of service design, practice and evaluation [21, 30]. Therefore, it is essential to build in action research into existing or newly developed integrated services to produce data on what models work well, what elements of the models make the most contribution to good outcomes, and what outcomes measures are more sensitive to service evaluation. Current evidence tended to focus on patient level but evidence for benefit at higher health system, and national levels are also required in order to support wider adoption of service integration practices [30, 86]. Moreover, the current preponderance of evidence for integrated services from HICs needs to be balanced with more research on LMICs in order to produce good quality evidence that is relevant to a wider section of the world.

## Continuity of Support

Integrated services are organic entities that have the capacity for growth or remodelling and, if not looked after, can fail [84]. Thus, the energy and enthusiasm that go into starting an integrated service need to be maintained to keep improving and growing it for even better benefit for users and the professionals working in the service. The growth and nurturing of the service require strategic leadership, which is informed by use of new research data, user feedback, and changes in the epidemiology and profiles of local health needs of CYP with NDEBIDs and MH disorders [22]. However, the goals need to be pragmatic, realistic, and fit into the wider health policy for service integration to be sustainable. While enthusiasm to embrace service integration is important, logistical constraints must be acknowledged, and trade-offs may need to be made in order to properly calibrate expectations in workload to avoid overloading the professionals delivering the service with the risk of burnout.

## Effective and Motivated Strong Leadership

Effective leadership at the most senior management levels is one of the indispensable requirements for successfully integrated care services [22]. Many attempts at successful integrated services have often been led and championed by highly motivated and dedicated leadership. These services are often at risk of not being sustained once the leader has retired or moved into other areas. Integrated services need to be carefully managed by a lead clinician or manager rather than allowed to drift along, providing nurture, and developing joint identity, involving the whole staff members to increase connectedness and effectiveness of the integrated service. This requires essential leadership skills in relationship-maintenance, diplomacy, consultation and negotiation [87].

In the wider context of public health, changes in the pattern of health and social care delivery across the UK provide the context for an increased alignment between social services and the NHS in the treatment of NDEBIDs [88]. Local authorities have Health and Well Being Boards (HWBB) which are responsible for the integration of public health and social care services. Child public health considers the wider picture of the health of a child, placing the health of children and their families in their full social, economic and political context [89]. This viewpoint will enable paediatricians and MH practitioners firstly, to better understand the context of a particular patient. For example, the relationship between a child's risky behaviours and the degree of engagement with services, against the backdrop of their individual lifestyle factors, social and community networks and wider socioeconomic, cultural and environmental conditions. Secondly, the clinicians are able to positively engage with the health of the wider population of CYP through each individual patient [90]. In addition, a clinician might need to reflect on, engage and deal with causal and upstream factors of a disease to address some of the issues that affect their patients. As an example, the national obesity observatory has gathered evidence to demonstrate the early impacts of obesity on emotional and behavioural problems, as well as other long-term predictors of adult health and mortality [91, 92]. Paediatric and MH clinicians are in a unique position to identify individual risk factors which, if they became embedded, would confer significant cumulative health risks, and thereby, modify the progression of behaviour and emotional disorders among children, adolescents and their families [90].

In a non-integrated service, the traditional role of the paediatrician involves assessing CYPs physical health before referring them to mental health clinicians. This sequencing of access rather than joint access can delay the process of addressing the CYPs MH problem, which prevents holistic care for CYP's physical and mental health needs. For example, in CYP with recurrent abdominal pain, which is associated with mental health issues in around 80% of cases, their quality of life, adherence to therapy and overall outcome can be severely negatively impacted, if emotional and behavioural factors are not addressed early as contributory to the original pathology [93]. This consideration is equally valid for other conditions like diabetes, asthma, constipation and epilepsy [94].

## Professional Training and Continuous Development

Ongoing staff training is crucial for the success of integrated services [39, 70]. Different professional groups need to come together to operate an integrated service. While each group brings its own specific expertise, the opportunity for synergy will be maximized by additional training before starting the service and ongoing [22]. The training would help staff to understand and support existing areas of overlap and areas of necessary specialized skill sets. This type of training could help to promote more realistic expectations and reduce unhelpful assumptions about different professional groups. Additional training could also be used to encourage extension of existing skills across professional boundaries where this is safe and appropriate for the benefit of users. The latter can improve task-sharing which is not only good for the professional development of the clinicians but also provides a wider pool of skill sets to meet the complex needs of the CYP who use the service.

In the UK, there are a number of online e-learning courses written by specialists for a general audience such as MindEd (http://www.minded.org.uk), which constitute an excellent starting point for professionals' training. MindEd also includes the "specialist CAMHS module" which paediatricians may find useful in extending their MH knowledge. Other websites such as Mental Elf (http://www.thementalelf.net) and the Royal College of Paediatrics and Child Health (RCPCH)'s Healthy Child Programme (http://www.rcpch.ac.uk/hcp) have content on mental health. Other specialist-comprehensive online modules in the field of NDEBIDs are available at websites such as Doctors.net.uk [95].

However, E-learning alone is not enough, and this is the reason why the RCPCH and the paediatric mental health association are working together on a number of face-to-face courses on mental health aspects of paediatrics (https://www.rcpch.ac.uk/education-careers/courses). It is essential to emphasize that paediatricians cannot offer the integrated care that CYP deserve without incorporating mental health routinely into their practice, although they will always need the assistance of mental health specialists around them [94]. As medical knowledge is constantly changing and new information becomes available, changes in treatment, procedures, equipment and use of medications necessary for integrated care of CYP will also be evolving.

In LMICs, use of existing programs such as world health organization mhGAP intervention guide can be a ready resource for training paediatric and child health professionals in relation to CYP with NDEBIDs and co-morbid MH difficulties [96].

**Parents' Training and Psychoeducation**

Psychoeducation involves health care professionals providing information about NDEBIDs, including their causes and impact, advice on parenting strategies and additional support. Psychoeducation is defined as an intervention with systematic, structured and didactic knowledge transfer for an illness and its treatment, integrating emotional and motivational aspects to enable patients to cope with the illness and to improve its treatment adherence and efficacy. With psychoeducation, families can feel empowered to determine their own best course of treatment from the available range of non-pharmacological and pharmacological interventions [97].

With increasing recognition and diagnosis of children with NDEBIDs, there is a need for the PCHS and MH services to develop innovative interventions to meet the needs of the large number of diagnosed CYP with their families for relevant specialist education. With recognition that many NDEBIDs, particularly ASD and ADHD, are lifelong conditions, integrated services need to be equipped with resources and information to support these families who may experience difficulties at different transitions points in the child's development [98].

Studies from HICs have shown that a variety of behaviour problems among CYP can be effectively managed with parent-delivered behaviour interventions [99 - 101]. In a Canadian study conducted in a community day-care centre over 12 weeks, Jocelyn *et al* taught 35 parents the use of functional analysis to understand challenging behaviour in children with ASD and developed treatment strategies for managing such behaviours. The authors showed that there was significant improvement in post-test behaviour measures [99]. In studies using reinforcement, antecedent-based techniques and environmental manipulations, there was a reduction in aggression to near zero level among children with autism aged 1-3 years [102, 103]. Similarly, Frea and colleagues [104] reported an immediate and rapid reduction in aggression in children with NDEBIDs through the use of Picture Exchange Communication Systems (PECS).

In the United States, a large-scale randomized clinical trial, among 180 children aged 3-7 years with NDEBIDs and behaviour problems, investigated effects of either parent training or education on disruptive behaviour in children with ASD. Significant reduction in disruptive behaviour was reported among the intervention parent group [105]. Similar findings were reported by other researchers in LMIC, including a pilot study involving 20 mothers of children with ASD who completed five sessions of weekly manualized group-based interventions which included functional behaviour analysis management strategies [106]. The robustness of this evidence underlines its recommendation in guidelines for management of children with ASD in the UK [107].

In the United Kingdom, several researchers have highlighted the importance of parent-directed psychoeducation in the management of CYP recently diagnosed with ASD) [108]. An evaluation of CYGNET training program which was developed for parents of children with ASD was evaluated in an integrated neurodevelopmental service in South-Eastern England found significant improvement in parents' knowledge, and as well as an increase in their confidence on how to deal with challenging behaviour of their CYP with ASD [109]. City and Hackney MH services in the UK have devised two sessions of psychoeducation group training for parents of children recently diagnosed with ASD to increase their understanding of the condition and support them to help them develop practical strategies to manage their child with the ASD. Feedback from these groups was generally positive, and found to be very helpful. However, many parents reported the need for further advice and support from a range of professionals including occupational, speech and language therapists and psychologists, who are more likely to be accessed in an integrated multidisciplinary service [98].

Similarly, psychoeducation training programs for parents and their children who are diagnosed with ADHD have been recommended as first-line treatment by different international clinical guidelines [110, 111], regardless the age of the patients [112]. assessed the outcomes of structured parenting training program which was offered to parents of children recently diagnosed with ADHD, and found it to be effective in significantly improving the level of knowledge and understanding of parents regarding several aspects of ADHD including diagnosis, symptom identification and behaviour control. Findings from a recent comprehensive systematic review study indicated that psychoeducation is an effective strategy, not only for the reduction of ADHD symptoms, but it also improves important secondary outcomes over the lifespan of people with ADHD. Importantly, psychoeducation also complements and enhances other treatment approaches, potentially through its promotion of treatment adherence and ability to help empower parents and give them more confidence in their own knowledge when choosing between treatment options for their child [113].

## SUCCESSFUL EXAMPLES OF INTEGRATED SERVICES FOR OTHER CHRONIC DISORDERS

It is worthy of note that integrated services have been successfully implemented for holistic care of other chronic physical problems and associated MH difficulties, including diabetes, cancers, heart diseases and stroke [114]. These innovative services in the UK and elsewhere are giving primary care an enhanced role at the interface between mental and physical health, in particular for people with long-term conditions through evidence-based "Collaborative Care" approach. This involves central roles of specially trained psychological wellbeing practitioners in the assessment and treatment of the patients while receiving regular supervision from MH specialists [86, 115]. A similar approach could be used to integrate PCHS with the tertiary level MH services for CYP with NDEBID and co-morbid MH problems.

It is unfortunate that the model of liaison psychiatry (or psychology) services which have existed in many paediatric/child health departments in the United Kingdom for several decades are not being sustained due to dwindling funding, inadequate human resources within CAMH services and lack of statutory underpinning policies [116].

## CONCLUSION

This chapter has presented a review of the literature on the integration of services for CYP with NDEBIDs and co-morbid MH difficulties. Service integration is an intuitively positive approach to meet the complex needs of these vulnerable CYP. The World Health Organization has identified it as a priority, and there is research evidence to support its benefits to the individual CYP and their families, including shorter waiting times, more comprehensive and holistic profiling of their needs and improved satisfaction. Benefits to the wider health system include efficiency gains and cost-saving. There are also benefits to professional groups such as PCHS and CAMH professionals because more joined up working and joint ownership of the goals to provide holistic services can lead to skills extension, less inter-professional rivalry and improved job satisfaction.

Despite the benefits of integrated care, this system of care provision is still not widely adopted due to several barriers starting with insufficient impetus at higher strategic levels where health policies are still dominated by the focus on acute care and less so on long-term conditions. Additional barriers arise from local commissioning and funding remits that still appear, perhaps unwittingly, to favour disjointed and disparate service provision. More proximal barriers include difficulties with staff culture and training, as well as stigma against mental illness.

Overcoming these barriers will require fundamental system and culture change at all levels of healthcare. This will require policymakers to pay more attention to long-term conditions such as NDEBIDs and co-morbid MH difficulties in order to facilitate support for service integration. Service commissioners and funders at local levels need to mandate the integration of services, and introduce outcomes that are user-led and explicitly measure integration as a key matrix.

The challenges of poorly integrated services exist at varying levels all over the world but maybe particularly difficult in LMICs. The additional challenges in LMICs include lack of system preparedness due to limited number of professionals, especially clinicians with expertise in CAMH, difficulty with training and funding challenges, including need in some cases for families of CYP with NDEBIDs and MH difficulties to make out-of-pocket payment for services. The evidence base for service integration in LMICs is also limited which makes it difficult to create service models that can be adapted to other settings in LMICs. Thus, there remains a continuing need for research to provide better evidence to guide implementation of service integration, especially in LMICs where the current evidence is more limited.

It is notable that of the available models of care for CYP with NDEBIDs and MH difficulties, none has better face value and evidence base than integrated services. Integrated care makes sense, and when practiced, it produces better outcomes for individual CYP and their families. The benefits can be even more critical for CYP with additional vulnerabilities such as children "Looked After" by the State, refugees and those seeking asylum. Integrated care has additional benefits to the wider health system and professionals.

It is noteworthy that while evidence base for integrated holistic services for CYP with NDEBIDs and co-morbid MH difficulties is still emerging, there are ample examples of successful implementation of integrated services for other chronic physical problems and associated MH difficulties.

There is a great and urgent need to overcome the inertia currently holding back the implementation of integrated services for CYP with NDEBIDs, and MH difficulties in many countries to realize the inherent wide-ranging benefits.

## CONSENT FOR PUBLICATION

Not applicable.

## CONFLICT OF INTEREST

The authors declare no conflict of interest, financial or otherwise.

## ACKNOWLEDGEMENT

Declared none.

## REFERENCES


[1]   Ayyash HF, Preece PM. Evidence-based treatment of motor co-ordination disorder. Curr Paediatr 2003; 13(5): 360-4.
[http://dx.doi.org/10.1016/S0957-5839(03)00058-7]

[2]   Ayyash H, Barrett E, Ogundele M. 243 Sensory Processing of Children with Autism: Uniting Evidence and Practice. Arch Dis Child 2012; 97 (Suppl. 2): A70-1.
[http://dx.doi.org/10.1136/archdischild-2012-302724.0243]

[3]   Mona , Endowed EDL. Autism Worldwide: Prevalence, Perceptions, Acceptance, Action. J Soc Sci 2012; 8(2): 196-201.
[http://dx.doi.org/10.3844/jssp.2012.196.201]

[4]   Willcutt EG. The prevalence of DSM-IV attention-deficit/hyperactivity disorder: a meta-analytic review. Neurotherapeutics 2012; 9(3): 490-9.
[http://dx.doi.org/10.1007/s13311-012-0135-8] [PMID: 22976615]

[5]   Gillberg C, Fernell E, Minnis H. Early symptomatic syndromes eliciting neurodevelopmental clinical examinations.     Scientific     World     Journal     2014;     2014(Jan):     710570.
https://www.ncbi.nlm.nih.gov/pmc/articles/PMC3886270/ [Internet].
[PMID: 24453934]

[6]   Ogundele MO. Behavioural and emotional disorders in childhood: A brief overview for paediatricians. World J Clin Pediatr 2018; 7(1): 9-26.
[http://dx.doi.org/10.5409/wjcp.v7.i1.9] [PMID: 29456928]

[7]   Ogundele MO, Ayyash HF. Review of the evidence for the management of co-morbid Tics disorders in children and adolescents with attention deficit hyperactivity disorder. World J Clin Pediatr 2018; 7(1): 36-42.
[http://dx.doi.org/10.5409/wjcp.v7.i1.36] [PMID: 29456930]

[8]   Parsons S, Platt L. Disability among young children: Prevalence, heterogeneity and socio-economic disadvantage. 2013; 28.

[9]     Eapen V. Developmental and mental health disorders: Two sides of the same coin. Asian J Psychiatr 2014; 8: 7-11.
[http://dx.doi.org/10.1016/j.ajp.2013.10.007] [PMID: 24655619]

[10]    Ogundele MO. A Profile of Common Neurodevelopmental Disorders Presenting in a Scottish Community Child Health Service –a One Year Audit (2016/2017). HR 2018; 2(1): 1.

[11]    Ogundele MO. Co-occurrence and co-morbidities among children and adolescents with ADHD and ASD in a scottish local authority. Arch Dis Child 2018; 103 (Suppl. 1): A192-2.

[12]    Ogundele MO. A multidisciplinary approach to the assessment and management of pre-school age neuro-developmental disorders: A local experience. 2017. https://www.heighpubs.org/hjncp/cjncp-aid1001.php

[13]    Ayyash HF, Preece P, Morton R, Cortese S. Melatonin for sleep disturbance in children with neurodevelopmental disorders: prospective observational naturalistic study. Expert Rev Neurother 2015; 15(6): 711-7.
[http://dx.doi.org/10.1586/14737175.2015.1041511] [PMID: 25938708]

[14]    Mayes SD, Gorman AA, Hillwig-Garcia J, Syed E. Suicide ideation and attempts in children with autism. Res Autism Spectr Disord 2013; 7(1): 109-19.
[http://dx.doi.org/10.1016/j.rasd.2012.07.009]

[15]    DeFilippis M. Depression in Children and Adolescents with Autism Spectrum Disorder. Children (Basel) 2018; 5(9): 112.
[http://dx.doi.org/10.3390/children5090112] [PMID: 30134542]

[16]    Hossain MM, Khan N, Sultana A, *et al.* Prevalence of comorbid psychiatric disorders among people with autism spectrum disorder: An umbrella review of systematic reviews and meta-analyses. Psychiatry Res 2020; 287: 112922.
[http://dx.doi.org/10.1016/j.psychres.2020.112922] [PMID: 32203749]

[17]    Verity R, Omran A, Ayyash H. A Transitional and Adult Service for Patients With ADHD. Responding To The NSF. Arch Dis Child 2006; 91 (Suppl. 1): A39-41.

[18]    Fitzgerald C, Dalsgaard S, Nordentoft M, Erlangsen A. Suicidal behaviour among persons with attention-deficit hyperactivity disorder. Br J Psychiatry 2019; 215(4): 615-20.
[http://dx.doi.org/10.1192/bjp.2019.128] [PMID: 31172893]

[19]    Agnew-Blais JC, Polanczyk GV, Danese A, Wertz J, Moffitt TE, Arseneault L. Young adult mental health and functional outcomes among individuals with remitted, persistent and late-onset ADHD. Br J Psychiatry 2018; 213(3): 526-34.
[http://dx.doi.org/10.1192/bjp.2018.97] [PMID: 29957167]

[20]    Bronfenbrenner U. Ecological systems theory.Six theories of child development: Revised formulations and current issues. London, England: Jessica Kingsley Publishers 1992; pp. 187-249.

[21]    Cooper M, Evans Y, Pybis J. Interagency collaboration in children and young people's mental health: a systematic review of outcomes, facilitating factors and inhibiting factors. Child Care Health Dev 2016; 42(3): 325-42.
[http://dx.doi.org/10.1111/cch.12322] [PMID: 26860960]

[22]    Ogundele M, Ayyash H, Ani C. Integrated Services for Children and Young People with Neurodevelopmental and Co-Morbid Mental Health Disorders: Review of the Evidence. Journal of Psychiatry & Mental Disorders 2020; 5(3): 1027.

[23]    Ani C, Ayyash HF, Ogundele MO. Community paediatricians' experience of joint working with child and adolescent mental health services: Findings from a British national survey. bmjpo 2022; 6(1): e001381.

[24]    Male I, Farr W, Reddy V. Should clinical services for children with possible ADHD, autism or related conditions be delivered in an integrated neurodevelopmental pathway? Integ Health J 2020; 2(1):

e000037.

[25]   World Health Organization (WHO). Integrated health services - what and why? 2008. https://www.who.int/healthsystems/technical_brief_final.pdf

[26]   Curry N, Ham C. Clinical and service integration: the route to improved outcomes. 2010. https://www.kingsfund.org.uk/publications/clinical-and-service-integration

[27]   Klaber RE, Blair M, Lemer C, Watson M. Whole population integrated child health: moving beyond pathways. Arch Dis Child 2017; 102(1): 5-7.
[http://dx.doi.org/10.1136/archdischild-2016-310485] [PMID: 27217582]

[28]   Wolfe I, Lemer C, Cass H. Integrated care: a solution for improving children's health? Arch Dis Child 2016; 101(11): 992-7.
[http://dx.doi.org/10.1136/archdischild-2013-304442] [PMID: 27052949]

[29]   World Health Organization (WHO). Framework on integrated people-centred health services. 2016. Available from: http://www.who.int/servicedeliverysafety/areas/people-centred-care/en/

[30]   Thornicroft G, Ahuja S, Barber S, *et al.* Integrated care for people with long-term mental and physical health conditions in low-income and middle-income countries. Lancet Psychiatry 2019; 6(2): 174-86.
[http://dx.doi.org/10.1016/S2215-0366(18)30298-0] [PMID: 30449711]

[31]   Hollis C, Hall CL, Guo B, *et al.* The impact of a computerised test of attention and activity (QbTest) on diagnostic decision-making in children and young people with suspected attention deficit hyperactivity disorder: single-blind randomised controlled trial. J Child Psychol Psychiatry 2018; 59(12): 1298-308.
[http://dx.doi.org/10.1111/jcpp.12921] [PMID: 29700813]

[32]   Ogundele MO, Ayyash HF, Banerjee S. Role of computerised continuous performance task tests in ADHD. Prog Neurol Psychiatry 2011; 15(3): 8-13.
[http://dx.doi.org/10.1002/pnp.198]

[33]   Kirby A, Thomas M. The whole child with developmental disorders. Br J Hosp Med (Lond) 2011; 72(3): 161-167, 164-167.
[http://dx.doi.org/10.12968/hmed.2011.72.3.161] [PMID: 21475097]

[34]   Levy SE, Giarelli E, Lee LC, *et al.* Autism spectrum disorder and co-occurring developmental, psychiatric, and medical conditions among children in multiple populations of the United States. J Dev Behav Pediatr 2010; 31(4): 267-75.
[http://dx.doi.org/10.1097/DBP.0b013e3181d5d03b] [PMID: 20431403]

[35]   Ødegård A. Exploring perceptions of interprofessional collaboration in child mental health care. Int J Integr Care 2006; 6(4): e25. https://www.ncbi.nlm.nih.gov/pmc/articles/PMC1762090/
[http://dx.doi.org/10.5334/ijic.165] [PMID: 17211492]

[36]   Widmark C, Sandahl C, Piuva K, Bergman D. Barriers to collaboration between health care, social services and schools. Int J Integr Care 2011; 11(3): e124.
http://www.ijic.org/articles/abstract/10.5334/ijic.653/
[http://dx.doi.org/10.5334/ijic.653] [PMID: 22125502]

[37]   Barr H, Koppel I, Reeves S, Hammick M, Freeth DS. Effective interprofessional education: Argument, assumption and evidence (promoting partnership for health). 2005. https://www.wiley.com/en-us/Effective+Interprofessional+Education%3A+Argument%2C+Assumption+and+Evidence+%28Promoting+Partnership+for+Health%29-p-9781405116541

[38]   Mossialos E, Wenzl M, Osborn R, Anderson C. International Profiles of Health Care Systems 2015: Commonwealth Fund 2016. https://www.commonwealthfund.org/publications/fund-reports/2016/jan/international-profiles-health-care-systems-2015

[39]   Ayyash H, Sankar S, Merriman H, *et al.* Engagement of commissioners, primary and secondary care for developing successful ADHD services. Eur Child Adolesc Psychiatry 2013; 22(1): 45-6.
[http://dx.doi.org/10.1007/s00787-012-0321-6] [PMID: 23179414]

[40]    Ayyash HF, Ogundele MO, Lynn RM, Schumm TS, Ani C. Involvement of community paediatricians in the care of children and young people with mental health difficulties in the UK: implications for case ascertainment by child and adolescent psychiatric, and paediatric surveillance systems. BMJ Paediatr Open 2021; 5(1): e000713.
[http://dx.doi.org/10.1136/bmjpo-2020-000713] [PMID: 33614992]

[41]    Hernandez M, Hodges S, Cascardi M. The ecology of outcomes: System accountability in children's mental health. J Behav Health Serv Res 1998; 25(2): 136-50.
[http://dx.doi.org/10.1007/BF02287476] [PMID: 9595878]

[42]    Hudson B. Integrated Commissioning: New Contexts, New Dilemmas, New Solutions? J Integr Care 2010; 18(1): 11-9.
[http://dx.doi.org/10.5042/jic.2010.0082]

[43]    Schrijvers G, van Hoorn A, Huiskes N. The care pathway: concepts and theories: An introduction. Int J Integr Care 2012; 12(Spec Ed Integrated Care Pathways): e192.
[http://dx.doi.org/10.5334/ijic.812]

[44]    McIntosh B, Sheppy B, Cohen I. Illusion or delusion – Lean management in the health sector. Int J Health Care Qual Assur 2014; 27(6): 482-92.
[http://dx.doi.org/10.1108/IJHCQA-03-2013-0028] [PMID: 25115051]

[45]    Embracing Complexity. Embracing Complexities in Diagnosis: Multi-diagnostic pathways for neurodevelopmental conditions. 2019. http://embracingcomplexity.org.uk/assets/documents/Embracing-Complexity-in-Diagnosis.pdf

[46]    Graham P, Jenkins S. Training of paediatricians for psychosocial aspects of their work. Arch Dis Child 1985; 60(8): 777-80.
[http://dx.doi.org/10.1136/adc.60.8.777] [PMID: 4037867]

[47]    Policy statement--The future of pediatrics: mental health competencies for pediatric primary care. Pediatrics 2009; 124(1): 410-21.
[http://dx.doi.org/10.1542/peds.2009-1061] [PMID: 19564328]

[48]    Henderson C, Noblett J, Parke H, et al. Mental health-related stigma in health care and mental health-care settings. Lancet Psychiatry 2014; 1(6): 467-82.
[http://dx.doi.org/10.1016/S2215-0366(14)00023-6] [PMID: 26361202]

[49]    Tungchama FP, Egbokhare O, Omigbodun O, Ani C. Health workers' attitude towards children and adolescents with mental illness in a teaching hospital in north-central Nigeria. J Child Adolesc Ment Health 2019; 31(2): 125-37.

[50]    Schulze B. Stigma and mental health professionals: A review of the evidence on an intricate relationship. Int Rev Psychiatry 2007; 19(2): 137-55.
[http://dx.doi.org/10.1080/09540260701278929] [PMID: 17464792]

[51]    Corrigan PW, Miller F. Shame, blame, and contamination: A review of the impact of mental illness stigma on family members. J Ment Health 2004; 13(6): 537-48.
[http://dx.doi.org/10.1080/09638230400017004]

[52]    Jenkins R, Mussa M, Haji SA, et al. Developing and implementing mental health policy in Zanzibar, a low income country off the coast of East Africa. Int J Ment Health Syst 2011; 5(1): 6.
[http://dx.doi.org/10.1186/1752-4458-5-6] [PMID: 21320308]

[53]    Fleury MJ, Mercier C. Integrated local networks as a model for organizing mental health services. Adm Policy Ment Health 2002; 30(1): 55-73.
[http://dx.doi.org/10.1023/A:1021227600823] [PMID: 12546256]

[54]    United Nations. Convention on the Rights of the Child 1990. https://www.ohchr.org/en/professionalinterest/pages/crc.aspx

[55]    Shaw MJ, Garrett P, MacSween M, et al. 'Doing Better Together': Developing a cross-agency

regional child health and wellbeing plan. Int J Integr Care 2017; 17(3): 36.
[http://dx.doi.org/10.5334/ijic.3148]

[56]   Ogundele MO. Profile of Neurodevelopmental and behavioural problems and associated psychosocial factors among a cohort of Looked-After children newly entering into the care of an England Local Authority. Adopt Foster In Press.

[57]   Ogundele M. Profile of neurodevelopmental and behavioural problems and associated psychosocial factors among a cohort of newly looked after children in an English local authority. Adopt Foster 2020; 44(3): 255-71.
[http://dx.doi.org/10.1177/0308575920945187]

[58]   Verity R, Coates J. Service innovation: transitional attention-deficit hyperactivity disorder clinic. Psychiatr Bull 2007; 31(3): 99-100.
[http://dx.doi.org/10.1192/pb.bp.105.008904]

[59]   Ogundele MO. Transitional care to adult ADHD services in a North West England district. Clin Gov 2013; 18(3): 210-9.
[http://dx.doi.org/10.1108/CGIJ-01-2013-0001]

[60]   Viner RM. Transition of care from paediatric to adult services: one part of improved health services for adolescents: Figure 1. Arch Dis Child 2008; 93(2): 160-3.
[http://dx.doi.org/10.1136/adc.2006.103721] [PMID: 17942588]

[61]   Ayyash H, Sankar S, Merriman H, *et al.* Multidisciplinary consensus for the development of ADHD services: the way forward. Clin Gov 2013; 18(1): 30-8.
[http://dx.doi.org/10.1108/14777271311297939]

[62]   Price A, Janssens A, Newlove-Delgado T, *et al.* Mapping UK mental health services for adults with attention-deficit/hyperactivity disorder: national survey with comparison of reporting between three stakeholder groups. BJPsych Open 2020; 6(4): e76.
https://www.ncbi.nlm.nih.gov/pmc/articles/PMC7443899/
[http://dx.doi.org/10.1192/bjo.2020.65] [PMID: 32723405]

[63]   Eke H, Ford T, Newlove-Delgado T, *et al.* Transition between child and adult services for young people with attention-deficit hyperactivity disorder (ADHD): findings from a British national surveillance study. Br J Psychiatry 2017; 217(5): 616-22.
[PMID: 31159893]

[64]   Ogundele MO, Ayyash HF. Evidence-based multidisciplinary assessment and management of children and adolescents with neurodevelopmental disorders. Arch Dis Child 2019; 104 (Suppl. 2): A268-8.

[65]   Corrigan P. How stigma interferes with mental health care. Am Psychol 2004; 59(7): 614-25.
[http://dx.doi.org/10.1037/0003-066X.59.7.614] [PMID: 15491256]

[66]   Gary FA. Stigma: barrier to mental health care among ethnic minorities. Issues Ment Health Nurs 2005; 26(10): 979-99.
[http://dx.doi.org/10.1080/01612840500280638] [PMID: 16283995]

[67]   Memon A, Taylor K, Mohebati LM, *et al.* Perceived barriers to accessing mental health services among black and minority ethnic (BME) communities: A qualitative study in Southeast England. BMJ Open 2016; 6(11): e012337.

[68]   Bradby H, Varyani M, Oglethorpe R, Raine W, White I, Helen M. British Asian families and the use of child and adolescent mental health services: A qualitative study of a hard to reach group. Soc Sci Med 2007; 65(12): 2413-24.
[http://dx.doi.org/10.1016/j.socscimed.2007.07.025] [PMID: 17766019]

[69]   Hickling FW, Robertson-Hickling H, Paisley V. Deinstitutionalization and attitudes toward mental illness in Jamaica: a qualitative study. Rev Panam Salud Publica 2011; 29(3): 169-76.
[PMID: 21484016]

[70]    Ventevogel P. Integration of mental health into primary healthcare in low-income countries: Avoiding medicalization. Int Rev Psychiatry 2014; 26(6): 669-79.
[http://dx.doi.org/10.3109/09540261.2014.966067] [PMID: 25553784]

[71]    Juengsiragulwit D. Opportunities and obstacles in child and adolescent mental health services in low- and middle-income countries: a review of the literature. WHO South-East Asia J Public Health 2015; 4(2): 110-22.
[http://dx.doi.org/10.4103/2224-3151.206680] [PMID: 28607309]

[72]    United Nations. World Population Prospects: The 2010 Revision. 2011. world-population-prospects-the-2010-revision.html

[73]    Serati M, Barkin JL, Orsenigo G, Altamura AC, Buoli M. Research Review: The role of obstetric and neonatal complications in childhood attention deficit and hyperactivity disorder - a systematic review. J Child Psychol Psychiatry 2017; 58(12): 1290-300.
[http://dx.doi.org/10.1111/jcpp.12779] [PMID: 28714195]

[74]    Galler JR, Bryce CP, Zichlin ML, Fitzmaurice G, Eaglesfield GD, Waber DP. Infant malnutrition is associated with persisting attention deficits in middle adulthood. J Nutr 2012; 142(4): 788-94.
[http://dx.doi.org/10.3945/jn.111.145441] [PMID: 22378333]

[75]    Blencowe H, Krasevec J, de Onis M, *et al.* National, regional, and worldwide estimates of low birthweight in 2015, with trends from 2000: a systematic analysis. Lancet Glob Health 2019; 7(7): e849-60.
[http://dx.doi.org/10.1016/S2214-109X(18)30565-5] [PMID: 31103470]

[76]    Ani C, Omigbodun O, Omigbodun O. The Sustainable Development Goals and Child and Adolescent Mental Health in Low- and Middle-Income Countries. The Routledge Handbook of International Development, Mental Health and Wellbeing Routledge. 2019; pp. 152-70.

[77]    Scott JG, Mihalopoulos C, Erskine HE, Roberts J, Rahman A. Childhood Mental and Developmental Disorders.Mental, Neurological, and Substance Use Disorders: Disease Control Priorities. 3rd ed. Washington, DC: The International Bank for Reconstruction and Development / The World Bank 2016; Vol. 4. [Internet] http://www.ncbi.nlm.nih.gov/books/NBK361938/

[78]    Lund C, Tomlinson M, De Silva M, *et al.* PRIME: a programme to reduce the treatment gap for mental disorders in five low- and middle-income countries. PLoS Med 2012; 9(12): e1001359.
[http://dx.doi.org/10.1371/journal.pmed.1001359] [PMID: 23300387]

[79]    World Health Organization (WHO). Mental Health Atlas 2014. 2015. http://www.who.int/mental_health/evidence/atlas/mental_health_atlas_2014/en/

[80]    Saxena S, Thornicroft G, Knapp M, Whiteford H. Resources for mental health: scarcity, inequity, and inefficiency. Lancet 2007; 370(9590): 878-89.
[http://dx.doi.org/10.1016/S0140-6736(07)61239-2] [PMID: 17804062]

[81]    Joshi R, Alim M, Kengne AP, *et al.* Task shifting for non-communicable disease management in low and middle income countries--a systematic review. PLoS One 2014; 9(8): e103754.
[http://dx.doi.org/10.1371/journal.pone.0103754] [PMID: 25121789]

[82]    Hanlon C, Luitel NP, Kathree T, *et al.* Challenges and opportunities for implementing integrated mental health care: a district level situation analysis from five low- and middle-income countries. PLoS One 2014; 9(2): e88437.
[http://dx.doi.org/10.1371/journal.pone.0088437] [PMID: 24558389]

[83]    Meads G, Ashcroft J, Barr H, Scott R, Wild A. The Case for Interprofessional Collaboration. In Health and Social Care. Oxford: Wiley-Blackwell 2005.

[84]    Hasse S, Austin MJ. Service Integration. Adm Soc Work 1997; 21(3-4): 9-29.
[http://dx.doi.org/10.1300/J147v21n03_02] [PMID: 10176511]

[85]    Ogundele MO, Ayyash HF, Banerjee S. ADHD management and disability register: an electronic aid

for the nice guideline implementation. Arch Dis Child 2011; 96 (Suppl. 1): A26-7.
[http://dx.doi.org/10.1136/adc.2011.212563.53]

[86]   Naylor C. Physical and Mental Health.Handbook Integrated Care. Cham: Springer International Publishing 2017; pp. 383-98. [Internet] http://link.springer.com/10.1007/978-3-319-56103-5_23
[http://dx.doi.org/10.1007/978-3-319-56103-5_23]

[87]   Sheaff R, Schofield J, Charles N, Mannion R, Reeves D. The management and effectiveness of professional and clinical networks. Plymouth: National Institute for Health Research 2011. http://www.netscc.ac.uk/hsdr/files/project/SDO_FR_08-1518-104_V01.pdf

[88]   Great Britain, Department of Health. Liberating the NHS. Norwich: TSO 2010.

[89]   Kohler L. Commentary. Child public health. A new basis for child health workers. Eur J Public Health 1998; 8(3): 253-5.
[http://dx.doi.org/10.1093/eurpub/8.3.253]

[90]   Weil LG, Lemer C, Cheung CR. The role of paediatricians in public health for children and young people. Arch Dis Child Educ Pract Ed 2016; 101(4): 181-6.
[http://dx.doi.org/10.1136/archdischild-2015-309958] [PMID: 27165173]

[91]   Griffiths LJ, Dezateux C, Hill A. Is obesity associated with emotional and behavioural problems in children? Findings from the Millennium Cohort Study. Int J Pediatr Obes 2011; 6(2-2): e423-432.
[http://dx.doi.org/10.3109/17477166.2010.526221]

[92]   Reilly JJ, Kelly J. Long-term impact of overweight and obesity in childhood and adolescence on morbidity and premature mortality in adulthood: Systematic review. International Journal of Obesity 2005; 35(7): 891-8.

[93]   Shapiro MA, Nguyen ML. Psychosocial stress and abdominal pain in adolescents. Ment Health Fam Med 2010; 7(2): 65-9.
[PMID: 22477924]

[94]   Davie M. Doing more for mental health. Arch Dis Child Educ Pract Ed 2016; 101(2): 77-81.
[http://dx.doi.org/10.1136/archdischild-2015-308344] [PMID: 26407732]

[95]   Ayyash HF, Karim K. Autism spectrum disorder in children and adolescents. Autism spectrum disorder in children and adolescents. 2020. Available From: http://www.doctors.net.uk/ecme/wfrmNewIntro.aspx?moduleid=1808

[96]   World Health Organization (WHO). mhGAP Intervention Guide for mental, neurological and substance use disorders in non-specialized health settings. 2010. Available From: http://www.who.int/mental_health/publications/mhGAP_intervention_guide/en/

[97]   Berge JM, Law DD, Johnson J, Wells MG. Effectiveness of a psychoeducational parenting group on child, parent, and family behavior: A pilot study in a family practice clinic with an underserved population. Fam Syst Health 2010; 28(3): 224-35.
[http://dx.doi.org/10.1037/a0020907] [PMID: 20939627]

[98]   Roughan LA, Parker JR, Mercer L. Improving interventions for parents of children and young people with autism spectrum disorder (ASD) in CAMHS. BMJ Open Qual 2019; 8(2): e000261.
[http://dx.doi.org/10.1136/bmjoq-2017-000261] [PMID: 31206044]

[99]   Jocelyn LJ, Casiro OG, Beattie D, Bow J, Kneisz J. Treatment of children with autism: a randomized controlled trial to evaluate a caregiver-based intervention program in community day-care centers. J Dev Behav Pediatr 1998; 19(5): 326-34.
[http://dx.doi.org/10.1097/00004703-199810000-00002] [PMID: 9809262]

[100]  Braithwaite KL, Richdale AL. Functional communication training to replace challenging behaviors across two behavioral outcomes. Behav Interv 2000; 15(1): 21-36.
[http://dx.doi.org/10.1002/(SICI)1099-078X(200001/03)15:1<21::AID-BIN45>3.0.CO;2-#]

[101]  Athens ES, Vollmer TR. An investigation of differential reinforcement of alternative behavior without extinction. J Appl Behav Anal 2010; 43(4): 569-89.
[http://dx.doi.org/10.1901/jaba.2010.43-569] [PMID: 21541145]

[102]  Mueller MM, Wilczynski SM, Moore JW, Fusilier I, Trahant D. Antecedent manipulations in a tangible condition: effects of stimulus preference on aggression. J Appl Behav Anal 2001; 34(2): 237-40.
[http://dx.doi.org/10.1901/jaba.2001.34-237] [PMID: 11421319]

[103]  Butler LR, Luiselli JK. Escape-Maintained Problem Behavior in a Child With Autism: Antecedent Functional Analysis and Intervention Evaluation of Noncontingent Escape and Instructional Fading. Journal of Positive Behavior Interventions 2007; 9(4): 195-202. https://journals.sagepub.com/doi/10.1177/10983007070090040201

[104]  Frea WD, Arnold CL, Vittimberga GL. A Demonstration of the Effects of Augmentative Communication on the Extreme Aggressive Behavior of a Child With Autism Within an Integrated Preschool Setting. J Posit Behav Interv 2001; 3(4): 194-8.
[http://dx.doi.org/10.1177/109830070100300401]

[105]  Bearss K, Johnson C, Smith T, *et al.* Effect of parent training *vs* parent education on behavioral problems in children with autism spectrum disorder: a randomized clinical trial. JAMA 2015; 313(15): 1524-33.
[http://dx.doi.org/10.1001/jama.2015.3150] [PMID: 25898050]

[106]  Bello-Mojeed M, Ani C, Lagunju I, Omigbodun O. Feasibility of parent-mediated behavioural intervention for behavioural problems in children with Autism Spectrum Disorder in Nigeria: a pilot study. Child Adolesc Psychiatry Ment Health 2016; 10(1): 28.
[http://dx.doi.org/10.1186/s13034-016-0117-4] [PMID: 27594900]

[107]  National Institute for Health and Care Excellence (NICE-UK). Autism spectrum disorder in under 19s: Recognition, referral and diagnosis. 2013. Available from: https://www.nice.org.uk/guidance/cg128

[108]  Gordon M, Chandratilake M, Baker P. Low fidelity, high quality: a model for e-learning. Clin Teach 2013; 10(4): 258-63.
[http://dx.doi.org/10.1111/tct.12008] [PMID: 23834573]

[109]  Ayyash HF, Ogundele MO, Cuff L, Azmi L, Weisblatt E. Effect of cygnet training programme at improving parents' knowledge and confidence in managing autistic children at an integrated neurodevelopmental service in south eastern england. Arch Dis Child 2019; 104 (Suppl. 2): A208-9.

[110]  Canadian ADHD Practice Guidelines (CADDRA). 2018. Available From: https://www.caddra.ca/canadian-adhd-practice-guidelines/

[111]  National Institute for Health and Clinical Excellence (NICE-UK). 2018. Available From: https://www.nice.org.uk/guidance/ng87

[112]  Ayyash H, Ogundele MO, Wisbey R, Weisblatt E, Cuff L, Reddy V. The outcome of an ADHD parenting group training programme (APEG) in the peterborough neurodevelopmental service (NDS). Clinical Journal of Nursing Care and Practice 2017; 1(1): 013-9.

[113]  Dahl V, Ramakrishnan A, Spears AP, *et al.* Psychoeducation Interventions for Parents and Teachers of Children and Adolescents with ADHD: a Systematic Review of the Literature. J Dev Phys Disabil 2020; 32(2): 257-92.
[http://dx.doi.org/10.1007/s10882-019-09691-3]

[114]  Scottish Executive Health Department (SEHD). Managed Clinical Networks: supporting and delivering the healthcare quality strategy. 2012. Available From: http://www.sehd.scot.nhs.uk/mels/CEL2012_29.pdf

[115]  Coventry P, Lovell K, Dickens C, *et al.* Integrated primary care for patients with mental and physical multimorbidity: cluster randomised controlled trial of collaborative care for patients with depression comorbid with diabetes or cardiovascular disease. BMJ 2015; 350: h638.

https://www.bmj.com/content/350/bmj.h638
[http://dx.doi.org/10.1136/bmj.h638] [PMID: 25687344]

[116]  Joint Commissioning Panel for Mental Health (JCPMH-UK). Guidance for commissioners of liaison mental health services to acute hospitals. 2003.

[117]  Souza I, Pinheiro MA, Mattos P. Anxiety disorders in an attention-deficit/hyperactivity disorder clinical sample. Arq Neuropsiquiatr 2005; 63(2b): 407-9.
[http://dx.doi.org/10.1590/S0004-282X2005000300008] [PMID: 16059589]

[118]  Blackman GL, Ostrander R, Herman KC. Children with ADHD and depression: a multisource, multimethod assessment of clinical, social, and academic functioning. J Atten Disord 2005; 8(4): 195-207.
[http://dx.doi.org/10.1177/1087054705278777] [PMID: 16110050]

[119]  Franke B, Michelini G, Asherson P, *et al.* Live fast, die young? A review on the developmental trajectories of ADHD across the lifespan. Eur Neuropsychopharmacol 2018; 28(10): 1059-88.
[http://dx.doi.org/10.1016/j.euroneuro.2018.08.001] [PMID: 30195575]

[120]  de Bruin EI, Ferdinand RF, Meester S, de Nijs PFA, Verheij F. High rates of psychiatric co-morbidity in PDD-NOS. J Autism Dev Disord 2007; 37(5): 877-86.
[http://dx.doi.org/10.1007/s10803-006-0215-x] [PMID: 17031447]

[121]  Hudson CC, Hall L, Harkness KL. Prevalence of Depressive Disorders in Individuals with Autism Spectrum Disorder: a Meta-Analysis. J Abnorm Child Psychol 2019; 47(1): 165-75.
[http://dx.doi.org/10.1007/s10802-018-0402-1] [PMID: 29497980]

[122]  Lai MC, Kassee C, Besney R, *et al.* Prevalence of co-occurring mental health diagnoses in the autism population: a systematic review and meta-analysis. Lancet Psychiatry 2019; 6(10): 819-29.
[http://dx.doi.org/10.1016/S2215-0366(19)30289-5] [PMID: 31447415]

[123]  Hirschtritt ME, Lee PC, Pauls DL, *et al.* Lifetime prevalence, age of risk, and genetic relationships of comorbid psychiatric disorders in Tourette syndrome. JAMA Psychiatry 2015; 72(4): 325-33.
[http://dx.doi.org/10.1001/jamapsychiatry.2014.2650] [PMID: 25671412]

[124]  Fryer SL, McGee CL, Matt GE, Riley EP, Mattson SN. Evaluation of psychopathological conditions in children with heavy prenatal alcohol exposure. Pediatrics 2007; 119(3): e733-41.
[http://dx.doi.org/10.1542/peds.2006-1606] [PMID: 17332190]

[125]  Lange S, Rehm J, Anagnostou E, Popova S. Prevalence of externalizing disorders and Autism Spectrum Disorders among children with Fetal Alcohol Spectrum Disorder: systematic review and meta-analysis. Biochem Cell Biol 2018; 96(2): 241-51.
[http://dx.doi.org/10.1139/bcb-2017-0014] [PMID: 28521112]

[126]  Blank R, Barnett AL, Cairney J, *et al.* International clinical practice recommendations on the definition, diagnosis, assessment, intervention, and psychosocial aspects of developmental coordination disorder. Dev Med Child Neurol 2019; 61(3): 242-85.
https://www.ncbi.nlm.nih.gov/pmc/articles/PMC6850610/
[http://dx.doi.org/10.1111/dmcn.14132] [PMID: 30671947]

[127]  Baker BL, Neece CL, Fenning RM, Crnic KA, Blacher J. Mental disorders in five-year-old children with or without developmental delay: focus on ADHD. J Clin Child Adolesc Psychol 2010; 39(4): 492-505.
[http://dx.doi.org/10.1080/15374416.2010.486321] [PMID: 20589561]

[128]  Emerson E. Prevalence of psychiatric disorders in children and adolescents with and without intellectual disability. J Intellect Disabil Res 2003; 47(1): 51-8.
[http://dx.doi.org/10.1046/j.1365-2788.2003.00464.x] [PMID: 12558695]

**CHAPTER 4**

# Epidemiological Evidence for Influences of Non-genetic Transgenerational Inheritance on Child and Adolescent Development



**Jean Golding**[1,*] and **Yasmin Iles-Caven**[1]

[1] *Centre for Academic Child Health, Population Health Sciences, Bristol Medical School, University of Bristol, Oakfield House, Oakfield Grove, Bristol BS8 2BN, UK*





**Abstract:** Our use of the term 'Non-genetic transgenerational inheritance' concerns the influence of environmental exposure to one generation on phenotypes in later generations in the absence of changes in the structure of the DNA. Although animal experiments have shown that the phenomenon exists in plants and animals, many scientists have expressed doubt as to whether this type of inheritance is detectable in humans. In this chapter, we describe the observational epidemiological data that has been published and evaluate the evidence for this type of inheritance. We mainly concentrate on the environmental exposures concerning famine, cigarette smoke and radiation, and chart the associations between pre-conception and prenatal exposures. We describe associations between these exposures and outcomes for the offspring and grandchildren. In general, we demonstrate frequent evidence of sex-specific differences in the likelihood of particular phenotypes, depending on whether it is the maternal or paternal ancestor who is exposed. We also show that the timing of the exposure is often important regarding specific outcomes, with particular emphasis on the 4-5 years before puberty for preconception exposures and the trimester of pregnancy for prenatal exposures. The evidence for non-genetic transgenerational inheritance is increasing. Interestingly, the consequences of exposures that are harmful to one generation often have a beneficial effect on a subsequent generation. It is important that future epidemiological studies are planned to collect information concerning previous and/or subsequent generations so that transgenerational consequences of exposures, such as medications or pesticides, can be charted.

**Keywords:** Asthma, Autism, Betel nut, Cognition, Diethylstilbestrol, DNA methylation, Endocrine disruptors, Environment, Epigenetic, Famine, Fat mass, Grandparental exposures, Hearing, Medications, Nutrition, Parental exposures, Radiation, Smoking, Taste, Transgenerational inheritance.



---



* **Corresponding author Jean Golding:** Centre for Academic Child Health, Population Health Sciences, Bristol Medical School, University of Bristol, Oakfield House, Oakfield Grove, Bristol BS8 2BN, UK, Tel: +44 (0)117 3310198; E-mail: jean.golding@bristol.ac.uk



**Nima Rezaei and Noosha Samieefar (Eds.)**
**All rights reserved-© 2023 Bentham Science Publishers**

## INTRODUCTION

There is international recognition of the importance of environmental factors such as diet, smoking, social circumstances, air pollution and stressful events, in influencing outcomes such as child growth, behavior and neurocognitive development. Such influences may continue throughout individuals' lives [1]. In parallel, though, there is considerable evidence from twin, adoption, and family studies that many outcomes have a strong familial component [2]. However, Genome-Wide Association Studies (GWAS) of DNA variants are often shown to explain relatively small proportions of this heritability [3], so other aspects of inheritance need to be considered. Non-genetic transgenerational inheritance is a major candidate. The phenomenon is currently recognized more among plant and animal rather than human research. It comprises the study of how exposure to an individual in one generation has a demonstrable effect on one or more later generations. Such effects may be beneficial or detrimental.

## NOMENCLATURE

Non-genetic inheritance has been known variously as intergenerational, multigenerational, or transgenerational, depending on whether the germline has been directly exposed or not (Fig. **1**). Intergenerational and multi-generational inheritance has been used synonymously, and it is assumed that the route of transmission is *via* a gonad. There are two possible scenarios for such a form of inheritance: (i) exposure of an individual boy/man or girl/woman (F0) prior to the conception of the next generation (F1); and (ii) the exposure of a pregnant woman (F0) with consequent (indirect) exposure of the embryo or fetus (F1) and thus of his/her developing gonads. These will be subsequently involved in the conception of the next generation (F2). Transgenerational inheritance has been defined as the consequence(s) of exposures to the initial generation (F0) on subsequent generations, excluding those covered by the definitions of inter- or multi-generational inheritance. Because these definitions can be confusing, the term epigenetic inheritance has started to be used to encompass any effect on a subsequent generation that does not involve a change in the DNA itself, such as a mutation.

## EXPERIMENTAL EVIDENCE

Non-genetic inheritance is known to exist in plants and insects, with evidence of environmental exposure to a single generation resulting in a phenotypic change that may be inherited for many generations in the absence of the exposure. For mammals, most experiments that are of possible relevance to human observations involve rodents. Many show sex-specific effects, and examples of effects on the fourth-generation or later have been published. Below are described two typical recent examples.

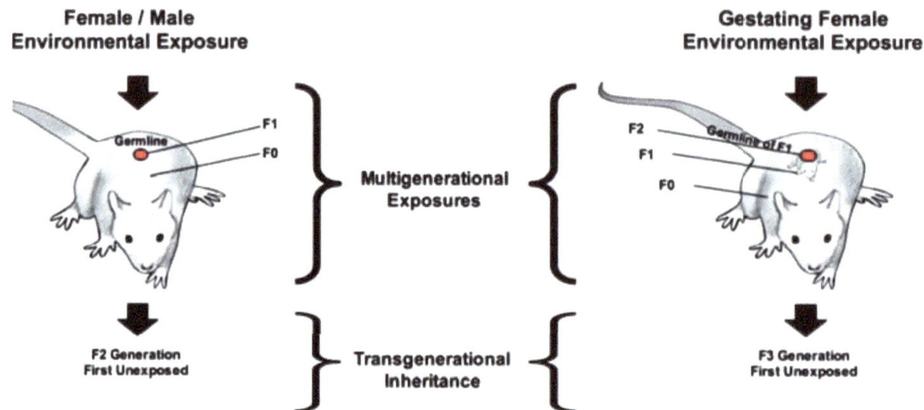



**Fig. (1).** Environmentally induced transgenerational epigenetic inheritance. Schematic of multigenerational versus transgenerational environmental exposures [4].

## Toxic Metal Exposure

A study by Camsari and colleagues [5] demonstrated that exposure of female mice to cadmium and mercury around the time of conception had adverse effects on the male but not female offspring in regard to increased adiposity and impaired glucose metabolism. Subsequent experiments where they continued to breed from the offspring (but with no further exposures) showed that the adverse adiposity and glucose phenotypes persisted in males down the female, but not the male line, even as far as the fourth generation when compared to controls [5].

## Endocrine Disruptors

There are many endocrine disruptors in the environment, but Bisphenol A (BPA) is one of the more ubiquitous. A recent study [6] has confirmed previous transgenerational studies and showed BPA administered in one pregnancy to be associated with patterns of social recognition in subsequent generations. The authors also showed that transmission was down the female line, and that the behavior was reflected in biomarkers in the brains of the third generation.

Many other animal experiments involving transgenerational associations are concerned with the impact of chemicals such as fungicides (*e.g.*, vinclozolin), pesticides and insecticides (*e.g.*, methoxychlor, DDT, and permethrin), and hazardous pollutants (*e.g.*, dioxin, phthalates, BPA, benzo(a)pyrene) on transgenerational outcomes such as disorders of the reproductive and renal systems, as well as on obesity and behavior changes (see Nilsson *et al.* [4] for a discussion).

## HUMAN OBSERVATIONAL STUDIES

Clearly, for ethical reasons, experimentation on humans is not possible, and detecting any transgenerational effects has to use observational data. There are two ways in which this has been undertaken.

### Prospective Pedigree

This starts with a group of ancestors, and follows their pedigrees forward in time, identifying their children, grandchildren, and even great-grandchildren. The result is varying numbers of grandchildren and great-grandchildren, especially as earlier generations tended to have large families. Researchers, including animal experimenters, often concentrate on particular inheritance lines (*e.g.*, the male line) or take the firstborn of each generation. However, this is likely to miss important lines of non-genetic inheritance.

### Retrospective Pedigree

This starts with a current set of individuals, and then traces their ancestors back in time (Fig. **2**). This results in more manageable pedigrees as each individual has just 2 parents, 4 grandparents and 8 great-grandparents. However, as can be seen, if the development of the index individual were to be influenced by exposure to a grandparent, there are four different pathways by which that could happen; if the influence is *via* exposure to a great-grandparent, there are eight different pathways to consider.

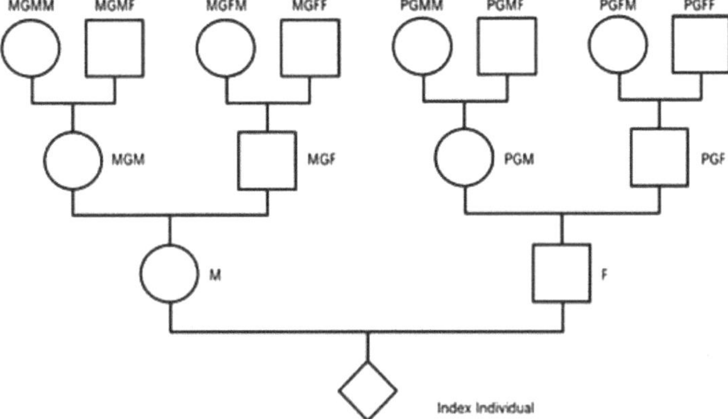


**Fig. (2).** Diagram of the structure of the generations from the index individual back to his/her great-grandparents. MGMM – Maternal GrandMother's Mother; MGMF – Maternal GrandMother's Father; MGFM - Maternal GrandFather's Mother; MGFF – Maternal GrandFather's Father; PGMM – Paternal GrandMother's Mother; PGMF – Paternal GrandMother's Father; PGFM – Paternal GrandFather's Mother; PGFF – Paternal GrandFather's Father. MGM/PGM – Maternal/Paternal GrandMother; MGF/PGF – Maternal/Paternal GrandFather; M – Mother; F – father.

## PRECONCEPTION EXPOSURES

### Famine and Glut

### *Överkalix and Uppsala*

The idea that environmental exposures of ancestors during childhood could influence the health of their grandchildren was not considered seriously (apart from the idea of cultural inheritance), until a major study from a research group led by Professor Lars Olle Bygren, focused on the town of Överkalix in Sweden.

Överkalix is an agricultural community in Norrbotten county on the edge of the Arctic Circle, north-east Sweden near the Finnish border. In the past, it remained cut off during the winter months by ice in the Baltic and the lack of a rail link with the rest of the country. In 2010, the population of Överkalix was just under 1000. From the late 18th century, detailed records had been kept of the gluts and famines experienced by the population. These records along with those of food prices were studied concerning longevity and causes of the grandchildrens' deaths.

Their first seminal paper was concerned with the exposure in the prepubertal period which they defined as years 9-12 for boys and 8-10 for girls, and which the authors labeled the 'Slow Growth' Period (SGP) [7]. The study design started by identifying individuals who had been born in Överkalix in 1905 and tracing their ancestors back as far as the four grandparents born in the late 18th and 19th centuries. The study showed that if the paternal grandfather had been exposed to a particularly lean harvest during this time, then the grandchildren lived an average of 15.8 years longer; however, if there had been a glut (and thus the 9-12-year-old grandfather had been likely to have overeaten), then the grandchild's age at death was reduced by 16.5 years.

Later analyses combined the data with two other cohorts of grandchildren born in 1890 and 1920 in Överkalix. This revealed a sex-specific mortality rate in the grandchildren. The mortality rate of the grandsons born in the target years was associated with their paternal grandfathers' food supply during the SGP, and the female mortality rate was associated with the paternal grandmother's food supply (Table **1**) [8]. The relative mortality rate ratio in grandsons was increased to 1.67 if their paternal grandfather had had a year with a food glut during their SGP, but it was decreased to 0.65 if there had been an extremely bad harvest during that period (these analyses had treated the grandparents with no extremes of food supply as the reference group). For granddaughters, the mortality rate ratio was increased to 2.13 if their paternal grandmother had experienced an exceptionally good harvest in their SGP, and a reduction to 0.72 if she had experienced a poor food supply. These risks persisted after taking account of the grandchild's early life circumstances [9]. Further analyses ascertaining the cohort-specific associations showed that the third cohort of grandchildren (born 1920) did not show such associations, but births in 1890 and 1905 both showed similar associations, suggesting the possibility that the grandparents with grandchildren born later in the 20th century may have had less severe contrasts between extremely good and very poor harvests [8].

**Table 1. Relationship between grandparents' exposures to famine or glut in their SGP and Mortality Risk Ratio (P-value) of their grandchildren; Överkalix births of grandchildren 1890, 1905 and 1920 [8].**

| Ancestor | Famine in SGP | | Glut in SGP | |
|---|---|---|---|---|
| - | **Grandsons** | **Granddaughters** | **Grandsons** | **Granddaughters** |
| PGF | 0.65 (0.025) | 1.17 (0.43) | 1.67 (0.009) | 0.81 (0.32) |
| PGM | 1.23 (0.27) | 0.72 (0.12) | 1.02 (0.93) | 2.13 (0.001) |
| MGF | 0.98 (0.90) | 1.05 (0.81) | 0.81 (0.22) | 1.23 (0.34) |
| MGM | 1.25 (0.24) | 1.30 (0.22) | 0.92 (0.62) | 0.79 (0.27) |

PGF Paternal GrandFather; PGM Paternal GrandMother; MGF Maternal GrandFather; MGM Maternal GrandMother.

An attempt to replicate these findings used the Uppsala Multigeneration Study [10]. The authors identified data from individuals born 1915-1929 (the study parents, F1), and traced their parents (the study grandparents, F0) and their offspring (the grandchildren, F2). They collected harvest data during the pre-pubertal period of grandparents (F0, n = 9,039) to examine its potential association with mortality in the parents (F1, n = 7,280), and analyzed the mortality rates of the grandchildren (F2, n = 11,561). Although only 10% of the grandchildren had died by 2015, this research supported the main Överkalix finding: paternal grandfather's food access pre-puberty predicted his grandson's, but not granddaughter's all-cause mortality. The authors did not replicate other aspects of the Bygren study, but that may not be surprising given that the Överkalix study had records of almost all deaths to the grandchildren who had been born 1895-1905. The Uppsala grandchildren had been born between 1932 and 1976.

### Other Famines

The Överkalix findings prompted several other studies based on exposure to famine during an ancestor SGP. One of these concerned the famine in Germany during 1916-1918. Germany imported large quantities of foodstuff and raw materials (mainly from the USA) to support its population prior to World War 1. Immediately at the onset of hostilities in August 1914, the British initiated a naval blockade of Germany while, concurrently, the French blockaded Austro-Hungarian ports in the Mediterranean. The blockade deprived Germany and the central powers of vital raw materials such as non-ferrous metals, coal and fertilizers. The latter impacted the nation's agricultural output, in particular: potatoes, grain, meat and dairy products. By 1916, food shortages were such that rioting and looting occurred in Germany, Vienna and Budapest. During the 1916-17 winter, the potato crop failed, which led to the population, in urban areas especially, having to survive on Swedish turnips (the so-called "Turnip Winter"). The blockade ended in June 1919 once Germany signed the Treaty of Versailles [11].

Van den Berg and Pinger [12] studied individuals who were exposed to this famine at ages 8-12 (F0) as well as their children (F1) and grandchildren (F2) with respect to a number of economic and health outcomes (height and BMI (Body Mass Index)). They found that F0 males living through the famine had larger families with higher proportions of daughters. In the F1 generation, those individuals whose mothers had been exposed during their SGP had worse health outcomes, particularly if they were male. In the third generation (F2), those grandsons whose paternal grandfathers had been exposed had larger families. Grandsons had higher (better) mental health scores if their paternal grandfather had been exposed to the famine during the SGP, and granddaughters had higher mental health scores if their maternal grandmother had experienced the famine during their SGP (Table **2**). There were no similar associations with height or educational abilities.

**Table 2. Relationship (P-value) between grandparents' exposure to famine in their SGP and mental health scores of their grandchildren: German Panel Research Data [13].**

| Ancestor exposed | Grandsons | Granddaughters |
|---|---|---|
| PGF | **+1.75 (0.04)** | +0.05 (0.96) |
| PGM | -0.08 (0.92) | +0.58 (0.59) |
| MGF | +0.39 (0.68) | +0.40 (0.74) |
| MGM | -0.48 (0.65) | **+2.14 (0.10)** |

(relationships with P<0.10 are in bold) PGF Paternal GrandFather; PGM Paternal GrandMother; MGF Maternal GrandFather; MGM Maternal GrandMother.

## *Nutrition in Guatemala*

A major study of childhood nutrition took place in four villages in Guatemala in 1969-1977. The children of two villages received a nutritious supplement (atole) and those in two other villages received a less nutritious supplement (fresco). Their offspring were contacted and examined in 2006 -2007. The results showed that if the mothers had received the atole supplements in childhood, their offspring had increased birthweight, head circumference and height when compared with the children of mothers who had received the fresco supplements in childhood. The differences were more pronounced for the sons rather than the daughters. There were no differences noted in the children of fathers who had received the different supplements [14].

## Preconception Smoking Effects

Following on from the Överkalix studies, the question was posed as to whether starting to smoke in the SGP also affected later generations. Data from the Avon Longitudinal Study of Parents and Children (ALSPAC) was used to address the question as to whether the age at the onset of regular smoking of the parents might have an association with their offspring's body fat. Information concerning the age at childhood-onset of regular smoking showed that the fathers who had started before age 11 had sons who gradually increased their body fat with time until by the age of 17, they contained 10.6 kg more fat than expected (Fig. **3a** [15];). Daughters of these men did not increase their body fat as consistently, but contained 5.8 kg more fat at 17 than expected (Fig. **3b**).

(a) Sons                                                          (b) Daughters

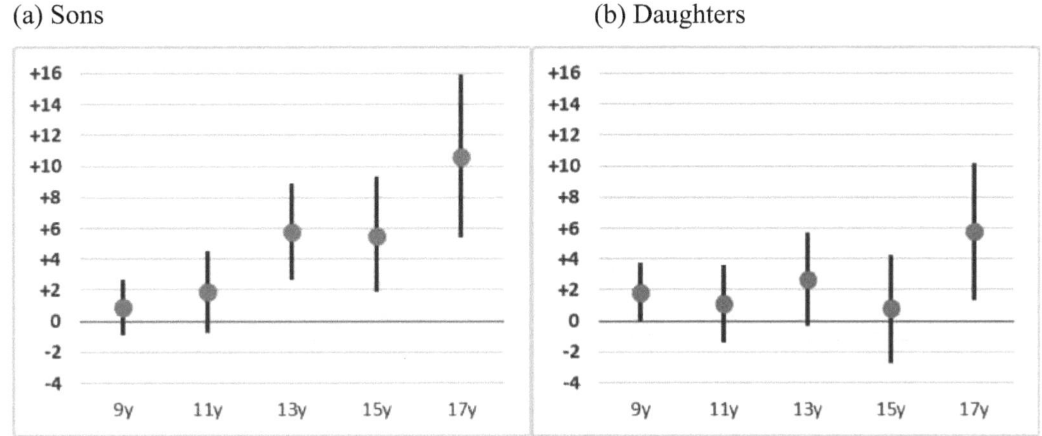


**Fig. (3).** The excess body fat in children whose fathers started smoking regularly before age 11 compared with all other children [15, 16].

A subsequent publication from this group analyzed ALSPAC data at age 24. This showed an excess of 13 kg of body fat in the sons and far less (5 kg) in daughters (Table 3). The authors also showed that if the mothers had started smoking regularly before the age of 16, their daughters (but not their sons) had a significantly increased amount of body fat [16].

**Table 3. Fat mass [95% CI (Confidence Interval)] of 24-year-old offspring related to the age at which their parents started smoking (from Golding *et al* [16]).**

| Parental history of starting smoking | Fat mass (kg) | |
|---|---|---|
| | Sons | Daughters |
| Father age <11 years | +13.2 [+4.8, +21.6] | +5.0 [-1.2, +11.2] |
| Mother age <16 years | +1.7 [-0.1, +3.5] | +2.5 [+1.1, +4.0] |

To our knowledge, the only other study that has linked paternal preconception smoking to a child outcome has been the large multinational Respiratory Health in Northern Europe (RHINE) study which has linked together information on the father starting to smoke in childhood with the likelihood of his offspring developing asthma. The authors [17, 18] demonstrated that offspring of fathers (but not mothers) who started to smoke at <15 years were at increased risk of asthma without nasal allergy, but not asthma with nasal allergy. Unfortunately, they did not publish information on whether the relationship differed between the sexes of the offspring. A published abstract also indicated that the offspring of fathers starting to smoke before age 15 had reduced lung function [19]. Further confirmation of the finding regarding asthma comes from a study analyzing English data [20]. The authors showed that the association between fathers starting to smoke at <15 years, and offspring asthma was repeated [OR (Odds Ratio) 1.71; 95% CI 1.23, 2.37], but was not found for non-biological fathers.

## Preconception Radiation Exposure

Strangely, there have been few studies that assess the relationship between radiation exposure of the grandparents prior to the conception of their offspring. One has compared 112 granddaughters whose grandparents were exposed to atomic bomb tests in the former Soviet Union with 53 controls. The authors showed that grandparental exposure (especially to the grandmothers) was associated with an increased risk of reproductive problems, including menstrual problems, miscarriage in the first trimester, pregnancy complications and preterm delivery. The women were also at increased risk of thyroid abnormalities, including autoimmune thyroiditis [21].

Occupational studies have determined the relationship between occupational exposure to radiation of the grandparents and shown no relationship with congenital malformations or other health issues in the first 7 years of the grandchild's life [22]. However, paternal exposure to radioactive isotopes has been associated with a greater risk of increased birth weight [23]. A population study in the UK [24] has documented paternal exposures to X-rays in which the radiation was likely to reach the fathers' gonads in the year before conception (but not earlier), and shown that these exposures were associated with a reduction in mean birthweight by 73g (P = 0.064).

## Other Preconception Exposures

Betel nut (*Areca catechu*) is used by 100s of millions of South and East Asian origin people, as a mild stimulant, breath freshener and as a component of Ayurvedic and traditional Chinese medicine. A few slices, wrapped in a betel leaf along with slaked lime, spices and other flavorings (sometimes including tobacco) are chewed. It has many negative effects on health, and is a known carcinogen in humans [25].

Transgenerational response to betel nut exposure in CD-1 mice has shown that paternal exposure is associated with an increased risk of obesity and hyperglycaemia, especially in first-generation male offspring [26]. Following on from such animal studies, Chen and colleagues [27] found a significant dose-response between the quantity and duration of exposure to paternal betel quid chewing and the risk of early metabolic syndrome in the offspring (when there was no indication of metabolic syndrome in the parents nor betel chewing in the offspring). Subsequently, a large Taiwanese study of betel-quid chewing and smoking (after childhood) reported that a longer duration of paternal betel-quid chewing and smoking pre-fatherhood, independently predicted the early occurrence of metabolic syndrome in their offspring [28].

## PRENATAL EXPOSURES

## Maternal Exposures in Pregnancy

### *Teratogens and Carcinogens*

There are four dramatic examples that illustrate the importance of prenatal environmental exposures to the developing fetus: (i) The thalidomide tragedy which resulted in very striking and unusual malformations, immediately recognizable at birth and mainly involving the absence of, or deformities of, the limbs [29]; (ii) antenatal exposure to rubella and increased prevalence of deafness and blindness in the affected child [30]; (iii) ionizing radiation: abdominal X-rays during pregnancy were shown to be linked to leukemia and other cancers in childhood, especially when the X-ray occurred in the first trimester [31], and exposure in utero to atomic bomb explosions before 18 weeks gestation was associated with small head circumference frequently accompanied by mental retardation [32]; (iv) the medication Diethylstilbestrol (DES) was prescribed to pregnant women to prevent miscarriage (even though randomized controlled trials had shown that it had no such effect); many years later a cluster of women presenting with a rare form of vaginal carcinoma prompted investigation as to the cause – exposure to DES was found to be the culprit [33]. Subsequently, examination of offspring of women who had taken the drug revealed several anomalies in the boys/men and the girls/women, particularly related to their reproductive systems [34].

The associations with thalidomide, rubella and DES were all discovered because they resulted in an unusual cluster of rare outcomes which prompted an investigation. These case reports were followed by epidemiological studies which demonstrated the validity of the early case studies [*e.g.*, 35,36]. These findings prompted the initiation of large studies monitoring the incidence of different defects over time with the aim of identifying unexpected increases for early investigation (*e.g.*, the EUROCAT studies (European network of population-based registries for the epidemiological surveillance of congenital anomalies)) [37]. Despite considerable effort, these studies have so far failed to identify any results as convincing or dramatic as those of thalidomide or rubella.

## *Famine*

Several studies have taken advantage of the Dutch Hunger Winter to assess the consequences of exposure to famine in pregnancy. The Netherlands was under Nazi occupation from May 1940 with increased food rationing. A general railroad strike by the Dutch population in support of the Allied invasion forces at Arnhem/Nijmegen in September 1944 resulted in retaliation: the occupying army stopped all food supplies from rural areas into the most heavily populated areas in the far west (where the main cities such as Amsterdam, Utrecht and Den Haag are situated) from September 22$^{nd}$, 1944, until liberation the following May. Coupled with a severe winter, the resulting famine (where individuals existed on 400-800 calories/day) resulted in ~22,000 deaths [38 - 40].

Retrospectively, Zena Stein and Mervyn Susser assembled national Dutch data concerning births between 1944-1946, their deaths, and examinations of those males who were conscripted into the military at age 19, and later supplemented this with data concerning their health in their 40s. Knowing their dates and places of birth enabled them to determine the stage of pregnancy and degree of exposure of each of this population's mothers to the famine. Their initial results are summarized in Table **4**. They were able to determine whether the outcomes were associated with different times of exposure. In particular, they determined that if the famine occurred around the time of conception, there were increased risks of neural tube defects, as well as psychiatric disorders such as antisocial personality and schizophrenia. Exposure in the first trimester was associated with preterm delivery, stillbirth, early neonatal death and obesity at age 19. Later exposures were related to lower mean birth weight, increased mortality in the first 3 months of life and a reduced risk of obesity at age 19 [41]. Subsequent study of 22,952 deaths, by age 63, who had been exposed to the famine in utero found no increase in deaths from cancer or cardiovascular disease, but an increase in deaths from external causes (*i.e.,* mainly accidents and self-harm) particularly associated with exposure in the first trimester [Hazard Ratio (HR) 1.46; 95% CI 1.09, 1.97] [42]. Another Dutch population study has linked maternal prenatal exposure to the famine with the national addiction register [43]; this demonstrated associations that differed by sex of the offspring and trimester of exposure: for males when the exposure was in the first trimester, the risk was greatest [OR 2.71; 95% CI 2.01, 3.65], whereas for females the most sensitive period was the third trimester [OR 1.89; 95% CI 1.34, 2.67].

**Table 4. Summary of notable outcomes to offspring of women exposed to the Dutch Hunger Winter during pregnancy (adapted from Susser and Stein [41]).**

| Outcome | Trimester Exposed | Result |
|---|---|---|
| Outcome of pregnancy | - | - |
| Organic brain defects | Pre-conception | Increase in neural tube defects |
| Preterm delivery | First | Increased risk |
| Stillbirth | First | Increased risk |
| Birthweight | $2^{nd}$- $3^{rd}$ trimester | Lower mean birthweight |
| Early childhood | - | - |
| Death in $1^{st}$ week | First | Marked increase |
| Death in $1^{st}$ 3 months | Third | Increased risk |
| Adulthood | - | - |
| Obesity at 19y | First | Increased risk |
| - | Third | Decreased risk |
| Schizoid personality at 19y | Periconception | Increased risk |
| Schizophrenia by 40+y | Periconception | Increased risk |
| Antisocial personality at 19y | Periconception | Increased risk |

There has been some controversy as to whether prenatal exposure to famine was associated with diabetes. Data from several famines have been compared by de Rooij and colleagues [44]; they concluded that, in general, prenatal exposure to such famines did increase the risk of developing diabetes in adulthood. Recent studies from China have shown that the adult women who had been exposed in utero to the famine were at increased risk of central obesity (OR 1.28; 95% CI 1.07, 1.53); but there was no such association with exposed men [45].

## Cigarette Smoking

Cigarette smoking was common among populations of Europe and North America in the 20th century, being as high as 90% among men in the UK in the 1920s. Only when the results of a longitudinal study of clinicians in Britain showed that smoking was associated with lung cancer [46]; and subsequently with large numbers of other outcomes including cardiovascular disease [47] were the adverse health effects of smoking taken seriously in Europe. Gradually, the proportion of the population that were smokers reduced over time.

From the early 1960s, it became clear that cigarette smoking during pregnancy influenced the growth of the fetus, the more the mother smoked the lower the mean birth weight [48]. Substantial evidence has accumulated since then to show that there were a large number of consequences to the offspring – Table **5** describes the published results of meta-analyses of systematic reviews looking at a variety of different outcomes to the child when the mother had smoked during pregnancy. It can be observed that the fetus is affected throughout, with an increased risk of miscarriage and congenital malformations, restricted growth (particularly of the head) and stillbirth. Among live-born infants, there is an increased risk of sudden unexpected infant death. The children are at increased risk of becoming overweight and obese, of developing asthma and behavioral problems such as ADHD (Attention Deficit Hyperactivity Disorder). Even among the adult offspring, there are associations with overweight and obesity as well as gestational diabetes (though not with Type 2 diabetes) [59]. Although no systematic reviews have yet been conducted on common psychiatric disorders such as depression and anxiety, an association has been shown with schizophrenia [58].

**Table 5. Selected results of meta-analyses, based on systematic reviews, showing the associations between maternal smoking in pregnancy and offspring outcome.**

| Outcome | No. of Studies | Results | Reference | Dose-response Tested |
|---|---|---|---|---|
| Outcome of pregnancy | - | - | - | - |
| Miscarriage | 25 | OR 1.32 [1.21, 1.44] | [49] | Dose response |
| Fetal head size 3rd Trim | 8 | -0.18SD [-.23, -.13] | [50] | Dose response |
| Femur length 3rd Trim | 8 | -0.27SD [-.32, -.21] | [50] | - |
| Stillbirth >19 weeks | 34 | OR 1.43 [1.32, 1.54] | [51] | Dose response |
| - | - | - | - | - |
| Congenital defects | - | - | - | - |
| Congenital heart disease | 43 | RR 1.11 [1.04, 1.18] | [52] | - |

*(Table 5) cont.....*

| Outcome | No. of Studies | Results | Reference | Dose-response Tested |
|---|---|---|---|---|
| Cryptorchidism | 20 | OR 1.18 [1.12, 1.24] | [53] | - |
| - | - | - | - | - |
| Childhood | - | - | - | - |
| Sudden unexpected infant death | a | OR 2.44 [2.31, 2.57] | [54] | Dose response |
| Overweight | 39 | OR 1.37 [1.28, 1.46] | [55] | - |
| Obesity | 39 | OR 1.55 [1.40, 1.73] | [55] | - |
| ADHD | 12 | RR 1.58 [1.33, 1.88] | [56] | - |
| Asthma < 3years | 5 | OR 1.85 [1.35, 2.53] | [57] | - |
| - | - | - | - | - |
| Adulthood | - | - | - | - |
| Schizophrenia | 7 | RR 1.34 [.90, 1.98] | [58] | - |
| Gestational diabetes | 3 | ES 1.38 [1.19, 1.61] | [59] | - |
| Overweight | 5 | ES 1.35 [1.16, 1.56] | [59] | - |
| Obese | 7 | ES 1.46 [1.39, 1.54] | [59] | - |

[a]Not based on a systematic review but a study of over 19,000 deaths and 20 million births.

## Effects of Grandmothers' Exposures in Pregnancy on the Grandchild

Although, as we have shown above, exposures occurring during pregnancy can have profound effects on the offspring, few studies have taken the subject further, and enquired as to whether there are effects on the grandchildren of the woman who was exposed during pregnancy. We describe below the results from some of the studies that are published.

### *The Example of DES*

As indicated earlier, the early monitoring for adverse effects of medication concerned the identification of congenital malformations, subsequently it came as a shock when a cluster of hitherto rare vaginal cancers was identified as being associated with the mother's use of synthetic estrogen. In the USA, from 1938 onwards, pregnant women have often been prescribed the synthetic hormone DES to prevent miscarriage and premature birth, apparently without adverse effects on the offspring. It was not until 1971 that a study was published highlighting the fact that girls exposed in utero to DES were at increased risk of a rare vaginal cancer (clear cell adenocarcinoma) [60]. The drug was withdrawn in the US in 1971, but later elsewhere. Subsequent studies have shown that it was not just the exposed mothers' offspring that were affected, but there is now evidence that the children of her exposed daughters (both boys and girls) were at increased risk of genital abnormalities [61, 62]. In addition, the granddaughters have been reported to have increased menstrual problems [33], and three times the risk of breast cancer [63].

## Famine during Grandmother's Pregnancy

### *The Dutch Hunger Winter*

The first study of the grandchildren of the women who had been exposed to this famine in pregnancy studied the birthweights of 1808 of their firstborn babies [64]. Those grandchildren whose grandmothers were exposed to the famine during the first and second trimesters had lower birth weights than babies of women who had not been exposed to famine. However, later prospective studies revealed a more complicated situation [65, 66], and in another set of births, no association was found between the grandmother's prenatal famine exposure and the grandchild's birthweight. A different study from the Netherlands studied the offspring of both men and women exposed in utero; they also showed no association with birthweight for either group, but did find a decrease in birth length and an increase in adiposity at the birth of the children born to the exposed mothers, but not to the exposed fathers [67].

A separate study of 360 adult offspring (F2) (mean age 37) of fathers who had been in utero during the famine (i.e. their paternal grandmothers were exposed prenatally) had a higher mean weight and higher BMI than the offspring of unexposed fathers (+4.9 kg, P = 0.03; +1.6 kg/m$^2$, $P$ = 0.006); this finding was not replicated in the F2 offspring of exposed mothers. There appeared to be no other differences in adult health at age 37 in the F2 generation [68].

### *The Chinese Famine 1959-61*

A major famine occurred in China between 1959 and 1961 resulting from the Great Leap Forward Economic & Social Plan, leaving an estimated 30 million dead [69]. A study of 449 women giving birth in 1993-1996 identified in which area they had been born and linked that information to the intensity of the famine in that area. The authors [70] showed that in rural areas, exposure of the grandmothers to famine when pregnant with a daughter was associated with larger birthweight of her grandchild (69 g; 95% CI 30, 108), as well as increased birth length (0.3 cm; 95% CI −0.0, 0.5) and birth body mass index (0.1 kg/m$^2$; 95% CI 0.0, 0.2). In urban areas, however, exposure to famine was not associated with offspring birth size. The authors concluded that their findings in rural areas (where the famine was worst) suggested that severe and prolonged famine leads to larger newborn size in the offspring of mothers exposed to famine in utero and during the first few years of life; less severe famine in urban areas, however, appeared to have no impact on the growth of the grandchild. The authors pointed out, however, that the findings may well be confounded by the large mortality rate, with the possibility that the results are biased by the fact that only the very fittest survived.

## Grandmother Smoked During Pregnancy

There have been several studies that have considered the consequence to the grandchildren of women who smoked during pregnancy, including our own. Here we describe the results of our analyses of various outcomes to the grandchildren, and of other studies that have also contributed to the topic. We analyzed data concerning whether either the Maternal GrandMother (MGM) or the Paternal GrandMother (PGM) smoked during the pregnancies that resulted in the study parent of the index grandchild (Fig. **4**). The data used are from the Avon Longitudinal Study of Parents and Children (ALSPAC), described in the Appendix. Information from 12,707 maternal and 9,677 paternal grandmothers of children concerned whether they had smoked while expecting the study parent.

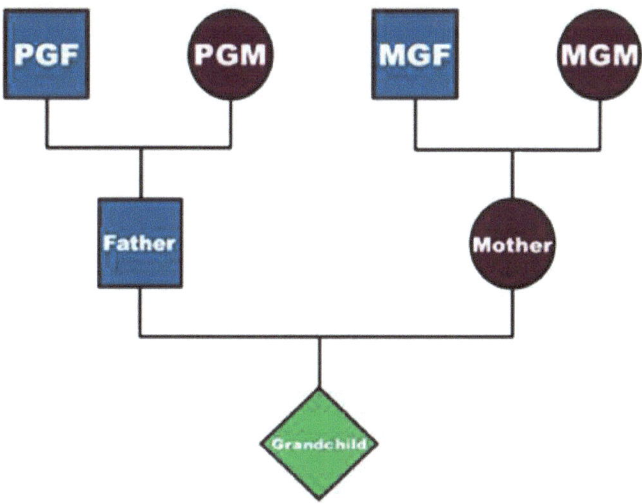


**Fig. (4).** Diagram of the family tree back to the grandparents.

## Grandchild's Growth

A study using data from the British National Cohort Study [71] has shown that non-smoking women whose own mothers (MGM) had smoked in pregnancy had children with greater mean birthweight than expected after adjustment. Using ALSPAC data we found that among grandchildren whose maternal grandmothers had smoked in pregnancy but who were born to non-smoking mothers, the average birthweight, birth length and birth BMI measurements of the grandsons (but not granddaughters) were greater after adjustment for parity, maternal education, partner smoking and gestation at delivery: birthweight = +61 [95% CI +30, +92] g; birth length = +0·19 [95% CI +0·02, +0·35] cm; BMI = +1·6 [95% CI +0·6, +2·6] g/m². Similar associations were seen in births to primiparas and multiparas. There were no fetal growth differences, however, if the paternal grandmother had smoked prenatally. The evidence from this study suggests that when the mother does not smoke during pregnancy the maternal grandmother's prenatal smoking habit is positively associated with her grandson's fetal growth [72].

A further ALSPAC study examined the birth measurements of the grandchildren when both the grandmother and the mother had smoked [73]. The authors showed that there was a strong negative association between the paternal grandmother having smoked prenatally and the head circumference at birth among her grandsons (adjusted mean difference −0.35 cm; 95% CI −0.57 to −0.14; p=0.001), but there was no such association with granddaughters (interaction p=0.006). Similar associations were found when primiparas and multiparas were analyzed separately.

### *Grandmother Smoking Prenatally and Childhood Anthropometry*

The ALSPAC children were followed up and measured on six occasions during childhood and adolescence (from 7 to 17 years). Measurements from 9 years onwards included DXA (Dual-Energy X-ray Absorptiometry) whole body scans, from which the fat mass, lean mass (mainly muscle) and bone mass were estimated. The results at P<0.05 of assessing the contributions of the prenatal smoking of the maternal and paternal grandmothers are indicated for the grandsons and granddaughters according to whether the mother herself smoked in Tables **6A** and **6B**.

It will be recalled that at birth if the maternal grandmother had smoked, but the mother had not, the grandsons were larger in regard to their weight, birth length and birth BMI. The granddaughters showed no such associations. As the children aged, the same pattern continued (Table **6A**), with the grandsons being heavier, having a greater BMI and waist circumference; the DXA scan revealed that their increased weight was related to increased lean mass not fat mass. There was no such association for the granddaughters during childhood. However, if the mother herself smoked, then there was no detectable association with the maternal grandmother smoking for the grandsons, but there were marked reductions in all the measurements (except BMI) for the granddaughters [74].

**Table 6A. Grandchildren's growth pattern comparing adjusted results of maternal grandmother smoking prenatally with maternal grandmothers not smoking prenatally, according to whether the mother herself smoked in pregnancy. Data was collected at ages 7, 9, 11, 13, 15 and 17. (adapted from [73]).**

| Measurement | MGM+M- v MGM-M- | | MGM+M+ v MGM-M+ | |
|---|---|---|---|---|
| - | **Grandsons** | **Granddaughters** | **Grandsons** | **Granddaughters** |
| Height | . | . | . | -ve |
| Weight | +ve | . | . | -ve |
| BMI | +ve | . | . | . |
| Waist circumference | +ve | . | . | -ve |
| Fat mass | . | . | . | -ve |
| Lean mass | +ve | . | . | -ve |
| Bone mass | . | . | . | -ve |

MGM+ Maternal GrandMother smoked in pregnancy; MGM- Maternal GrandMother did not smoke in pregnancy; M+ Mother smoked in pregnancy; M- mother did not smoke in pregnancy; A dot indicates no significant association.

A different overall pattern was shown when the paternal grandmother was considered (Table **6B**). If the mother had been a non-smoker, grandchildren of both sexes tended to be larger, but the body distribution of weight tended to differ. The grandsons weighed more, had a greater BMI, lean and bone mass, but not an increase in fat mass. In contrast, the granddaughters had increases in all measurements including fat mass. Contrary to the findings for the maternal grandmother smoking – when the mother herself smoked, there was no effect of the paternal grandmother smoking on the anthropometry of the grandchild of either sex [74].

The fat mass of the 24-year-old adult grandchildren was assessed using an exposome technique to determine the exposures to the grandparents and parents in childhood independently associated with their fat mass. As well as the father commencing to smoke before age 11, there was a strong association with the paternal grandmother having smoked in pregnancy; her adult granddaughters, but not grandsons had elevated mean fat mass (interaction with sex after adjustment, P = 0.001) [16].

## *Cognition and Developmental Traits*

The ALSPAC offspring had their IQ (Intelligence Quotient) tested at ages 8 and 15. There were no relationships with the smoking habits of the maternal grandmother, but some associations were found with that of the paternal grandmother. After adjustment for potential confounders, there were associations with reduced performance IQ points at age 8 (-2.67; 95% CI -4.00, -1.34), but no difference between the sexes. There were no associations between either grandmother smoking in pregnancy or IQ as measured at 15 [75].

**Table 6B. Grandchildren's growth pattern comparing adjusted results of paternal grandmother smoking prenatally with paternal grandmothers not smoking prenatally, according to whether the mother herself smoked in pregnancy. Data was collected at ages 7, 9, 11, 13, 15 and 17.**

| Measurement | PGM+M- v PGM-M- | | PGM+M+ v PGM-M+ | |
| --- | --- | --- | --- | --- |
| - | Grandsons | Granddaughters | Grandsons | Granddaughters |
| Height | . | +ve | . | . |
| Weight | +ve | +ve | . | . |
| BMI | +ve | +ve | . | . |
| Waist circumference | . | +ve | . | . |
| Fat mass | . | +ve | . | . |
| Lean mass | +ve | +ve | . | . |
| Bone mass | +ve | +ve | . | . |

PGM+ Paternal GrandMother smoked in pregnancy; PGM- Paternal GrandMother did not smoke in pregnancy; M+ Mother smoked in pregnancy; M- Mother did not smoke in pregnancy; A dot indicates no significant association.

Although ALSPAC had commenced before early measures of autistic traits had been identified, the study had collected many different quantitative traits annually, and a detailed set of analyses had identified four of them as predictive of the autism spectrum [76]. Of these, none were associated with the paternal grandmother smoking, but two of the traits were associated with the maternal grandmother smoking [77]. Table 7 shows the unadjusted and adjusted associations with these traits, one of which (the SCDC or Social and Communication Disorders Checklist [78]) showed an excess risk to granddaughters, which became stronger with adjustment for potential confounders. Similarly, the repetitive behavior scale also showed an association with granddaughters. Both traits showed a significant interaction between the sexes. Diagnosed autism, however, showed a different pattern – with increased adjusted OR for both sexes.

## *Other Conditions Associated with the Grandmother Smoking in Pregnancy*

### *Asthma*

Various cohorts specifically designed to study asthma have collected data on whether the maternal grandmother smoked during pregnancy. The publications have taken different asthma-related phenotypes, identified at different ages, making it difficult to compare. For reasons of economy, we have summarized only the significant results in Table **8**. Seven of the eight studies published so far are from Europe (Scandinavia (5) and England (2)), and just one from North America.

**Table 7. Autistic traits and diagnosed autism in regard to whether the maternal grandmother had smoked in pregnancy (excluding mothers who themselves had smoked in pregnancy) adjusted for the years of birth of the MGM and MGF, the age of the PGM at the birth of the father and the social class of the PGF – adapted from [77].**

| Autism spectrum | Unadjusted OR [95%CI] | | Adjusted OR [95%CI] | |
|---|---|---|---|---|
| | Grandson | Granddaughter | Grandson | Granddaughter |
| Traits | - | - | - | - |
| SCDC | 1.10 [0.91, 1.32] | 1.32 [1.06, 1.65] | 1.04 [0.81, 1.34] | 1.67 [1.25, 2.25]* |
| RB | 1.09 [0.94, 1.27] | 1.22 [1.02, 1.44] | 1.11 [0.88, 1.41] | 1.48 [1.12, 1.94]* |
| Diagnosed | - | - | - | - |
| ASD | 1.22 [0.82, 1.82] | 1.59 [0.74, 3.40] | 1.53 [1.02, 2.29] | 1.56 [0.68, 3.58] |

ASD = Autism Spectrum Disorder; RB = Repetitive Behaviour; SCDC = Social and Communications Disorders Checklist [77]; *sex interaction P<0.10.

**Table 8. The studies concerning grandparental smoking in pregnancy and asthma in the grandchild.**

| Study | n | MGM Result | PGM Result | Phenotype | Reference |
|---|---|---|---|---|---|
| ECRHS | 2233 | 1.25[1.02,1.55] | - | A with nasal allergies | [17] |
| - | 1964 | - | 1.60[.95,2.68] | A | - |
| South California | 338 A 570 Cl | 2.1 [1.4, 3.2] | NC | A | [79] |
| MoBa | 25,394 | 1.21 [1.07,1.37] | NC | A at 7 years | [80] |
| - | 45,607 | 1.15 [1.04, 1.26] | NC | A medications 7y | [80] |
| Sweden registries | 46,197 | Trend with amount smoked | NC | A medications | [81] |
| - | 10,762 | MGM+M- 1.45 [1.17,1.79] | NC | Early persistent wheeze | [81] |
| ALSPAC | 1723 | - | PGM+M- 1.17 [0.97,1.41]* | Doctor diagnosed asthma | [82] |
| - | 1689 | 1.26 [0.95, 1.67] | - | Persistent wheeze | [82] |
| Isle of Wight | 1536 | MGM+M+ 2.6 [0.9, 7.1] | NC | - | [83] |

A = Asthma; Cl = Controls; NC = Not Collected; * = sex interaction; ECRHS = European Community Respiratory Health Survey; MoBA = Norwegian Mother and Child Cohort Study.

All these studies had information on whether the maternal grandmother smoked or did not smoke during pregnancy. All showed a positive association with at least one asthma phenotype, varying from an early persistent wheeze to whether the child had been given asthma medications. Only two studies had collected data on whether the paternal grandmother had smoked, and they both found positive associations.

### *Sensory Phenotypes*

The ALSPAC study has considered three sensory attributes. The measure of vision was the development of myopia before the child was aged 7 [84]; this demonstrated a reduced risk if the paternal grandmother had smoked: (AOR (Adjusted Odds Ratio) 0.47 [95% CI 0.28, 0.79]), with even lower risk for grandsons (0.31 [0.14, 0.65]) than granddaughters (0.60 [0.33, 1.0]).

For hearing, a measure of sensitivity to sound at age 6 was used: maternal report of intolerance to loud noise was more likely in 6-year-old grandsons if the maternal grandmother had smoked [AOR 1.27; 95% CI 1.03,1.56; P = 0.025], but less likely in girls [AOR 0.82; 95% CI 0.63,1.07] $P_{interaction}$ <0.05. When the grandchildren were 11, they were tested using an objective measure of volume choice for music through headphones; this showed that grandsons of both maternal and paternal smoking grandmothers were less likely to choose high volumes compared with granddaughters (P<0.05) [85].

Comparison of PROP supertasters (a subset of the population who find the bitter taste of 6-*n*-propylthiouracil practically intolerable) showed that when their paternal grandmother had smoked prenatally, their grandchildren were more likely to be supertasters [OR 1.28; 95% CI 1.03, 1.59], and that this was somewhat more likely to be true of granddaughters [OR 1.42; 95% CI 1.03, 1.95] than grandsons [OR 1.18; 95% CI 0.88, 1.60] [86].

### *Radiation*

Meyer and Tonascia [87] found that the maternal grandchildren of women who had had diagnostic X-rays in pregnancy were more likely to be stillborn (3.5% of those exposed compared with 1.3% of control grandchildren; OR = 2.90; P = 0.004), but no other studies appear to have tried to replicate these findings, or to study the longitudinal development of such grandchildren.

A study in Norway identified the children and grandchildren of women who had been exposed to radiation fall-out from the testing of atomic bombs elsewhere. They have reported that the grandsons had a reduced level of IQ when either of their grandmothers had been exposed to elevated radiation at 3-4 months gestation (unfortunately, data were not available on the IQ of the granddaughters) [88].

## DISCUSSION

### General Results

We have considered the evidence from observational studies to support the likelihood of non-genetic inheritance among humans. It should be pointed out, however, that most of the results we have reported would be described as intergenerational/multigenerational rather than transgenerational. However, those concerning exposures of the grandfather to famine or glut in the SGP in Sweden [8 - 10] and Germany [12] are truly transgenerational (Fig. **1**).

Skinner [89] has suggested that the main environmental epigenetic impacts on biology and disease are to be found among conditions that include: (a) having a low frequency of a genetic component to disease as determined by GWAS; (b) having shown dramatic increases in frequency in recent years; and (c) having known environmental exposures that are associated with a disease. In this chapter, we have summarized results from observational studies mainly concerning generational outcomes after exposure, both preconception and prenatally to famine, cigarette smoking and radiation to grandparents or parents. From the results, it is clear that:

1. There are many associations between exposures to a grandparent, prior to or during pregnancy and outcomes in the grandchild.
2. The outcomes often differ depending on whether the exposed grandparent is in the male or female line.
3. The results often differ depending on the sex of the grandchild.
4. The age at exposure is often important in regard to whether a specific outcome is triggered. This was particularly noted for the gestation at exposure to the Dutch Hunger Winter [44], and that of radiation exposure in Norway from atomic bomb testing [88]. For the preconception exposures, the time before puberty was shown to be particularly important for exposures to famine (or glut) in Överkalix [7 - 9] and Germany [12, 13].
5. Results of non-genetic inheritance may not necessarily be disadvantageous. For example, (i) exposure of the grandfather to famine in his SGP is associated with improved mental health in his grandsons [13]; (ii) grandchildren had a lower risk of early myopia if their paternal grandmother had smoked prenatally [84].

The studies we have reviewed in this chapter may be considered preliminary in a relatively new field of epidemiological interest. Nevertheless, it is informative to examine the data so far available to assess whether there is evidence of causation. Therefore, we compare below, our observations to some of Bradford Hill's suggestions as to the criteria needed to interpret whether associations are causal [90]. These include consistency (*i.e.,* replication), specificity, temporality, biological gradient, plausibility, coherence and experimental evidence.

## *Consistency (Replication)*

We have shown that the biological responses to environmental exposures are complex. It could be argued that the study of human epigenetic inheritance is in its infancy, and therefore, there is too little replication or evidence from biological markers to substantiate the claims made by these studies. However, where similar conditions and outcomes are reported, there is frequent replication. For example, several studies have shown that when the maternal grandmother smokes during pregnancy: (a) the birthweight of the grandchild is greater [71, 72], and (b) the child is more likely to develop asthma-like symptoms (Table **8**). The Överkalix study started with one cohort of grandchildren (born in 1905) and then, for replication, used two others (cohorts born in 1895 and 1915). The 1895 cohort demonstrated the same associations as that of 1905, but 1915 did not. However, the much larger study from Uppsala showed a similar finding to the two early Överkalix ones concerning mortality [8 - 10].

## *Specificity*

Many, but not all, of the outcomes we have examined, are specific to either the male or female lines. If associations between an exposure to the grandparent were due to socioeconomic confounding, one would expect both the grandparental associations to be similar.

## *Temporality*

By definition, all non-genetic transgenerational inheritance associations are longitudinal proceeding down the generations.

## *Biological gradient*

By this term, Hill meant a dose-response relationship. With the data available, there is rarely exposure data that would allow such calculations when the data are obtained by retrospective recall (*e.g.,* amount smoked during pregnancy).

## *Plausibility*

The results we have described would likely be deemed implausible were it not for the experimental evidence from animal models, where similar effects are seen.

## Coherence

Here, Hill meant that "the cause-and-effect interpretation of the data should not seriously conflict with the generally known facts of the natural history and biology of the disease". Again, the experimental evidence, together with evidence from studies of DNA methylation below supports this.

## Experimental Evidence

As already noted, there is substantial evidence from animal experiments that the phenomenon of non-genetic inheritance exists.

Thus, there are various indications that many of the associations described above are likely to be causal using Bradford Hill's criteria.

## Evidence from Biomarkers

Epigenetic transgenerational inheritance has been shown in non-human experiments to be associated with biomarkers such as DNA methylation. This biomarker is the one that has been most studied among the human population, and environmental exposures as well as the development of medical conditions, have been shown to be associated with changes in DNA methylation. Several such changes have been shown to occur with the different patterns of human non-genetic inheritance. These include:

a. Differences in Differentially Methylated Regions (DMRs) related to insulin processing, adipose development and hypothalamus development in grandchildren whose grandparents had been exposed to different types of harvest in their SGP [91].
b. Analyses of the Dutch famine data [92] indicated that individuals who were exposed to famine prenatally had lower levels of DNA methylation of the imprinted *IGF2* gene compared with their unexposed, same-sex siblings 60 years later.
c. The same group found that persistent changes in DNA methylation associated with prenatal famine exposure were dependent on the gestational timing and the sex of the exposed individual [93].
d. Later, in genome-scale analysis of differential DNA methylation in whole blood after peri-conceptional exposure to the Dutch famine, Tobi and colleagues [94] analyzed six P-DMRs (Prenatal malnutrition-associated Differentially Methylated Regions), and showed that P-DMRs preferentially occurred at regulatory regions, and were characterized by intermediate levels of DNA methylation, and mapped to genes enriched for differential expression

during early development.

e. In the RHINESSA (Respiratory Health in Northern Europe, Spain and Australia) cohort six DMRs were identified in offspring of pre-adolescent smoking men. These were annotated to genes of the offspring involved in innate and adaptive immunity, fatty acid synthesis, development and function of neuronal systems and cellular processes [95].

We note, however, that these associations with DNA methylation do not suggest that DNA methylation is necessarily the mechanism of non-genetic inheritance. To show this, we would need to trace changes in DNA methylation in the germ cells of the exposed ancestors, and somehow link them to the DNA methylation associations in the descendants.

## CONCLUSION

The studies described here have pointed to the importance, in the study of any environmental exposure to parents, of following the offspring and their offspring throughout their lifespans to identify unexpected consequences. Although this has been admirably carried out in the follow-up of some of the exposures discussed in this chapter, especially for those exposed to the Dutch Hunger Winter, there are many gaps in the literature. For example, the demonstration of the linkage of prenatal abdominal X-rays to childhood cancer has not resulted in exploration as to what other positive or negative consequences there might be over the generations.

It is noteworthy that it was only the appearance of a very rare outcome that spurred the identification of DES as having an inter-generationally harmful effect. What chance is there for a common adverse outcome to a common exposure being suspected – especially if the relevant outcomes are in the third or fourth generation? This emphasizes the importance of developing longitudinal studies identifying environmental exposures and following subsequent generations over time.

## APPENDIX

The Avon Longitudinal Study of Parents and Children (ALSPAC) (n = 14,541 initial enrolment in 1991-1992) was designed to assess the ways in which the environment interacts with the genotype to influence health and development [96 - 98].

Information was elicited during pregnancy on the mothers and their partners' (F1) smoking histories as well as those of their parents (*i.e.,* the study grandparents (F0)). If the grandmothers (F0) had smoked, and if they had smoked whilst pregnant. If the parents reported their mother smoked but, were unsure whether she had smoked during her pregnancy, data were analyzed assuming that these women did smoke during pregnancy. This assumption has been validated by demonstrating that the mean birthweights of this group of study mothers were reduced when compared with those who reported that their mother had definitely not smoked during pregnancy [72]. Around 28 years later, both parents were asked again the same questions on whether their own parents (and also whether their grandparents had smoked), and whether the women had smoked during pregnancy. A validation exercise between these data and that collected around the time of birth of the index child showed a good correlation [99].

## ABBREVIATIONS

| | |
|---|---|
| **ADHD** | Attention Deficit Hyperactivity Disorder |
| **ASD** | Autism Spectrum Disorder |
| **ALSPAC** | Avon Longitudinal Study of Parents and Children |
| **AOR** | Adjusted Odds Ratio |
| **BMI** | Body Mass Index |
| **BPA** | Bisphenol A |
| **CD-1** | Strain of Mice |
| **CHSSC** | Children's Health Study in Southern California |
| **CI** | Confidence Interval |
| **DDT** | Dichlorodiphenyltrichloroethane (an insecticide) |
| **DES** | Diethylstilbestrol |
| **DMR** | Differentially-Methylated Regions |
| **DNA** | Deoxyribonucleic Acid |
| **DXA** | Dual-energy X-ray Absorptiometry (sometimes called 'DEXA') |
| **ECRHS** | European Community Respiratory Health Survey |
| **EUROCAT** | European Network of Population-Based Registries for the Epidemiological Surveillance of Congenital Anomalies |
| **F0** | 1st Generation (*e.g.* Grandparent) |
| **F1** | 2nd Generation (*e.g.* Parent) |
| **F2** | 3rd Generation (the offspring) |
| **GWAS** | Genome-Wide Association Studies |
| **HR** | Hazard Ratio |
| **IQ** | Intelligence Quotient |
| **MGF** | Maternal GrandFather |
| **MGM** | Maternal GrandMother |

| | |
|---|---|
| **MoBa** | Norwegian Mother and Child Cohort Study |
| **OR** | Odds Ratio |
| **P-DMRs** | Prenatal Malnutrition-Associated Differentially Methylated Regions |
| **PGF** | Paternal GrandFather |
| **PGM** | Paternal GrandMother |
| **PROP** | 6-$n$-Propylthiouracil |
| **RHINE** | Respiratory Health in Northern Europe Study |
| **RHINESSA** | Respiratory Health in Northern Europe, Spain and Australia |
| **SCDC** | Social and Communications Disorders Checklist |
| **SGP** | Slow Growth Period |

## CONSENT FOR PUBLICATION

Not applicable.

## CONFLICT OF INTEREST

The authors declare no conflict of interest, financial or otherwise.

## ACKNOWLEDGEMENTS

We are very grateful to Professor Marcus Pembrey and Dr. Matthew Suderman for helpful suggestions and comments, and to Steven Gregory for help with the illustrations. Yasmin Iles-Caven is currently funded by the John Templeton Foundation grant (60828).

## REFERENCES

[1]     Golding J, Jones R, Brune M-N & Pronczuk J. Why carry out a longitudinal birth survey? Paediatr Perinat Epidemiol 2009a; 23 (Suppl. 1): 1-14.
[http://dx.doi.org/10.1111/j.1365-3016.2008.01009.x] [PMID: 19490440]

[2]     Golding J. The importance of a genetic component in longitudinal birth cohorts. Paediatr Perinat Epidemiol 2009; 23 (Suppl. 1): 174-84. b
[http://dx.doi.org/10.1111/j.1365-3016.2009.01013.x] [PMID: 19490455]

[3]     Monaco AP. An epigenetic, transgenerational model of increased mental health disorders in children, adolescents and young adults. Eur J Hum Genet 2020; 18: 1-9.
[PMID: 32948849]

[4]     Nilsson EE, Sadler-Riggleman I, Skinner MK. Environmentally induced epigenetic transgenerational inheritance of disease. Environ Epigenet 2018; 4(2): dvy016.
[http://dx.doi.org/10.1093/eep/dvy016] [PMID: 30038800]

[5]     Camsari C, Folger JK, Rajput SK, McGee D, Latham KE, Smith GW. Transgenerational effects of periconception heavy metal administration on adipose weight and glucose homeostasis in mice at maturity. Toxicol Sci 2019; 168(2): 610-9.
[http://dx.doi.org/10.1093/toxsci/kfz008] [PMID: 30629257]

[6]     Wolstenholme JT, Drobná Z, Henriksen AD, *et al.* Transgenerational bisphenol A causes deficits in social recognition and alters postsynaptic density genes in mice. Endocrinology 2019; 160(8): 1854-67.
[http://dx.doi.org/10.1210/en.2019-00196] [PMID: 31188430]

[7]     Bygren LO, Kaati G, Edvinsson S. Longevity determined by paternal ancestors nutrition during their slow growth period. Acta Biotheor 2001; 49(1): 53-9.
[http://dx.doi.org/10.1023/A:1010241825519] [PMID: 11368478]

[8]     Pembrey ME, Bygren LO, Kaati G, *et al.* Sex-specific, male-line transgenerational responses in humans. Eur J Hum Genet 2006; 14(2): 159-66.
[http://dx.doi.org/10.1038/sj.ejhg.5201538] [PMID: 16391557]

[9]     Kaati G, Bygren LO, Pembrey M & Sjostrom M. Transgenerational response to nutrition, early life circumstances and longevity. Eur J Hum Genet 2007; 15(7): 784-90.
[http://dx.doi.org/10.1038/sj.ejhg.5201832] [PMID: 17457370]

[10]    Vågerö D, Pinger PR, Aronsson V, van den Berg GJ. Paternal grandfathers access to food predicts all-cause and cancer mortality in grandsons. Nat Commun 2018; 9(1): 5124.
[http://dx.doi.org/10.1038/s41467-018-07617-9] [PMID: 30538239]

[11]    Cox ME. Hunger games: or how the Allied blockade in the First World War deprived German children of nutrition, and Allied food aid subsequently saved them. Econ Hist Rev 2015; 68(2): 600-31.
[http://dx.doi.org/10.1111/ehr.12070]

[12]    van den Berg GJ, Pinger PR. Transgenerational effects of childhood conditions on third generation health and education outcomes. Econ Hum Biol 2016; 23: 103-20.
[http://dx.doi.org/10.1016/j.ehb.2016.07.001] [PMID: 27592272]

[13]    van den Berg GJ, Pinger PR. Transgenerational effects of childhood conditions on third generation health and education outcomes. SOEP papers on Multidisciplinary Panel Data Research 2014; 709.
[http://dx.doi.org/10.2139/ssrn.2539013]

[14]    Behrman JR, Calderon MC, Preston SH, Hoddinott J, Martorell R, Stein AD. Nutritional supplementation in girls influences the growth of their children: Prospective study in Guatemala. Am J Clin Nutr 2009; 90(5): 1372-9.
[http://dx.doi.org/10.3945/ajcn.2009.27524] [PMID: 19793851]

[15]    Northstone K, Golding J, Davey Smith G, Miller LL, Pembrey M. Prepubertal start of fathers smoking and increased body fat in his sons: further characterisation of paternal transgenerational responses. Eur J Hum Genet 2014; 22(12): 1382-6.
[http://dx.doi.org/10.1038/ejhg.2014.31] [PMID: 24690679]

[16]    Golding J, Gregory S, Northstone K, Iles-Caven Y, Ellis G, Pembrey M. Investigating possible trans/intergenerational associations with obesity in young adults using an exposome approach. Front Genet 2019; 10: 314.
[http://dx.doi.org/10.3389/fgene.2019.00314] [PMID: 31024624]

[17]    Accordini S, Calciano L, Johannessen A, *et al.* A three-generation study on the association of tobacco smoking with asthma. Int J Epidemiol 2018; 47(4): 1106-17.
[http://dx.doi.org/10.1093/ije/dyy031] [PMID: 29534228]

[18]    Svanes C, Koplin J, Skulstad SM, *et al.* Fathers environment before conception and asthma risk in his children: a multi-generation analysis of the Respiratory Health In Northern Europe study. Int J Epidemiol 2017; 46(1): 235-45.
[PMID: 27565179]

[19]    Accordini S, Johannessen A, Calciano L, *et al.* Three-generation effects of tobacco smoking on lung function within the paternal line. Eur Respir J 2017; 50 (Suppl. 61): PA1178.

[20]    Potts J, Svanes C, Accordini S, Jarvis D. Adolescent smoking by parents and asthma in their children: repeat cross-sectional surveys in England. Eur Respir J 2018; 52: PA3916.

[http://dx.doi.org/10.1183/13993003.congress-2018.PA3916]

[21]   Dudareva YA, Gureva VA, Nemtseva GV. Prevalence and risk of reproductive disorders in descendants depending on grandparents irradiation. Ekologiya Cheloveka (Hum Ecol) 2018; 15(11): 16-9.
[http://dx.doi.org/10.33396/1728-0869-2018-11-16-19]

[22]   Petrushkina NP, Musatkova OB, Okladnikova ND. Health status of children whose grandparents had been subjected to occupational external gamma-exposure. Sci Total Environ 1994; 142(1-2): 111-8.
[http://dx.doi.org/10.1016/0048-9697(94)90079-5] [PMID: 8178129]

[23]   Magnusson LL, Bodin L, Wennborg H. Adverse pregnancy outcomes in offspring of fathers working in biomedical research laboratories. Am J Ind Med 2006; 49(6): 468-73.
[http://dx.doi.org/10.1002/ajim.20317] [PMID: 16691607]

[24]   Shea KM, Little RE, Team AS. Is there an association between preconception paternal x-ray exposure and birth outcome? The ALSPAC Study Team. Am J Epidemiol 1997; 145(6): 546-51.
[http://dx.doi.org/10.1093/oxfordjournals.aje.a009143] [PMID: 9063345]

[25]   World Health Organization. Review of areca (betel) nut and tobacco use in the Pacific: A technical report. Manila: WHO Regional Office for the Western Pacific 2012.

[26]   Boucher BJ, Ewen SWB, Stowers JM. Betel nut (Areca catechu) consumption and the induction of glucose intolerance in adult CD1 mice and in their F1 and F2 offspring. Diabetologia 1994; 37(1): 49-55.
[http://dx.doi.org/10.1007/BF00428777] [PMID: 8150230]

[27]   Chen THH, Chiu YH, Boucher BJ. Transgenerational effects of betel-quid chewing on the development of the metabolic syndrome in the Keelung Community-based Integrated Screening Program. Am J Clin Nutr 2006; 83(3): 688-92.
[http://dx.doi.org/10.1093/ajcn.83.3.688] [PMID: 16522918]

[28]   Yen AMF, Boucher BJ, Chiu SYH, *et al.* Longer duration and earlier age of onset of paternal betel chewing and smoking increase metabolic syndrome risk in human offspring, independently, in a community-based screening program in Taiwan. Circulation 2016; 134(5): 392-404.
[http://dx.doi.org/10.1161/CIRCULATIONAHA.116.021511] [PMID: 27448815]

[29]   Lenz W. A short history of thalidomide embryopathy. Teratology 1988; 38(3): 203-15.
[http://dx.doi.org/10.1002/tera.1420380303] [PMID: 3067415]

[30]   Sheridan MD. Final report of a prospective study of children whose mothers had rubella in early pregnancy. BMJ 1964; 2(5408): 536-9.
[http://dx.doi.org/10.1136/bmj.2.5408.536] [PMID: 14174515]

[31]   Gilman EA, Kneale GW, Knox EG, Stewart AM. Pregnancy x-rays and childhood cancers: effects of exposure age and radiation dose. J Radiol Prot 1988; 8(1): 3-8.
[http://dx.doi.org/10.1088/0952-4746/8/1/301]

[32]   Miller R, Blot W. Small head size after in-utero exposure to atomic radiation. Lancet 1972; 300(7781): 784-7.
[http://dx.doi.org/10.1016/S0140-6736(72)92145-9] [PMID: 4116229]

[33]   Titus-Ernstoff L, Hatch EE, Hoover RN, *et al.* Long-term cancer risk in women given diethylstilbestrol (DES) during pregnancy. Br J Cancer 2001; 84(1): 126-33.
[http://dx.doi.org/10.1054/bjoc.2000.1521] [PMID: 11139327]

[34]   Stillman RJ. In utero exposure to diethylstilbestrol: Adverse effects on the reproductive tract and reproductive performance in male and female offspring. Am J Obstet Gynecol 1982; 142(7): 905-21.
[http://dx.doi.org/10.1016/S0002-9378(16)32540-6] [PMID: 6121486]

[35]   Smithells RW. Thalidomide and malformations in Liverpool. Lancet 1962; 279(7242): 1270-3.
[http://dx.doi.org/10.1016/S0140-6736(62)92367-X] [PMID: 13914462]

[36]    Peckham CS. Clinical and laboratory study of children exposed in utero to maternal rubella. Arch Dis Child 1972; 47(254): 571-7.
[http://dx.doi.org/10.1136/adc.47.254.571] [PMID: 5046774]

[37]    Dolk H. EUROCAT: 25 years of European surveillance of congenital anomalies. Arch Dis Child Fetal Neonatal Ed 2005; 90(5): F355-8.
[http://dx.doi.org/10.1136/adc.2004.062810] [PMID: 16113149]

[38]    Dols MJL, van Arcken DJAM. Food supply and nutrition in the Netherlands during and immediately after World War II. Milbank Mem Fund Q 1946; 24(4): 319-58.
[http://dx.doi.org/10.2307/3348196] [PMID: 20282873]

[39]    Burger GCE, Drummond JC, Sandstead HR. Malnutrition and Starvation in Western Netherlands, September 1944 to July 1945 Part 1 & 2. s-Gravenhage: Staatsuitgeverij 1948.

[40]    Trienekens G. The food supply in the Netherlands during the Second World War.Food, Science, Policy and Regulation in the Twentieth Century International and Comparative Perspectives. London: Routledge 2000; pp. 117-33.

[41]    Susser M, Stein Z. Timing in prenatal nutrition: A reprise of the dutch famine study. Nutr Rev 1994; 52(3): 84-94.
[http://dx.doi.org/10.1111/j.1753-4887.1994.tb01395.x] [PMID: 8015751]

[42]    Ekamper P, van Poppel F, Stein AD, Bijwaard GE, Lumey LH. Prenatal famine exposure and adult mortality from cancer, cardiovascular disease, and other causes through age 63 years. Am J Epidemiol 2015; 181(4): 271-9.
[http://dx.doi.org/10.1093/aje/kwu288] [PMID: 25632050]

[43]    Franzek EJ, Akhigbe KO, Willems EI. Prenatal Malnutrition and Its Devastating Consequences on Mental Health Later in Life. Open J Nutr Food Sci 2019; 1(1): 1004.

[44]    de Rooij SR, Roseboom TJ, Painter RC. Famines in the last 100 years: implications for diabetes. Curr Diab Rep 2014; 14(10): 536.
[http://dx.doi.org/10.1007/s11892-014-0536-7] [PMID: 25173690]

[45]    Song C, Wang M, Chen Z, *et al.* Fetal exposure to Chinese famine increases obesity risk in adulthood. Int J Environ Res Public Health 2020; 17(10): 3649.
[http://dx.doi.org/10.3390/ijerph17103649] [PMID: 32456074]

[46]    Doll R, Hill AB. Lung cancer and other causes of death in relation to smoking; a second report on the mortality of British doctors. BMJ 1956; 2(5001): 1071-81.
[http://dx.doi.org/10.1136/bmj.2.5001.1071] [PMID: 13364389]

[47]    Doll R. Uncovering the effects of smoking: historical perspective. Stat Methods Med Res 1998; 7(2): 87-117.
[http://dx.doi.org/10.1177/096228029800700202] [PMID: 9654637]

[48]    Goldstein H, Goldberg ID, Frazier TM, Davis GE. Cigarette smoking and prematurity. Public Health Rep 1964; 79(7): 553-60. 1
[http://dx.doi.org/10.2307/4592188] [PMID: 14177783]

[49]    Pineles BL, Park E, Samet JM. Systematic review and meta-analysis of miscarriage and maternal exposure to tobacco smoke during pregnancy. Am J Epidemiol 2014; 179(7): 807-23.
[http://dx.doi.org/10.1093/aje/kwt334] [PMID: 24518810]

[50]    Abraham M, Alramadhan S, Iniguez C, *et al.* A systematic review of maternal smoking during pregnancy and fetal measurements with meta-analysis. PLoS One 2017; 12(2): e0170946.
[http://dx.doi.org/10.1371/journal.pone.0170946] [PMID: 28231292]

[51]    Marufu TC, Ahankari A, Coleman T, Lewis S. Maternal smoking and the risk of still birth: systematic review and meta-analysis. BMC Public Health 2015; 15(1): 239.
[http://dx.doi.org/10.1186/s12889-015-1552-5] [PMID: 25885887]

[52]   Zhang D, Cui H, Zhang L, Huang Y, Zhu J, Li X. Is maternal smoking during pregnancy associated with an increased risk of congenital heart defects among offspring? A systematic review and meta-analysis of observational studies. J Matern Fetal Neonatal Med 2017; 30(6): 645-57.
[http://dx.doi.org/10.1080/14767058.2016.1183640] [PMID: 27126055]

[53]   Yu C, Wei Y, Tang X, *et al.* Maternal smoking during pregnancy and risk of cryptorchidism: a systematic review and meta-analysis. Eur J Pediatr 2019; 178(3): 287-97.
[http://dx.doi.org/10.1007/s00431-018-3293-9] [PMID: 30465272]

[54]   Anderson LM, Riffle L, Wilson R, Travlos GS, Lubomirski MS, Alvord WG. Preconceptional fasting of fathers alters serum glucose in offspring of mice. Nutrition 2006; 22(3): 327-31.
[http://dx.doi.org/10.1016/j.nut.2005.09.006] [PMID: 16500559]

[55]   Rayfield S, Plugge E. Systematic review and meta-analysis of the association between maternal smoking in pregnancy and childhood overweight and obesity. J Epidemiol Community Health 2017; 71(2): 162-73.
[http://dx.doi.org/10.1136/jech-2016-207376] [PMID: 27480843]

[56]   He Y, Chen J, Zhu LH, Hua LL, Ke FF. Maternal smoking during pregnancy and ADHD: results from a systematic review and meta-analysis of prospective cohort studies. J Atten Disord 2020; 24(12): 1637-47.
[http://dx.doi.org/10.1177/1087054717696766] [PMID: 29039728]

[57]   Burke H, Leonardi-Bee J, Hashim A, *et al.* Prenatal and passive smoke exposure and incidence of asthma and wheeze: systematic review and meta-analysis. Pediatrics 2012; 129(4): 735-44.
[http://dx.doi.org/10.1542/peds.2011-2196] [PMID: 22430451]

[58]   Hunter A, Murray R, Asher L, Leonardi-Bee J. The effects of tobacco smoking, and prenatal tobacco smoke exposure, on risk of schizophrenia: a systematic review and meta-analysis. Nicotine Tob Res 2020; 22(1): 3-10.
[http://dx.doi.org/10.1093/ntr/nty160] [PMID: 30102383]

[59]   Kataria Y, Gaewsky L, Ellervik C. Prenatal smoking exposure and cardio-metabolic risk factors in adulthood: a general population study and a meta-analysis. Int J Obes 2019; 43(4): 763-73.
[http://dx.doi.org/10.1038/s41366-018-0206-y] [PMID: 30232417]

[60]   Herbst AL, Ulfelder H, Poskanzer DC. Adenocarcinoma of the Vagina. N Engl J Med 1971; 284(16): 878-81.
[http://dx.doi.org/10.1056/NEJM197104222841604] [PMID: 5549830]

[61]   Kalfa N, Paris F, Soyer-Gobillard MO, Daures JP, Sultan C. Prevalence of hypospadias in grandsons of women exposed to diethylstilbestrol during pregnancy: a multigenerational national cohort study. Fertil Steril 2011; 95(8): 2574-7.
[http://dx.doi.org/10.1016/j.fertnstert.2011.02.047] [PMID: 21458804]

[62]   Newbold RR. Lessons learned from perinatal exposure to diethylstilbestrol. Toxicol Appl Pharmacol 2004; 199(2): 142-50.
[http://dx.doi.org/10.1016/j.taap.2003.11.033] [PMID: 15313586]

[63]   Fénichel P, Brucker-Davis F, Chevalier N. The history of Distilbène® (Diethylstilbestrol) told to grandchildren-the transgenerational effect. Ann d'Endocrinol (Paris) 2015; 76(3): 253-9.
[http://dx.doi.org/10.1016/j.ando.2015.03.008] [PMID: 25934356]

[64]   Lumey LH. Decreased birthweights in infants after maternal in utero exposure to the Dutch famine of 1944-1945. Paediatr Perinat Epidemiol 1992; 6(2): 240-53.
[http://dx.doi.org/10.1111/j.1365-3016.1992.tb00764.x] [PMID: 1584725]

[65]   Lumey LH, Stein AD, Ravelli ACJ. Timing of prenatal starvation in women and offspring birth weight: an update. Eur J Obstet Gynecol Reprod Biol 1995; 63(2): 197.
[http://dx.doi.org/10.1016/0301-2115(95)02240-6] [PMID: 8903779]

[66]   Lumey LH, Stein AD. Offspring birth weights after maternal intrauterine undernutrition: a comparison

within sibships. Am J Epidemiol 1997; 146(10): 810-9.
[http://dx.doi.org/10.1093/oxfordjournals.aje.a009198] [PMID: 9384201]

[67]   Painter RC, Osmond C, Gluckman P, Hanson M, Phillips DIW, Roseboom TJ. Transgenerational effects of prenatal exposure to the Dutch famine on neonatal adiposity and health in later life. BJOG 2008; 115(10): 1243-9.
[http://dx.doi.org/10.1111/j.1471-0528.2008.01822.x] [PMID: 18715409]

[68]   Veenendaal MVE, Painter RC, de Rooij SR, *et al.* Transgenerational effects of prenatal exposure to the 1944-45 Dutch famine. BJOG 2013; 120(5): 548-54.
[http://dx.doi.org/10.1111/1471-0528.12136] [PMID: 23346894]

[69]   Smil V. China's great famine: 40 years later. BMJ 1999; 319(7225): 1619-21.
[http://dx.doi.org/10.1136/bmj.319.7225.1619] [PMID: 10600969]

[70]   Huang C, Li Z, Venkat Narayan KM, Williamson DF, Martorell R. Bigger babies born to women survivors of the 1959-1961 Chinese famine: a puzzle due to survival selection? J Dev Orig Health Dis 2010; 1(6): 412-8.
[http://dx.doi.org/10.1017/S2040174410000504] [PMID: 25142012]

[71]   Hyppönen E, Smith GD, Power C. Effects of grandmothers smoking in pregnancy on birth weight: intergenerational cohort study. BMJ 2003; 327(7420): 898.
[http://dx.doi.org/10.1136/bmj.327.7420.898] [PMID: 14563745]

[72]   Miller LL, Pembrey M, Davey Smith G, Northstone K, Golding J. Is the growth of the fetus of a non-smoking mother influenced by the smoking of either grandmother while pregnant? PLoS One 2014; 9(2): e86781. a
[http://dx.doi.org/10.1371/journal.pone.0086781] [PMID: 24504157]

[73]   Pembrey M, Northstone K, Gregory S, Miller LL, Golding J. Is the growth of the child of a smoking mother influenced by the fathers prenatal exposure to tobacco? A hypothesis generating longitudinal study. BMJ Open 2014; 4(7): e005030. b
[http://dx.doi.org/10.1136/bmjopen-2014-005030] [PMID: 25015471]

[74]   Golding J, Northstone K, Gregory S, Miller LL, Pembrey M. The anthropometry of children and adolescents may be influenced by the prenatal smoking habits of their grandmothers: A longitudinal cohort study. Am J Hum Biol 2014; 26(6): 731-9.
[http://dx.doi.org/10.1002/ajhb.22594] [PMID: 25130101]

[75]   Golding J, van den Berg G, Northstone K, *et al.* Grandchild's IQ is associated with grandparental environments prior to the birth of the parents. Wellcome Open Res 2020; 5(198): 198.

[76]   Steer CD, Golding J, Bolton PF. Traits contributing to the autistic spectrum. PLoS One 2010; 5(9): e12633.
[http://dx.doi.org/10.1371/journal.pone.0012633] [PMID: 20838614]

[77]   Golding J, Ellis G, Gregory S, *et al.* Grand-maternal smoking in pregnancy and grandchilds autistic traits and diagnosed autism. Sci Rep 2017; 7(1): 46179.
[http://dx.doi.org/10.1038/srep46179] [PMID: 28448061]

[78]   Skuse DH, Mandy WPL, Scourfield J. Measuring autistic traits: heritability, reliability and validity of the Social and Communication Disorders Checklist. Br J Psychiatry 2005; 187(6): 568-72.
[http://dx.doi.org/10.1192/bjp.187.6.568] [PMID: 16319410]

[79]   Li YF, Langholz B, Salam MT, Gilliland FD. Maternal and grandmaternal smoking patterns are associated with early childhood asthma. Chest 2005; 127(4): 1232-41.
[http://dx.doi.org/10.1016/S0012-3692(15)34472-X] [PMID: 15821200]

[80]   Magnus MC, Haberg SE, Karlstad O, Nafstad P, London SJ, Nystad W. Grandmothers smoking when pregnant with the mother and asthma in the grandchild: the Norwegian Mother and Child Cohort Study. Thorax 2015; 70(3): 237-43.
[http://dx.doi.org/10.1136/thoraxjnl-2014-206438] [PMID: 25572596]

[81]    Lodge CJ, Braback L, Lowe AJ, Dharmage SC, Olsson D, Forsberg B. Grandmaternal smoking increases asthma risk in grandchildren: A nationwide Swedish cohort. Clin Exp Allergy 2018; 48(2): 167-74.
[http://dx.doi.org/10.1111/cea.13031] [PMID: 28925522]

[82]    Miller LL, Henderson J, Northstone K, Pembrey M, Golding J. Do grandmaternal smoking patterns influence the etiology of childhood asthma? Chest 2014; 145(6): 1213-8. b
[http://dx.doi.org/10.1378/chest.13-1371] [PMID: 24158349]

[83]    Arshad SH, Karmaus W, Zhang H, Holloway JW. Multigenerational cohorts in patients with asthma and allergy. J Allergy Clin Immunol 2017; 139(2): 415-21.
[http://dx.doi.org/10.1016/j.jaci.2016.12.002] [PMID: 28183434]

[84]    Williams C, Suderman M, Guggenheim JA, *et al.* Grandmothers smoking in pregnancy is associated with a reduced prevalence of early-onset myopia. Sci Rep 2019; 9(1): 15413.
[http://dx.doi.org/10.1038/s41598-019-51678-9] [PMID: 30626917]

[85]    Hall A, Northstone K, Iles-Caven Y, *et al.* Intolerance of loud sounds in childhood: Is there an intergenerational association with grandmaternal smoking in pregnancy? PLoS One 2020; 15(2): e0229323.
[http://dx.doi.org/10.1371/journal.pone.0229323] [PMID: 32092095]

[86]    Pembrey ME, Gregory S, Suderman M, Iles-Caven Y, Northstone K, Golding J. Extreme sensitivity to bitter taste: a possible transgenerational association. Proc Natl Acad Sci USA 2021.

[87]    Meyer MB, Tonascia J. Long-term effects of prenatal x-ray of human females. I. Reproductive experience. Am J Epidemiol 1981; 114(3): 304-16.
[http://dx.doi.org/10.1093/oxfordjournals.aje.a113196] [PMID: 7304566]

[88]    Black SE, BA1/4tikofer A, Devereux PJ, Salvanes KG. This is only a test? Long-run and intergenerational impacts of prenatal exposure to radioactive fallout. Rev Econ Stat 2019; 101(3): 531-46.
[http://dx.doi.org/10.1162/rest_a_00815]

[89]    Skinner MK. Endocrine disruptor induction of epigenetic transgenerational inheritance of disease. Mol Cell Endocrinol 2014; 398(1-2): 4-12.
[http://dx.doi.org/10.1016/j.mce.2014.07.019] [PMID: 25088466]

[90]    Hill AB. The environment and disease: association or causation? Proc R Soc Med 1965; 58(5): 295-300.
[http://dx.doi.org/10.1177/003591576505800503] [PMID: 14283879]

[91]    Bygren LO, Müller P, Brodin D, Kaati G, Gustafsson JA, Kral JG. Paternal grandparental exposure to crop failure or surfeit during a childhood slow growth period and epigenetic marks on third generations growth - glucoregulatory and stress genes. bioRxiv 2018; 215467.

[92]    Heijmans BT, Tobi EW, Stein AD, *et al.* Persistent epigenetic differences associated with prenatal exposure to famine in humans. Proc Natl Acad Sci USA 2008; 105(44): 17046-9.
[http://dx.doi.org/10.1073/pnas.0806560105] [PMID: 18955703]

[93]    Tobi EW, Lumey LH, Talens RP, *et al.* DNA methylation differences after exposure to prenatal famine are common and timing- and sex-specific. Hum Mol Genet 2009; 18(21): 4046-53.
[http://dx.doi.org/10.1093/hmg/ddp353] [PMID: 19656776]

[94]    Tobi EW, Goeman JJ, Monajemi R, *et al.* DNA methylation signatures link prenatal famine exposure to growth and metabolism. Nat Commun 2014; 5(1): 5592.
[http://dx.doi.org/10.1038/ncomms6592] [PMID: 25424739]

[95]    Mørkve Knudsen GT, Rezwan FI, Johannessen A, *et al.* Epigenome-wide association of fathers smoking with offspring DNA methylation: a hypothesis-generating study. Environ Epigenet 2019; 5(4): dvz023.
[http://dx.doi.org/10.1093/eep/dvz023] [PMID: 31827900]

[96]     Golding J. The Avon Longitudinal Study of Parents and Children (ALSPAC)--study design and collaborative opportunities. Eur J Endocrinol 2004; 151 (Suppl. 3): U119-23.
[http://dx.doi.org/10.1530/eje.0.151u119] [PMID: 15554896]

[97]     Boyd A, Golding J, Macleod J, *et al.* Cohort Profile: the children of the 90s--the index offspring of the Avon Longitudinal Study of Parents and Children. Int J Epidemiol 2013; 42(1): 111-27.
[http://dx.doi.org/10.1093/ije/dys064] [PMID: 22507743]

[98]     Fraser A, Macdonald-Wallis C, Tilling K, *et al.* Cohort profile: the Avon Longitudinal Study of Parents and Children: ALSPAC mothers cohort. Int J Epidemiol 2013; 42(1): 97-110.
[http://dx.doi.org/10.1093/ije/dys066] [PMID: 22507742]

[99]     Golding J, Gregory S, Matthews S, *et al.* Ancestral childhood environmental exposures occurring to the grandparents and great-grandparents of the ALSPAC study children. Wellcome Open Res 2020; 5: 207.
[http://dx.doi.org/10.12688/wellcomeopenres.16257.1] [PMID: 33043146]

# CHAPTER 5

# Clinical Approaches to Genetic Epilepsies in Children

**Mario Mastrangelo**[1,2,*]

[1] *Department of Maternal, Infantile, and Urological Sciences, Sapienza University of Rome, Rome, Italy*

[2] *Child Neurology and Psychiatry Unit, Department of Neurosciences/Mental Health, Azienda Ospedaliero-Universitaria Policlinico Umberto I, Rome, Italy*

**Abstract:** A genetic etiology is determined in more than 30% of all diagnosed cases of epilepsy with onset at the pediatric age. About 210 single disease-causing genes and 400 chromosomal imbalances are associated with epilepsy, and a presumed pathogenic role has been suggested for about 7000 different genes.

Genetic epilepsies can be divided, according to the main correlated epileptogenic mechanisms, into the following groups: a) channelopathies, b) transportopathies, c) disorders of the intermediate metabolism, d) disorders of the neuronal cellular cycle and signaling, e) disorders of synaptic vesicles trafficking and release, f) disorders involving neuronal structural proteins, g) disorders of synaptic secreted proteins and h) chromosomopathies and pathogenic copy number variants.

A careful diagnostic work-up should be focused on the exclusion of acquired causes of seizures, the analysis of family history, the definition of seizure semiology and epileptic syndromes, and the characterization of associated neurological and non-neurological manifestations.

Traditional genetic techniques (karyotype, array CGH, and Sanger sequencing) remain useful for known epilepsy phenotypes (*e.g.* Dravet syndrome) and for various syndromes including neurodevelopmental impairment.

Next-generation sequencing (NGS) includes different techniques (targeted gene panels and whole genome sequencing) that allow a simultaneous sequencing of exons belonging to a selected group of genes organized in panels or to the whole exome or genome.

* **Corresponding author Mario Mastrangelo:** Department of Maternal, Infantile, and Urological Sciences, Sapienza University of Rome, Rome, Italy and Child Neurology and Psychiatry Unit, Department of Neurosciences/Mental Health, Azienda Ospedaliero-Universitaria Policlinico Umberto I, Rome, Italy; Tel: +39649972939; Fax: +3964440232; E-mail: mario.mastrangelo@uniroma1.it

Advantages of NGS include: a) the identification of new disease-causing genes associated with epilepsy, b) an expansion of the known phenotypes associated with previously discovered disease-causing genes, c) an improvement of genetic counseling, d) a reduction of the times for the diagnosis, and e) a reduction of economic costs.

**Keywords:** brain, bioinformatic tools, cortical excitability, children, developmental delay, developmental encephalopathies, Epilepsy, epileptic encephalopathies, epileptogenesis, genotype, gene, genetic counselling, intellectual disability, infants, neurogenetic disorders, neurometabolic disorders, next-generation sequencing, phenotype, newborns, seizures.

## INTRODUCTION

Epilepsy is the most common neurologic disorder at the pediatric age with an incidence of about 70 per 100.000 cases in children under the age of 2 [1].

The complex landscape of genetic etiologies of epilepsies has largely expanded in the last decades. About 7000 genes with a presumed pathogenic role and more than 150 genes with a known associated clinical phenotype were reported in the literature (about 30% of the whole diagnosed epilepsies) [2]. Most of the genetic epilepsies were prominently studied in subjects in which an early or very early onset of seizures and a very severe developmental and neurological impairment occurred [3]. In this context, the OMIM database has currently reported 99 diseases that were classified as "developmental and epileptic encephalopathies" [4]. Other common associated clinical presentations include facial dysmorphisms, abnormalities of head circumference (microcephaly or macrocephaly), movement disorders, and malformations in other organs such as the heart, eye, skeleton, or kidney [5].

Most of the reported genes encode ion channel subunits, membrane receptors/transporters and proteins involved in the transduction of neuronal signaling or enzymes of the intermediate metabolism. Pathogenic variants of these genes result in dysfunctions of different stages of neuronal development and functioning, including synaptogenesis, pruning, neuronal migration and differentiation, and neurotransmitter synthesis and release.

Epilepsy phenotypes and severity, degree of developmental impairment, and concurrent neurological and non-neurological manifestations are extremely variable according to the functions of the different involved genes and their role in epileptogenic mechanisms. Several studies also evidenced a remarkable heterogeneity in terms of different clinical conditions resulting from variants of the same genes (*e.g. SCN2A* causes both familial benign neonatal infantile epilepsy and severe epileptic encephalopathy; *KCNQ2* was initially associated with familial benign neonatal seizures and, subsequently, with an early onset epileptic encephalopathy) or similar clinical syndromes caused by different genes (*e.g.* Dravet syndrome can be caused by pathogenic variants of *SCN1A, PCDH 19, STXBP1 or GABRA1*).

About 400 different chromosomal imbalances associated with epilepsy have been reported, including several Copy Number Variants (CNVs) [3]. In this context, physicians should always consider the involvement of genes in the deleted or duplicated region that could have a known or presumed link with epileptogenic mechanisms [1, 2].

## CLINICAL AND DIAGNOSTIC APPROACH

The suspect of a genetic etiology in a child with epilepsy should be primarily suggested by four main steps: the exclusion of acquired causes of seizures, the careful analysis of family history, the characterization of seizure semiology and epileptic syndromes and the evaluation of associated neurological and non-neurological signs and symptoms [6].

Acquired causes of epilepsy seizures include hypoxic-ischemic encephalopathy or other neonatal disorders, infectious or autoimmune encephalitis, traumatic brain injuries, stroke, neoplasm, vasculitis, drug withdrawal or toxicity, metabolic disturbances (including those conditions resulting in hypoglycemia, hyponatremia, or hypomagnesemia).

Family history should be investigated regarding recurrent epilepsy phenotypes in different family members and the mode of inheritance of specific disturbances. Family history of different seizures and EEG patterns might suggest either a genetic condition with variable phenotypes or the possibility of different causes of seizures among the involved family members [1].

Clinical presentation of genetic epilepsy can be differentiated into two main patterns, including seizures as prominent/ unique symptoms or seizures associated with a syndromic phenotype, even if the variability is high, and several diseases may present with both clinical patterns.

In patients presenting with the first pattern, seizures are the most evident and characterizing feature, and other neurological symptoms include a cognitive and developmental delay that could precede or follow the onset of epilepsy. Among newborns and infants belonging to this group and presenting with intractable seizures, a therapeutic trial for vitamin-dependent epilepsies (mainly through the administration of pyridoxine, pyridoxal phosphate or folinic acid) should always be considered, because it also has a diagnostic role for the characterization of treatable early onset epileptic and developmental encephalopathies (*e.g.,* *ALDH7A1, PNPO or FOLR1* deficiency). In other cases, a long list of monogenic diseases or chromosomal abnormalities should be adequately studied through the available genetic methods [2 - 6]. Some conditions in which a specific seizure semiology is strongly related to single gene disorders should be considered (*e.g.* sleep-related hypermotor epilepsy due to pathogenic variants of CHRNA*4* or genes belonging to GATOR1 complex) [1, 2].

In several cases, such as Down, Rett, Angelman, Miller-Dieker or Menkes syndrome and facial dysmorphisms allow a gestaltic diagnosis.

Abnormalities of occipito-frontal circumference could address the diagnostic suspect towards specific metabolic or monogenic non-metabolic conditions. Acquired microcephalies are usually linked to metabolic dysfunction (apart from children with maternal phenylketonuria in which microcephaly can be detected during the pregnancy), while congenital ones are due to monogenic non-metabolic diseases (apart from phosphoglycerate dehydrogenase deficiency). Macrocephaly is typically associated with genetic non-metabolic diseases apart from Canavan disease and Glutaric aciduria type 1.

Movement disorders associated with epilepsy are mainly represented by dystonia and different forms of dyskinesia. In some genetic diseases, they are largely prominent over epileptic manifestations (*e.g.,* GLUT1 deficiency).

Multiorgan involvement may include skin signs in neurocutaneous disorders (*e.g.* tuberous sclerosis and Sturge Weber syndrome), septic-like symptoms in various metabolic disorders associated with a risk of life-threatening derangement (*e.g.* organic acidurias, some aminoacidopathies or mitochondriopathies), visceral enlargement/malformations in some chromosomopathies (*e.g.* Down syndrome) or in other metabolic disorders (*e.g.* lysosomal storage diseases or congenital defects of glycosylation) [6].

EEG abnormalities correlate more closely with the seizure types than with the underlying etiology. Even if some specific patterns are more suggestive of a genetic etiology, especially in newborns and infants (*e.g.* suppression burst pattern and hypsarrhytmia). Early onset photosensitivity, at low frequencies, is addressed towards specific etiologies (neuronal ceroid lipofuscinosis, Dravet syndrome or progressive myoclonic epilepsies). Fig. **1** shows some EEG patterns that are frequently observed in genetically determined epilepsies.

Brain MRI is extremely useful for the exclusion of non-genetic etiologies, but it is also important for the detection of epileptogenic cortical or posterior fossa malformations [1, 6]. In other cases, some suggestive but non-specific abnormalities (cortical or cerebellar atrophy, callosal dysgenesis/absence and white matter lesions) could suggest the following diagnostic steps. Illustrative brain MRIs for some neurogenetic disorders presenting with epileptic seizures are provided in Fig. (2).

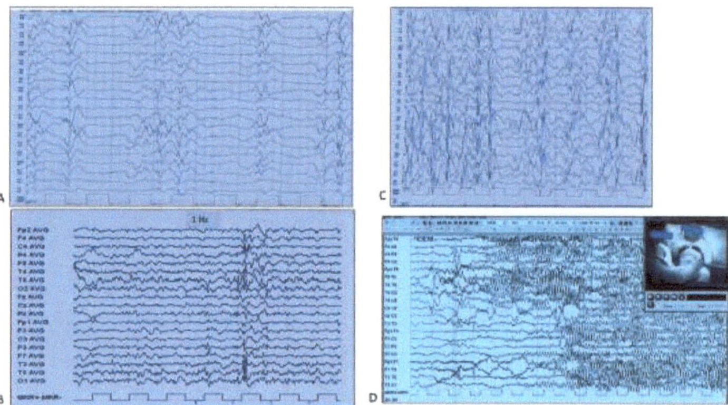

**Fig. (1).** Some illustrative EEG patterns that are detectable in genetic epilepsies of childhood: A) Suppression-burst pattern in a newborn with ALDH7A1 deficiency; B) Hypsarrhytmia in a patient with Down syndrome presenting with a West syndrome; C) A photo paroxysmal response at a very low frequency (1Hz) in a patient with neuronal ceroid lipofuscinosis type 2; D) Focal secondarily generalized epileptic discharges starting from right frontotemporal region in a patient with tuberous sclerosis during a versive seizure.

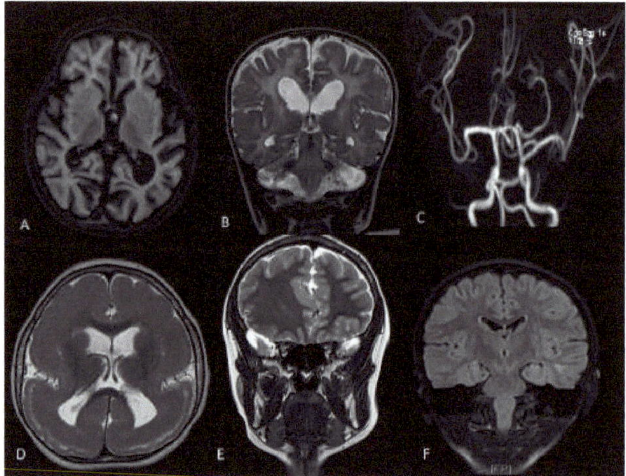

**Fig. (2).** Examples of MRI abnormalities in patients with genetically determined epilepsies: A) A diffuse cortical atrophy in a patient with neuronal ceroid lipofuscinosis type 10; B) A diffuse hypomyelination, especially in frontal regions, in a patient with Canavan disease; C) Tortuous cerebral blood vessels in a patient with Menkes disease; D) Lissencephaly in a patient with Miller-Dieker syndrome; E) Hemimegalencephaly in a patient carrying a PTEN gene variant; F) A subcortical tuber in a patient with tuberous sclerosis.

In some circumstances, brain magnetic resonance spectroscopy may identify metabolic abnormalities (*i.e.* lack of creatine peak in defects of creatine metabolism, lactate elevation in mitochondrial disorders, or in Menkes disease and N-acetyl aspartate elevation in Canavan disease). Positron emission tomography may show evident or subtle metabolic abnormalities of selected and diffuse cortical areas, especially in surgically treatable epilepsies or in specific diseases such as GLUT1 deficiency syndrome [6].

## MOLECULAR GENETIC WORK-UP

In Table **1**, the objectives, and the indications of all the molecular genetics diagnostic tests are summarized.

**Table 1. Diagnostic aims and indications of available molecular genetic methods for the study of pediatric patients with epilepsy.**

| Diagnostic Tests | Diagnostic Aim | Indications |
|---|---|---|
| **Karyotype** | Analysis of all chromosomes for large duplications/deletions. | Patients with suggestive facial dysmorphism and/or multiorgan involvement (*i.e.* Down syndrome). |
| **Array CGH** | To identify single nucleotide polymorphisms (SNP arrays) or to characterize chromosomal rearrangements (array-CGH) as copy number variants (CNVs). | Patients with epilepsy associated with developmental delay, Dysmorphism or autism spectrum disorder. |
| **Sanger sequencing** | Single gene sequencing (detection of changes in the gene and the correlated amino acid alterations). | Suspected single-gene defect or peculiar epilepsy syndrome (i..e. SCN1A-related Dravet syndrome). |
| **Multiplex ligation-dependent probe amplification (MLPA)** | Detection of duplication/deletion of a single gene. | Suspicious of a single gene defect when sequencing is inconclusive. |
| **Research of a specific mutation** | Sequencing of a specific mutation. | Research on parents of a mutation detected in a proband to understand if it is inherited and/or pathogenic. |
| **Targeted - resequencing** | Sequencing and duplication/deletion research of a gene panel for a specific disease (*e.g.* epilepsy). | Diseases with more genes involved. |
| **Fluorescent *in situ* hybridization (FISH)** | Analysis of specific chromosome's portions *via* ad hoc probes. | Confirmation of a duplication/deletion. |
| **Whole-exome and genome sequencing** | Sequencing of all DNA only for codifying regions (exons) or all regions (genome). | Suspected genetic etiology with otherwise normal investigations. |

During the pre-next-generation sequencing era, patients who were suspected to have single gene-related epilepsy underwent a prolonged diagnostic odyssey, including gene by gene Sanger sequencing and complex biochemical and laboratory work-up [3, 5].

Next-generation sequencing (NGS) includes different techniques that allow a simultaneous sequencing of exons belonging to a selected group of genes organized in panels or to the whole exome or genome.

Whole-Exome Sequencing (WES) involves the encoding part of the human genome (about 20,000 disease-causing genes). Whole Genome Sequencing (WGS) involves both the encoding and non-encoding parts of the human genome [2].

NGS methods identify gene variants and analyze their possible pathogenic role through a comparison with the non-pathogenic variants that are distributed in the general population. The putative pathogenic mutations are subsequently characterized in terms of de novo occurrence (when variants are not detected in the parents) or patterns of inheritance [6]. In epileptic children, recently published next generation sequencing studies have evidenced a detection rate for pathogenic or likely pathogenic variants ranging between 18,3% and 40% according to different extensions of the specific gene panels that were built [7 - 15]. A recent WGS study in 197 subjects highlighted the role of several new genes in the pathogenesis of both epileptic and developmental encephalopathies with a clear prevalence of de novo point mutation if compared with other mechanisms of inheritance [16].

A suggestion for a possible diagnostic algorithm including NGS is included in Fig. **3**. Although every form of pediatric epilepsy can be diagnosed by NGS, a more useful applicability of these techniques was reported for patients without gestaltic facial dysmorphisms or structural abnormalities in the neuroimaging. Gene panels, WES and WGS do not identify non-coding regulatory sequences and deletions/duplications of exons that can be studied through array CGH and other cytogenetic techniques.

NGS approaches have resulted in remarkable advantages including: a) the discovery of an increasing number of new genes responsible for rare forms of monogenic epilepsies; b) an expansion of the known phenotypes associated with previously reported disease-causing genes c) an improvement of genetic counseling with an increase of molecular genetic diagnosis, and the demonstration that most of the pathogenic variants in childhood epilepsies are de novo; d) an optimization of diagnostic work-up and therapeutic choices through a reduction of diagnostic delays; e) a remarkable reduction of economic costs [2, 6].

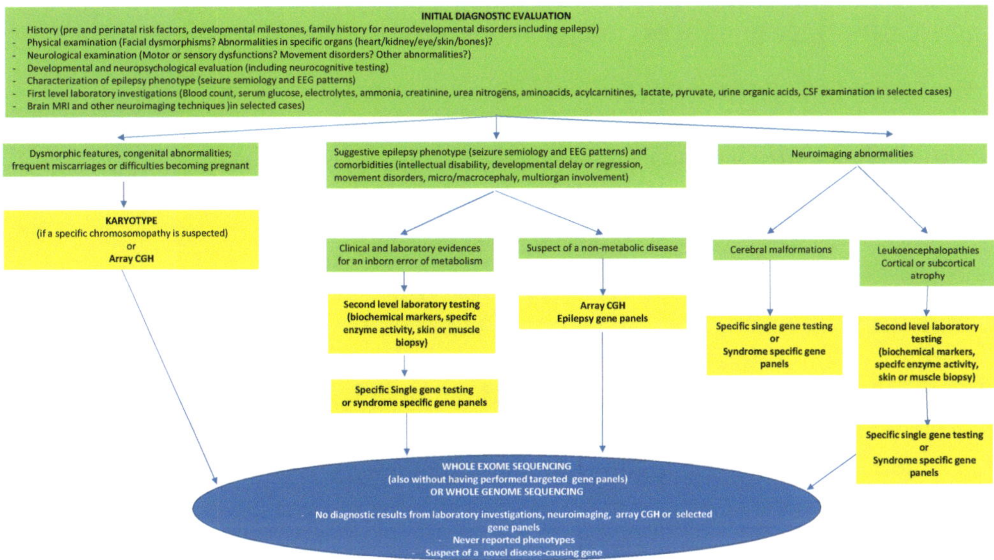


**Fig. (3).** Suggested algorithm for the diagnostic work-up in pediatric epilepsies with a probable genetic etiology.

The possibility of analyzing concurrently a wider group of disease-causing genes, and the faster gene-sequencing was counterbalanced by: a) the availability of a large amount of data that often complicate genotype-phenotype correlations; b) the frequent detection of variants of uncertain significance; c) the frequent need for functional studies to assess the real pathogenic effect of the detected variants; d) a limited epidemiological impact (most of the known disease-causing genes associated with epilepsy accounts for a limited quote of cases).

The interpretation of functional effects and pathogenicity of the detected variants can be supported by several bioinformatics tools. The ExAC (http://exac.broadinstitute.org), the gnomAD (http://gnomad.broadinstitute.org) or the 1000 Genomes Project (http://www.internationalgenome.org) databases list the different variants and their alleles frequencies in the population. The ClinVar database (https://www.ncbi.nlm.nih.gov/clinvar/), the Human Gene Mutation Database (HGMD) (http://www.hgmd.cf.ac.uk/ac/index.php) or several locus-specific databases correlate genomic variants with clinical presentations that were reported in the literature [7].

A positive correlation can be assessed between the number of genes included in an NGS panel and its diagnostic yield [2, 7]. The number of sequenced genes should be continuously updated according to the progression of knowledge, even if frequent changes in the composition of the panels result in a contemporary increase of the identified variants and, subsequently, in increasing complexity of bioinformatics filtering process and genotype–phenotype correlations [6].

## ILLUSTRATIVE DISEASES

A detailed description of all the genetic epilepsies is beyond the scope of this chapter, but a section focusing on some valuable examples of illustrative diseases could be useful for the definition of a pragmatic approach to this complex subject.

Genetic epilepsies can be divided, according to the main epileptogenic mechanisms, into the following groups: a) channelopathies, b) transportopathies, c) disorders of the intermediate metabolism, d) disorders of the neuronal cellular cycle and signaling, e) disorders of synaptic vesicles trafficking and release, f) disorders involving neuronal structural proteins, g) disorders of synaptic secreted proteins and h) chromosomopathies and pathogenic copy number variants.

## Channelopathies

### *General Aspects*

Ion channels are pore-forming membrane proteins that are essential for different regulatory mechanisms of neuronal excitability: a) the establishment of action potentials, b) the maintenance of homeostasis by gating the ionic flow traversing the cell membrane, c) the management of the ionic flow across cells and d) the regulation of cell volume [17]. Table **2.** summarizes these ion channels and their main physiological functions.

**Table 2. Ion channels involved in human diseases.**

| Ion Channels | Gene (Protein) | Physiologic Function |
|---|---|---|
| **POTASSIUM CHANNELS**<br>**Voltage gated**<br>**Calcium-activated**<br>**Sodium-activated** | *KCNA2* (KV1.2), *KCNB1* (KV2.1), *KCNC1* (KV3.1), *KCND2* (KV4.2), *KCND3* (KV4.3), *KCNH2* (KV11.1), *KCNH5* (KV10.2), *KCNQ2* (KV7.2), *KCNQ3* (KV7.3), *KCNV2* (KV8.2) *KCNMA1* (KCa1.1) *KCNT1* (KCa4.1) | Modulation of outward K currents and action potentials, modulation of neurotransmitter release. Modulation of neuronal firing properties and circuit Excitability. Modulation of delayed outward $IK_{Na}$ currents and contribution to adaptation of firing rate |

*(Table 2) cont.....*

| Ion Channels | Gene (Protein) | Physiologic Function |
|---|---|---|
| **SODIUM CHANNELS** | *SCN1A* (NaV1.1), *SCN1B* (NaVb1), *SCN2A* (NaV1.2), *SCN3A* (NaV1.3), *SCN8A* (NaV1.6), *SCN9A*(NaV1.7) | Generation and propagation of action potentials. |
| **CHLORIDE CHANNELS** | *CLCN2* (CLC-2), *CLCN4* (CLC-4) | Maintenance of resting membrane potential and modulation of cell volume. |
| **CALCIUM CHANNELS** | *CACNA1A* (CaV2.1), *CACNA1H* (CaV3.2), *CACNA2D2* (CaVa2d-2), *CACNB4* (CaVb4), | React to membrane potential depolarization by opening and provide an elevation of Calcium ions to modulate many processes. |
| **HYPERPOLARIZATION-ACTIVATED CYCLIC NUCLEOTIDE-GATED CHANNELS** | *HCN1* (HCN1), *HCN2* (HCN2) | Permeation of Na and K fluxes. |
| **NICOTINIC ACETYLCHOLINE RECEPTORS** | *CHRNA2* (nAChRa2), *CHRNA4* (nAChRa4), *CHRNA7* (nAChRa7), *CHRNB2* (nAChRb2) | Permeation of Na and K and modulation of neurotransmitter release. |
| **IONOTROPIC GLUTAMATE RECEPTORS** | *GRIN1* (GluN1), *GRIN2A* (GluN2A), *GRIN2B* (GluN2B), *GRIN2D* (GluN2D) | Excitatory synaptic transmission, plasticity, and excitotoxicity of the central nervous system. |
| **C-AMINOBUTYRIC ACID TYPE A RECEPTOR** | *GABRA1* (GABAAa1), *GABRA6* (GABAAa6), *GABRB1*(GABAAb1), *GABRB2* (GABAAb2), *GABRB3* (GABAAb3), *GABRD* (GABAAd), *GABRG2* (GABAAc2) | Regulation of major inhibitory functions in neurotransmission. |

Mutations of genes encoding for ion channels subunits are the most frequent cause of genetic epilepsies [3]. A recent analysis of several online databases identified 60 ion channel genes with a proved (28 genes) or a potential role (32 genes) in human epilepsies and more than 1600 pathogenic or likely pathogenic variants of these genes [17].

## Illustrative Disease: Dravet Syndrome

Dravet syndrome (OMIM 607208) is the most frequent epileptic channelopathy. Mutations involving sodium channel neuronal type 1a subunit (*SCN1A*) account for about 85% of patients with this epileptic and developmental encephalopathy

[3, 18]. A minority of patients carried mutations in other genes, including *PCDH19* or *STXBP1*, while various Dravet-like phenotypes were associated with *CN2A, SCN8A, SCN9A, SCN1B, GABRA1, GABRG2, HCN1, CHD2,* and *KCNA2.*

The clinical phenotype includes prolonged generalized or hemiclonic seizures triggered by fever, photo-stimulation or hot water, myoclonic seizures, atypical absences, and partial seizures. Developmental milestones are usually normal before the onset of epilepsy but are gradually impaired by recurrent epileptic episodes (also including life-threatening status epilepticus), resulting in mental delay, spasticity, or ataxia [3].

Antiepileptic treatment usually includes polytherapy, including valproate, clobazam and/or stiripentol, even if encouraging results have been recently obtained in trials with fenfluramine and cannabidiol [18].

## Transportopathies

### *General Aspects*

Membrane transporters are proteins involved in the transport of molecules across the blood-brain barrier or between cytosol and the internal parts of various organelles such as mitochondria or endoplasmic reticulum. The molecules involved in transport are usually represented by glucose, amino acids (*e.g.* GABA, glutamate), creatine, vitamins (*e.g.* thiamine, folate), or trace elements (*e.g.* copper, manganese).

Pathogenic variants involving genes encoding for membrane transporters activate epileptogenic mechanisms *via* the depletion of substrates for neuronal energy reactions (*e.g.* glucose in GLUT 1 deficiency syndrome) and cofactors for several biochemical processes, including glycosylation of neuronal membrane proteins (*e.g.* manganese in *SLC39A8* deficiency), and the biosynthesis of inhibitory or excitatory neurotransmitter (*e.g.* glutamate in *SLC25A22* deficiency syndrome, folate in *FOLR1* deficiency syndrome, thiamine in *SLC22A1* deficiency syndrome, creatine in *SLC6A8* deficiency and copper in Menkes disease).

Common phenotypic features of these disorders often include a catastrophic and life-threatening neonatal epileptic encephalopathy associated with suppression bursts on the EEG (*e.g.* in *SLC25A22* deficiency syndrome) and a severe developmental impairment in the less severe cases (Glut 1 deficiency syndrome). Movement disorders (*e.g.* paroxysmal kinesigenic dyskinesia in Glut 1 deficiency syndrome) or autistic spectrum disorder (*e.g. FOLR1* deficiency syndrome) characterize some diseases [3].

## *Illustrative Disease: GLUT1 Deficiency Syndrome*

GLUT1 deficiency syndrome (OMIM 138140) is a valuable example of the possible phenotypic heterogeneity in epileptic transportopathies.

GLUT1 is a membrane glucose transporter that is expressed in the brain (across the blood-brain barrier), placenta and erythrocytes.

GLUT1 deficiency syndrome is caused by *SCL2A1* gene mutations (de novo mutations or autosomal dominant inheritance) [19].

Its clinical presentation includes a classical phenotype (early-onset epileptic encephalopathy, acquired microcephaly, developmental delay and movement disorders including dystonia and ataxia, hypotonia or spasticity) and different atypical phenotypes (paroxysmal exercise-induced dystonia with or without seizures, choreoathetosis, intermittent ataxia, early-onset absences, migraine, alternating hemiplegia, different degree of cognitive or language delay, expressive language or learning difficulties).

Electroencephalogram (EEG) abnormalities are variable and often non-specific even if some of them decrease after a meal [20]. Positron-emission tomography often detects a decreased glucose uptake in the mesial temporal regions and thalamus. Other neuroimaging techniques, including brain MRI, do not play a relevant role in the diagnostic work-up [19].

The main biochemical hallmark for GLUT1 deficiency syndrome is a glycorrhachia lower than the third percentile for age [19]. Cerebrospinal fluid-t--blood glucose ratio levels lower than 0.35 is strongly suggestive even if the ratio can be higher than 0.59 in milder phenotypes [19]. Pediatricians should consider that other more frequent causes of hypoglycorrachia should be excluded (meningitis, status epilepticus, mitochondrial diseases, hypoglycemic states, subarachnoid hemorrhage and meningeal carcinomatosis). After having excluded these diseases, second-level investigations for GLUT1 deficiency, including tests for the uptake of 3-*O*-methylglucose into erythrocytes and *SLC2A1* gene sequencing, could be performed.

A ketogenic diet is the therapeutic gold standard because it provides an alternative source of energy for cerebral structures [20]. It includes a high proportion of fats and a restriction of carbohydrates, and it mimics the metabolic state of fasting with increased production of ketones [19]. Ketones are considered strong stabilizers of neuronal membranes with a subsequent inhibitory effect on cellular excitability and epileptogenesis. A ketogenic diet in patients with GLUT1 deficiency induces optimal seizure control and a reduction of movement disorders [20].

## Disorders of the Intermediate Metabolism

### *General Aspects*

This group includes a wide number of diseases involving genes encoding for enzymes belonging to different metabolic pathways. Epileptogenic mechanisms in these diseases include: a) reduced availability of substrates (disorders of serine metabolism, disorders of molybdenum cofactor biosynthesis and biotinidase deficiency), b) reduced availability of enzyme cofactors involved in the synthesis of neurotransmitter (*e.g.* vitamin B6-dependant epilepsies due to mutations in *ALDH7A1, PNPO, ALDH4A1 or PLPBP*), c) neurotoxic effects of intermediate compounds (*e.g.* urea cycle disorders or organic acidurias and some aminoacidopathies such as maple syrup urine disease), d) abnormal storage of metabolites (lysosomal storage disorders such as Niemann Pick type C disease), e) altered production of energy substrates (*e.g.* mitochondrial disorders, such as pyruvate dehydrogenase deficiency or defects of creatine metabolism), f) disturbances in neuronal membrane permeability (*e.g.* holocarboxylase synthetase deficiency) and g) dysregulation of intracellular/extracellular ions (organic acidurias).

An important quote about these diseases includes treatable conditions with effective available therapies that allow good seizure control: a) vitamin B6-dependent epilepsies, b) cerebral folate deficiency, c) congenital disorders of serine metabolism, d) biotinidase deficiency, e) inborn errors of creatine metabolism and f) molybdenum cofactor deficiency [19].

### *Illustrative Disease: ALDH7A1 Deficiency*

Pyridoxine-dependent epilepsy due to *ALDH7A1* mutations represented the first historical example of a treatable vitamin-dependent epilepsy. *ALDH7A1* encodes an enzyme involved in lysine catabolism (alpha-aminoadipic semialdehyde dehydrogenase deficiency or antiquitin) [20]. The deficient or absent activity of this enzyme results in the accumulation of two precursors: α-aminoadipic semialdehyde (α-AASA) and Δ1-1-piperideine-6-carboxylate (P6C). P6C induces a Knoevenagel condensation product with the activated form of pyridoxine (pyridoxal-5′-phosphate or PLP). PLP is an essential cofactor for different enzymes involved in more than 140 neuronal intracellular processes. The above-mentioned chemical reaction removes PLP from several cellular processes with the subsequent activation of different epileptogenic mechanisms [19].

The classical clinical presentation of *ALDH7A1* deficiency is represented by a neonatal or early infantile onset epileptic and developmental encephalopathy [20]. Other clinical manifestations include neurological (abnormal fetal movements, signs of hypoxic-ischemic encephalopathy, dystonia, increased startle response, irritability, and intellectual disability) and non-neurological (respiratory distress, abdominal distension, hepatomegaly, bilious vomiting, shock, hypothermia and metabolic acidosis) signs and symptoms [19]. EEG patterns vary from suppression bursts or hypsarrhythmia to focal or multifocal epileptic discharges. Brain MRI may evidence hemispheric hypoplasia or atrophy, cerebellar or cortical dysplasia, intracerebral hemorrhage or periventricular hyperintensities [20]. A therapeutic trial with an intravenous (100 mg) or an oral/enteral (30 mg/kg/day) administration of pyridoxine can be an important step also for the diagnosis. Acute intravenous administration of 100 mg of pyridoxine should be followed by a long-term oral/enteral administration at the dosage of 15–30 mg/kg/day in responding patients. Lysine-restricted diet or L-arginine supplementation could represent possible therapeutic alternatives [21].

## Disorders of Neuronal Cellular Cycle and Signaling

### *General Aspects*

This group of diseases is caused by mutations in genes encoding for proteins that are implicated in different phases of anchoring the synaptic machinery, neuronal cellular cycle, subcellular signaling pathways and, subsequently, in the regulation of neuronal excitability [3]. The correlated phenotypes include catastrophic early infantile onset epileptic encephalopathies associated with severe developmental delay and/or movement disorders (*e.g. ARX, CDKL5, PLCβ1, MAGI1, DOCK7, GNAO1, ARHGEF 9, ST3GalIII and WWOX encephalopathies*) but also less severe clinical presentations (*e.g.* disorders of GATOR1 complex) [3].

### *Illustrative Diseases: Disorders of mTOR and GATOR1 Pathways*

The first studied subcellular cascade involved in focal epilepsies was represented by the mammalian target of the rapamycin (mTOR) neuronal transduction signal pathway. The mTOR pathway has a pivotal role in synaptic protein synthesis and in the integrations of inputs resulting from NMDA and metabotropic glutamate receptors. The mTOR pathway is also a regulator of the synaptic excitation / inhibition balance. Abnormal recruitment of the mTOR cascade occurs in the tuberous sclerosis complex, which is a genetic multiple-organ system disease, characterized by localized cellular overgrowth leading to benign tumor-like lesions. Tuberous sclerosis is a developmental disorder resulting from the loss of function of either hamartin or tuberin because of pathogenic mutations in *TSC1* and *TSC2* genes. TSC1 and TSC2 act as negative modulators of mTORC1 (one of the two complexes forming the mTOR pathway). Variants of these genes produce a hyperactivation of the mTOR pathway, resulting in a downstream kinase signaling cascade that can consequently lead to alterations in cellular excitation/inhibition balance, therefore, to abnormalities in several cell processes, including cell cycle progression, transcription, translation and metabolic control. These events are involved in the pathogenesis of the clinical hallmarks of tuberous sclerosis, including epileptic seizures, formation of dysplastic areas ("tubers"), cutaneous manifestations and benign tumors involving organs such as the kidney or heart [22].

Germline mutations have been found in genes encoding for the proteins involved in the GATOR1 complex (*DEPDC5, NPRL2, NPRL3*), another repressor system of mTORC1. These mutations are implicated in a wide spectrum of focal epilepsy syndromes with and without cortical structural abnormalities. Patients carrying mutations in *DEPDC5, NPRL2,* and *NPRL3* have a similar epilepsy phenotype. They usually present with focal epilepsy without predilection for a specific cortical area, even if sleep-related hypermotor epilepsy with a frontal focus is extremely frequent. The age of seizure onset is variable. Ictal EEG may evidence focal (frontal, temporal, more rarely parietal or occipital) epileptiform abnormalities. Brain MRI can be normal or may show focal cortical dysplasia, hemimegaloencephaly, or polymicrogyria. Developmental milestones are usually normal even if intellectual disability or other neuropsychiatric manifestations can be observed. Drug resistance rates may be higher than in other focal epilepsies [23].

**Disorders of Synaptic Vesicles Trafficking and Release**

*General Aspects*

The neurotransmitter release machinery includes various modulators of the synaptic vesicle formation, fusion and recycling. The more studied proteins belonging to this group include: a) SV2A and Synapsins (involved in synaptic vesicle formation), b) t-SNARE proteins (Syntaxin 1B and SNAP25), c), SNARE-associated protein or STXBP1/MUNC18-1, and voltage-dependent P/Q-type calcium channel subunit a-1A or CACNA1A (involved in synaptic vesicle fusion), and d) Dynamin 1 (involved in synaptic vesicle recycling) [3]. Epilepsy is a remarkable phenotypic feature in patients with pathogenic variants of all these proteins.

## *Illustrative Disease: STXBP1 Encephalopathy*

Syntaxin binding protein 1 modulates the release of synaptic vesicles and vesicular docking *via* interactions with syntaxin A (Stx1a) and with the soluble N-ethylmaleimide-sensitive factor attachment protein receptor complex [3].

The phenotypic spectrum of *STXBP1* encephalopathy has expanded from a severe neonatal/ early infantile epileptic and developmental encephalopathy to a less severe Dravet-like pattern. Epileptic spasms or tonic seizures are part of the clinical presentations in most patients. Additional neurologic symptoms include intellectual disability, autistic traits, and movement disorders.

EEG features include focal or multifocal spikes and wave discharges, while burst suppression or hypsarrhythmia are reported in about 30% of patients. MRI detects no abnormalities in 50% of patients, even if cortical atrophy, delayed myelination, and thin corpus callosum are frequently reported [24].

## Disorders Involving Neuronal Structural Proteins

### *General Aspects*

These disorders are caused by mutations of genes encoding for proteins involved in neuronal structural integrity and in trans-synaptic adhesion.

The prototype of structural proteins, that are essential for neuronal integrity, and are involved in early-onset epilepsies, is represented by Non-erythrocytic alpha-spectrin-1 (*SPTAN 1*). *SPTAN 1* gene maps to 9q33-q34 and encodes a filamentous cytoskeletal protein that regulates the stability of the axonal structure. Clinical presentation of patients with mutations in this gene mainly includes intractable seizures with hypsarrhythmia, mental retardation, spastic quadriplegia, and progressive microcephaly [3].

Adhesion molecules are essential for trans-synaptic communication and, subsequently, for synapse development and synaptic transmission and plasticity. Recent studies have identified various synaptic adhesion molecules (presynaptic Neurexins and postsynaptic Neuroligins, IL1RAPL1, TrkC, Slitrks, NGLs, LRRTMs, Dystroglycan, and SALMs). Knowledge about the linkage between these proteins and epilepsy remains limited, probably due to their functional redundancies. Examples of human epilepsy mutations include compound heterozygous deletion of *NRXN1*, a microdeletion encompassing *IL1RAPL1,* and mutations of *CNTNAP2* (Caspr2) [25].

### *Illustrative Disease: PCDH19-Related Epilepsy*

Protocadherin 19 (*PCDH19*) gene maps to Xq22 and encodes a transmembrane protein that controls calcium-dependent cell-cell adhesion. *PCDH19* may be involved in specific synaptic networks and its impairment results in abnormal neuronal excitability.

The role of *PCDH* in epilepsy was described for the first time in the so-called "epilepsy and mental retardation limited to females" or EFMR (OMIM 300088) and then, in patients with SCN1A-negative Dravet syndrome [3].

EFMR phenotype includes a seizure onset between 6 and 36 months, a combination of febrile and afebrile seizures, and variable degrees of psychomotor and cognitive dysfunctions [3, 26]. The typical prominent expression in females of EFMR, notwithstanding the *PCDH19* gene is on the X chromosome, has been explained through two possible mechanisms: the existence of compensatory factors in males with mutated *PCDH19* (such as Protocadherin 19Y gene) and the presence of tissue mosaicism including *PCDH19*-positive and *PCDH19*-negative cells with subsequent impaired interactions between the two cellular populations [3].

## Disorders of Synaptic Secreted Proteins

### *General Aspects*

This group of disorders results from the deficient synthesis of proteins acting as extracellular synaptic organizers. The most important proteins with this role include C1q family proteins and *SRPX2*. C1q complement regulates synapse elimination during development, and in mice models' loss of C1q causes failure in the pruning of excessive excitatory synapses in the retinogeniculate and neocortical neurons, leading to atypical absences. *SRPX2* pathogenic mutations were reported in patients with temporal seizures and speech impairment [25].

### *Illustrative Disease: LGI1-Related Epilepsy*

*LGI1* mutations cause autosomal dominant lateral temporal lobe epilepsy. The encoded protein LGI1 binds to ADAM22 transmembrane protein that is anchored by a postsynaptic PSD-95 scaffold. Loss of LGI1 or ADAM22 reduces AMPA-receptor mediated synaptic transmission and causes life-threatening epilepsy in mice models. In the absence of LGI1, PSD-95 is unable to modulate AMPA receptor-mediated synaptic transmission with an increase in neuronal excitability. In addition, LGI1 autoantibodies observed in patients with limbic encephalitis, which is characterized by seizures and amnesia, inhibit the LGI1-ADAM22 interaction, reducing the number of synaptic AMPA receptors [25].

## Chromosomopathies and Pathogenic Copy Number Variants

### General Aspects

In the past decade, the introduction of array-Comparative Genomic Hybridization (array-CGH) technology expanded the number of chromosomal imbalances associated with epilepsy that was characterized in the karyotype era (1p36 deletion, 4p16.3 deletion/Wolf–Hirschhorn syndrome, 15q11-q13 deletion/Angelman syndrome, 17p13.3 deletion/Miller–Dieker syndrome and ring chromosome 20) [27].

Clinically relevant CNVs involve about 5–10% of the examined populations in pediatric neurology tertiary centers, and up to 30% when seizures are co-morbid with other neurodevelopmental disorders [1, 2]. An increased risk of pathogenic CNV was observed in patients with concurrent intellectual disability, dysmorphic features, autism spectrum disorder, drug resistance or other comorbidities [28]. Deletions up to 2MB are the most common chromosomal mutations that are reported in clinical practice [5]. The most involved chromosomal regions are 15q11.2, 15q13.3, and 16p13.15 [28].

### Illustrative Disease: 15q13.2–13.3 Microdeletion Syndrome

The 15q13.2–13.3 microdeletion was one of the most studied CNVs in the last decade. The main suggested correlated epileptogenic mechanism involves haploinsufficiency of *CHRNA7* (a gene encoding for the α7-subunit of the acetylcholine receptor and included in the deleted region).

The clinical presentation may include generalized epilepsy (mainly absences and myoclonic seizures) associated with intellectual disability, severe neurodevelopmental impairment, or autism spectrum disorder. Epilepsy usually persists during adulthood, and its pharmacological control is usually difficult. Facial dysmorphisms are not always present, and the most frequent are represented by hypertelorism, up-slanting palpebral fissures, prominent philtrum with full everted lips and clinodactyly [29]. Behavioral disturbances are common, and include poor attention span, hyperactivity, mood disorder and aggressive and/or impulsive behavior [29].

## CONCLUSION

*De novo* monogenic variants and, in a minority of the cases, large deletion/duplication of genes involved in epileptogenesis represent frequent etiologies for pediatric-onset epilepsies. The diagnostic yield of available genetic techniques is generally higher in developmental encephalopathy with epilepsy and in subjects with an onset of seizures under the age of 2. The early use of next-generation sequencing tools for the study of patients with epilepsy results in economic advantages and cuts the prolonged diagnostic pathways of the past decades. Careful clinical phenotyping improves the detection rate of pathogenic variants and eases pharmacological planning. The achievement of these aims requires close collaboration between epileptologists and geneticists to ensure the proper management of genetic investigations. This collaboration is crucial for both pediatric and adult patients toward the aim of a personalized (precision) medicine

## LIST OF ABBREVIATIONS

**CGH**     Comparative Genome Hybridization;

**NGS**     Next Generation Sequencing;

**CNV**     Copy Number Variants;

**SCN2A**     Sodium Channel, Neuronal Type II Alpha Subunit;

**KCNQ2**     Potassium Channel, Voltage-gated, kqt-like Subfamily, Member 2;

**SCN1A**     Sodium Channel, Neuronal Type I, Alpha Subunit;

**PCDH 19**     Protocadherin 19;

**STXBP1**     Syntaxin Binding Protein 1 ;

**GABRA1**     Gamma-aminobutyric Acid Receptor, Alpha-1;

**ALDH7A1**     Aldehyde Dehydrogenase 7 Family, Member A1;

**PNPO**     Pyridoxamine Phosphate Oxydase;

**FOLR1**     Folate Receptor 1;

**ALDH4A1**     Aldehyde Dehydrogenase 4 Family, Member A1;

**PLPBP**     Pyridoxal Phosphate Binding Protein;

**CHRNA4**     Cholinergic Receptor, Neuronal Nicotinic, Alpha Polypeptide 4;

**GATOR1**     GAP Activity Toward Rags 1;

**mTOR**     Mammalian Target of Rapamycin;

**GLUT1**     Glucose Transporter 1;

**WES**     Whole Exome Sequencing;

**WGS**     Whole Genome Sequencing;

**HGMD**     Human Gene Mutation Database;

| | |
|---|---|
| **SCN8A** | Sodium Channel, Neuronal Type 8 Alpha Subunit; |
| **SCN9A** | Sodium Channel, Neuronal Type 9 Alpha Subunit; |
| **SCN1B** | Sodium Channel, Neuronal type I, Beta Subunit; |
| **GABRG2** | Gamma-aminobutyric Acid Receptor, Gamma-2; |
| **HCN1** | Hyperpolarization-Activated Cyclic Nucleotide-gated Potassium Channel 1; |
| **CHD2** | Chromodomain Helicase Dna-Binding Protein 2; n |
| **KCNA2** | Potassium Channel, Voltage-gated, Shaker-Related Subfamily, Member 2; |
| **SLC39A8** | Solute Carrier Family 39, Member 8; |
| **SLC25A22** | Solute Carrier Family 25 Member 22; SLC2A1= Solute Carrier Family 2 Member 1; PLP=Pyridoxal 5 Phosphate; $\alpha$-AASA=$\alpha$-aminoadipic Semialdehyde; |
| **P6C** | $\Delta$1-1-Piperideine-6-Carboxylate; |
| **NMDA** | N-methyl-D-aspartate; |
| **TSC1** | Tuberous Sclerosis Complex 1; |
| **TSC2** | Tuberous Sclerosis Complex 2; |
| **ARX** | Aristaless Homeobox Gene; |
| **CDKL5** | Cyclin-dependent Kinase-like 5; |
| **PLCβ1** | Phospholipase C β1; |
| **MAGI1** | Membrane-associated Guanylate Kinase, ww and pdz Domains-containing, 1; DOCK7=dedicator of Cytokinesis 1; |
| **GNAO1** | Guanine Nucleotide-Binding Protein, Alpha-activating Activity Polypeptide o; |
| **ARHGEF 9** | rho Guanine Nucleotide Exchange Factor 9; |
| **ST3GalIII** | st3 Beta-Galactoside Alpha-2,3-Sialyltransferase 3; |
| **WWOX** | ww Domain-Containing Oxidoreductase; |
| **DEPDC5** | dep Domain-Containing Protein 5; |
| **NPRL2** | npr2-Like Protein, Gator1 Complex Subunit; |
| **NPRL3** | npr3-Like Protein, Gator1 Complex Subunit; |
| **mTORC1** | Mammalian Target of Rapamycin Complex 1; |
| **SV2A** | Synaptic Vesicle Glycoprotein 2A; |
| **SNARE** | SNAP(Soluble NSF Attachment Protein) Receptor; |
| **SNAP25b** | Synaptosomal-Associated Protein, 25kDa, Protein b; |
| **CACNA1A** | Voltage-Dependent P/Q-type Calcium Channel Subunit a-1A; |
| **SPTAN 1** | Nonerythrocytic Alpha-Spectrin-1; |
| **IL1RAPL1** | X-Linked Interleukin-1 Receptor Accessory Protein-Like 1; |
| **TrkC** | Tropomyosin Receptor Kinase C; |
| **Slitrks** | SLIT and NTRK-like Family Proteins; NGLs= netrin-G Ligand Proteins; LRRTMs=leucine-rich Repeat Transmembrane Neuronal Proteins; |

| | |
|---|---|
| **SALMs** | Synaptic Adhesion-like Molecules; |
| **NRXN1** | Neurexin 1; |
| **CNTNAP2** | Contactin Associated Protein Like 2; LGI1= Leucine Rich Glioma Inactivated 1; ADAM22= Disintegrin and Metalloproteinase Domain-containing Protein 22; |
| **PSD-95** | Postsynaptic Density 95; |
| **AMPA** | α-amino-3-hydroxy-5-methyl-4-isoxazolepropionic Acid; |
| **CHRNA7** | Cholinergic Receptor, Neuronal Nicotinic, Alpha Polypeptide 7. |

## CONSENT FOR PUBLICATION

Not applicable.

## CONFLICT OF INTEREST

The authors declare no conflict of interest, financial or otherwise.

## ACKNOWLEDGEMENT

Declared none.

## REFERENCES


[1] Shorvon S, Guerrini R, Schachter S, Trinka E, Eds. The Causes of Epilepsy: Common and Uncommon Causes in Adults and Children. Cambridge: Cambridge University Press 2019.
[http://dx.doi.org/10.1017/9781108355209]

[2] Guerrini R, Balestrini S, Wirrell EC, Walker MC. Monogenic Epilepsies. Neurology 2021; 97(17): 817-31.
[http://dx.doi.org/10.1212/WNL.0000000000012744] [PMID: 34493617]

[3] Mastrangelo M, Leuzzi V. Genes of early-onset epileptic encephalopathies: from genotype to phenotype. Pediatr Neurol 2012; 46(1): 24-31.
[http://dx.doi.org/10.1016/j.pediatrneurol.2011.11.003] [PMID: 22196487]

[4] OMIM - Online Mendelian Inheritance in Man.

[5] Mastrangelo M. Novel genes of early epileptic encephalopathies. Pediatr Neurol 2015; 53: 119-29.
[http://dx.doi.org/10.1016/j.pediatrneurol.2015.04.001] [PMID: 26073591]

[6] Mastrangelo M, Celato A, Leuzzi V. A diagnostic algorithm for the evaluation of early onset genetic-metabolic epileptic encephalopathies. Eur J Paediatr Neurol 2012; 16(2): 179-91.
[http://dx.doi.org/10.1016/j.ejpn.2011.07.015] [PMID: 21940184]

[7] Foo JN, Liu J, Tan EK. Next-generation sequencing diagnostics for neurological diseases/disorders: from a clinical perspective. Hum Genet 2013; 132(7): 721-34.
[http://dx.doi.org/10.1007/s00439-013-1287-2] [PMID: 23525706]

[8] Parrini E, Marini C, Mei D, *et al.* Diagnostic Targeted Resequencing in 349 Patients with Drug-Resistant Pediatric Epilepsies Identifies Causative Mutations in 30 Different Genes. Hum Mutat 2017; 38(2): 216-25.
[http://dx.doi.org/10.1002/humu.23149] [PMID: 27864847]

[9] Gokben S, Onay H, Yilmaz S, *et al.* Targeted next generation sequencing: the diagnostic value in early-onset epileptic encephalopathy. Acta Neurol Belg 2017; 117(1): 131-8.

[http://dx.doi.org/10.1007/s13760-016-0709-z] [PMID: 27734276]

[10]   Ortega-Moreno L, Giráldez BG, Soto-Insuga V, *et al.* Molecular diagnosis of patients with epilepsy and developmental delay using a customized panel of epilepsy genes. PLoS One 2017; 12(11): e0188978.
[http://dx.doi.org/10.1371/journal.pone.0188978] [PMID: 29190809]

[11]   Bevilacqua J, Hesse A, Cormier B, *et al.* Clinical utility of a 377 gene custom next-generation sequencing epilepsy panel. J Genet 2017; 96(4): 681-5.
[http://dx.doi.org/10.1007/s12041-017-0791-x] [PMID: 28947717]

[12]   Rim JH, Kim SH, Hwang IS, *et al.* Efficient strategy for the molecular diagnosis of intractable early-onset epilepsy using targeted gene sequencing. BMC Med Genomics 2018; 11(1): 6.
[http://dx.doi.org/10.1186/s12920-018-0320-7] [PMID: 29390993]

[13]   Ko A, Youn SE, Kim SH, *et al.* Targeted gene panel and genotype-phenotype correlation in children with developmental and epileptic encephalopathy. Epilepsy Res 2018; 141: 48-55.
[http://dx.doi.org/10.1016/j.eplepsyres.2018.02.003] [PMID: 29455050]

[14]   Peng J, Pang N, Wang Y, *et al.* Next☐generation sequencing improves treatment efficacy and reduces hospitalization in children with drug☐resistant epilepsy. CNS Neurosci Ther 2019; 25(1): 14-20.
[http://dx.doi.org/10.1111/cns.12869] [PMID: 29933521]

[15]   Liu J, Tong L, Song S, *et al.* Novel and de novo mutations in pediatric refractory epilepsy. Mol Brain 2018; 11(1): 48.
[http://dx.doi.org/10.1186/s13041-018-0392-5] [PMID: 30185235]

[16]   Hamdan FF, Myers CT, Cossette P, *et al.* High Rate of Recurrent De Novo Mutations in Developmental and Epileptic Encephalopathies. Am J Hum Genet 2017; 101(5): 664-85.
[http://dx.doi.org/10.1016/j.ajhg.2017.09.008] [PMID: 29100083]

[17]   Wei F, Yan LM, Su T, *et al.* Ion Channel Genes and Epilepsy: Functional Alteration, Pathogenic Potential, and Mechanism of Epilepsy. Neurosci Bull 2017; 33(4): 455-77.
[http://dx.doi.org/10.1007/s12264-017-0134-1] [PMID: 28488083]

[18]   Wheless JW, Fulton SP, Mudigoudar BD. Dravet Syndrome: A Review of Current Management. Pediatr Neurol 2020; 107: 28-40.
[http://dx.doi.org/10.1016/j.pediatrneurol.2020.01.005] [PMID: 32165031]

[19]   Mastrangelo M. Actual Insights into Treatable Inborn Errors of Metabolism Causing Epilepsy. J Pediatr Neurosci 2018; 13(1): 13-23.
[PMID: 29899766]

[20]   Koch H, Weber YG. The glucose transporter type 1 (Glut1) syndromes. Epilepsy Behav 2019; 91: 90-3.
[http://dx.doi.org/10.1016/j.yebeh.2018.06.010] [PMID: 30076047]

[21]   Mastrangelo M, Cesario S. Update on the treatment of vitamin B6 dependent epilepsies. Expert Rev Neurother 2019; 19(11): 1135-47.
[http://dx.doi.org/10.1080/14737175.2019.1648212] [PMID: 31340680]

[22]   Baulac S. mTOR signaling pathway genes in focal epilepsies. Prog Brain Res 2016; 226: 61-79.
[http://dx.doi.org/10.1016/bs.pbr.2016.04.013] [PMID: 27323939]

[23]   Baldassari S, Licchetta L, Tinuper P, Bisulli F, Pippucci T. GATOR1 complex: the common genetic actor in focal epilepsies. J Med Genet 2016; 53(8): 503-10.
[http://dx.doi.org/10.1136/jmedgenet-2016-103883] [PMID: 27208208]

[24]   Stamberger H, Nikanorova M, Willemsen MH, *et al.* *STXBP1* encephalopathy. Neurology 2016; 86(10): 954-62.
[http://dx.doi.org/10.1212/WNL.0000000000002457] [PMID: 26865513]

[25]   Fukata Y, Fukata M. Epilepsy and synaptic proteins. Curr Opin Neurobiol 2017; 45: 1-8.

[http://dx.doi.org/10.1016/j.conb.2017.02.001] [PMID: 28219682]

[26]    Smith L, Singhal N, El Achkar CM, *et al. PCDH19* -related epilepsy is associated with a broad neurodevelopmental spectrum. Epilepsia 2018; 59(3): 679-89.
[http://dx.doi.org/10.1111/epi.14003] [PMID: 29377098]

[27]    Battaglia A, Guerrini R. Chromosomal disorders associated with epilepsy. Epileptic Disord 2005; 7(3): 181-92.
[PMID: 16162426]

[28]    Helbig I, Swinkels MEM, Aten E, *et al.* Structural genomic variation in childhood epilepsies with complex phenotypes. Eur J Hum Genet 2014; 22(7): 896-901.
[http://dx.doi.org/10.1038/ejhg.2013.262] [PMID: 24281369]

[29]    van Bon BWM, Mefford HC, Menten B, *et al.* Further delineation of the 15q13 microdeletion and duplication syndromes: a clinical spectrum varying from non-pathogenic to a severe outcome. J Med Genet 2009; 46(8): 511-23.
[http://dx.doi.org/10.1136/jmg.2008.063412] [PMID: 19372089]

CHAPTER 6

# Medical and Social Outcomes in the Management of Cardiac Diseases in Children

**Josephat M. Chinawa**[1,*] and **Fortune A. Ujunwa**[1]

[1] *College of Medicine, Department of Pediatrics, University of Nigeria Teaching Hospital (UNTH), Ituku-Ozalla, Enugu State, Nigeria*

**Abstract:** Children with cardiovascular diseases, especially congenital heart diseases are exposed to socioeconomic burdens ranging from poverty, economic difficulties, and emotional breakdown to parental schism.

There are various ways by which cardiac diseases affect children. These include the effect of the disease on the child, the family and the nation as a whole. Management of cardiovascular diseases in children comprises diagnosis, investigations, medical and surgical rehabilitation/ergonomics and follow-up. All these steps in management have both medical and social implications on the child.

The effects of cardiovascular diseases are not limited to health, but can seep into social life, as well. Affected individuals tend to forgo a lot of things, including restrictions in their life, depression and even family structure disintegration, decrease life expectancy and family disharmony in some cultures.

The socio-economic burden of pediatric cardiovascular diseases is quite huge both for the individual, household and society. The impact includes loss in financial resources, productivity, increased disability-adjusted life years, decreased quality of life, catastrophic expenditure and premature death. These burdens are more in the low and middle-income countries. This chapter aims at eliciting the various social and economic burdens that children with heart diseases encounter in the course of their illness.

**Keywords:** Cardiovascular, Catastrophic, Children, Congenital, Death, Disease, ergonomics, Family, Financial, Follow-up, Heart, Investigations, Management, Medical, Parental, Poverty, Rehabilitation, Schism, Socio-economic, Surgical.

---

* **Corresponding Author Josephat M. Chinawa:** College of Medicine, Department of Pediatrics, University of Nigeria Teaching Hospital (UNTH), Ituku-Ozalla, Enugu State, Nigeria; Tel: +2348063981403; E-mail: josephat.chinawa@unn.edu.ng

**Nima Rezaei and Noosha Samieefar (Eds.)**
**All rights reserved-© 2023 Bentham Science Publishers**

# INTRODUCTION

Cardio-Vascular Diseases (CVDs) are the leading cause of mortality worldwide [1, 2]. Mortalities by CVDs could be acquired or congenital in origin. The acquired type occurs mainly due to Coronary Heart Disease (CHD), stroke, Rheumatic Heart Disease (RHD) and Myocardial Infarction (MI), while the congenital variety stems from cyanotic and acyanotic congenital heart defects. Cardiovascular disease (CVD) accounts for nearly half of noncommunicable diseases (NCDs) and is the leading global cause of death, accounting for 17.3 million deaths per year; this will double by 2030. In children, the bane of cardiac diseases is structural heart diseases, which are mostly congenital [3].

## EPIDEMIOLOGY OF CARDIAC DISEASES IN CHILDREN

In Nigeria, a multi-center study on the variable prevalence of congenital heart disease exists. For instance, Sadoh *et al*, in their study in southeast Nigeria, among 605 children, noted Ventricular Septal Defect (VSD; 46.6%) as the commonest congenital heart defect. Other heart defects in order of frequency were Patent Ductus Arteriosus (PDA;12.1%), Atrial Septal Defect (ASD;8.7%), and Atrio-Ventricular Septal Defect (AVSD;8.2%). Tetralogy of Fallot (TOF;7.8%) was the commonest cyanotic congenital heart defect seen in their study [4].

In the study of Miyague *et al.* [5] in Brazil, among 4,538 children in a pediatric hospital over a three-year period, 44.4% of the children were diagnosed with congenital heart diseases, with 4.4% being acquired, and 1.2% presented with arrhythmias. Congenital heart diseases were noted in 71.5% of the cases. In their series, VSD was seen as the most frequent acyanotic anomaly, and TOF was the most frequent cyanotic anomaly.

In China, Liu *et al.* [6] in their study among 1,817 children with CHD noted the overall prevalence of 16.4 per 1,000 live births with boys being higher with the prevalence of 24.1 per 1,000 live births and females with 20.0 per 1,000 live births. Males presented with a higher prevalence of ASD with a prevalence of 10.6 per 1,000 live births. They noted that a variety of maternal antenatal correlates such as pregnancy infections, older age, pregnancy-induced hypertension, family history of CHD, gestational diabetes and lower education level are implicated as a causal effect of congenital heart disease [6].

Chinawa *et al.* [7], in Enugu, Nigeria, in their work among 31,795 children that attended children outpatient clinics of the hospital over 5 years, noted an overall prevalence of children with cardiac disease as 0.22%. The commonest congenital heart disease seen in their study was VSD, followed by TOF. They also noted some extra-cardiac anomalies that were associated with these defects, such as

Downs's syndrome and VACTERL (Vertebral defects, Anal atresia, Cardiac defects, Tracheoesophageal fistula, Renal anomalies and Limb abnormalities).

In a meta-analysis of the world prevalence of congenital heart diseases, Denise *et al.* [8] noted that CHD accounts for almost a third of all major congenital anomalies. They opined a varying birth prevalence of CHD worldwide. In the systematic review of 114 papers involving 24,091,867 live births with CHD, they identified 164,396 children with congenital heart defect. They noted an increase in prevalence from 0.6 per 1,000 live births from 1930 to 1934 to 9.1 per 1,000 live births after 1995. They found very significant geographical differences in their study. For instance, in Asia, they found the highest CHD birth prevalence, at 9.3 per 1,000 live births, and pulmonary outflow obstructions as a predominant cardiac lesion. Their report from Europe was significantly higher than in North America with 8.2 per 1,000 live births and 6.9 per 1,000 live births, respectively [8 - 13].

Rheumatic heart disease is the commonest cause of acquired heart disease. Paar *et al.* [14], noted the high morbidity and mortality of children with heart disease which is disproportionate among children in developing countries when compared with their Western counterparts. In their study among 3,150 children aged 5 to 15 years and 489 adults aged 20 to 35 years from urban and rural areas, they noted an overall prevalence in children of 48 in 1,000 while the prevalence in urban children was 34 in 1,000, and in rural settings, this was 80 in 1,000. Poor socio-economic class, poverty, and very poor political will have been implicated as the causes of this rise in prevalence.

Saxena *et al.* [15], among children between the age of 5-15 years from randomly selected schools in four regions, noted that among 16,294 children, RHD was detected using echocardiography in 125 children giving a prevalence of 7.7/1000.

Finally, cardiomyopathy, another acquired cardiac disease in children afflicts about 100,000 children worldwide. One in every 100,000 children who are less than 18 years is affected in the United States. It is commoner in children less than one-year-old, with very high morbidity and mortality. It is documented that about 40% of children with cardiomyopathy undergo heart transplantation or die within 2 years [16].

Dilated Cardiomyopathy (DCM) is the commonest cardiomyopathy seen in children. It causes heart failure in both children. Other types of cardiomyopathy are Left Ventricular Non-Compaction cardiomyopathy (LVNC), Arrhythmogenic Right Ventricular Dysplasia (ARVD), Hypertrophic Cardiomyopathy (HCM) or Restrictive Cardiomyopathy (RCM), as well as a mixed phenotypic disease *e.g.* dilated-hypertrophic cardiomyopathy. Dilated Cardiomyopathy is usually progressive, and is a leading indication for cardiac transplantation in adults and children [17 - 21].

A study noted the annual incidence of dilated cardiomyopathy in children younger than 18 years of age as 0.57 cases per 100,000. It also found that annual incidence was higher in boys than girls. The majority of children had an idiopathic disease, with the most common causes being myocarditis and neuromuscular disease [22 - 27].

## MEDICAL AND SOCIAL OUTCOMES

The objectives of this section are to explain the various ways by which cardiac diseases affect the child, to understand the effect of the disease on the family, to explain the medical and social outcomes of cardiovascular diseases, and to explain various ways by which the outcomes will be improved.

## EFFECTS OF MANAGEMENT

Management of cardiovascular diseases in children comprises diagnosis, investigations, medical and surgical rehabilitation/ergonomics, and follow-up. All these steps in management have both medical and social implications [28].

The effects of cardiovascular diseases are not limited to health but can seep into social life, as well. Heart diseases are usually chronic illnesses, and the outcome affects patients holistically. Affected individuals tend to forgo a lot of things, including restrictions in their life *e.g.*, strenuous exercises and lifestyles. This limitation of physical, social, and unstable health leads to depression. The rate of depression in the USA is 10% but the rate among CVD patients is 27% [29].

Management of children with cardiac diseases affects the society and overall well-being of the child. It affects the family structure and decreases life expectancy and causes family disharmony in some cultures [29].

A cross-sectional study in Saudi Arabia on the impact on family-scale questionnaires showed a higher impact on family social scale among those that underwent complex procedures than families with minor heart diseases. They also noted that congenital heart diseases impacted negatively all the aspects of the Quality Of Life (QOL) of patients and their families, with associated high comorbidities.

Patients and their caregivers are psychologically affected by the scar of the surgery, stigma, and the fear of going back to the hospital [30].

## MENTAL HEALTH

Families and patients with cardiac diseases tend to become depressed and withdrawn following the diagnosis of heart disease [31]. The gamut of the investigations tends to create a lot of anxiety among these patients and caregivers [31]. The cost of investigations and treatment is usually catastrophic, especially in a set-up with no social security system. This tends to lead to delayed intervention with worsening outcomes [31]. Allabadi *et al.*, using a total of 1,053 patients with a cardiac disease noted that symptoms of anxiety and depression were seen more among females and less educated children. Symptoms of post-traumatic stress disorder, psycho-somatic symptoms, low physical and mental health component scores, active smoking, low level of self-esteem, physical inactivity and longer disease duration are seen as proponents of psycho-social disorder.

## THE SOCIAL OUTCOMES OF CARDIAC DISEASES MANAGEMENT

The treatment of cardiovascular diseases in children is usually prolonged. The social outcomes could be negative or positive, and this correlates with the severity of the disease or condition. In the course of treatment, children need their parents to cater to them; this leads to work and school absenteeism, loss of job, separation, sibling rivalry, child abuse and neglect, burnt-out syndrome, parental guilt and poverty due to catastrophic spending, especially among the poor and poorest of the poor [32]. Other social outcomes of the management of cardiac diseases in children include fear of re-hospitalization, especially in complex anomalies with initial palliative treatment and cardiac lesions with progressive sequel *e.g.*, aortic stenosis.

## THE POSITIVE SOCIAL OUTCOMES OF MANAGEMENT

Following adequate management of cardiac diseases; families tend to have relief from the trauma of the diagnosis [33]. There is a social re-integration into society with less rate of internalizing disorders such as withdrawal, depression, somatoform disorders and aggression. Improved concentration and focus on activities by the caregivers are now appreciated. There is also a notable improvement in self-esteem. Caregivers/parents tend to be more informed about the diseases and help in educating other parents [33].

## MORBIDITY AND MORTALITY

Over the years, advanced therapies and surgical techniques have improved the survival of children with cardiac diseases [34]. More children are surviving into adolescence and adulthood with an increased risk of complications of inherent cardiac diseases. Improved care and survival have made transitional care an integral part of cardiovascular medicine, not overemphasizing that most cardiovascular diseases track from childhood to adulthood [35]. Cardiac diseases in children are mostly structural heart defects with the end pathway being recurrent heart failure, respiratory infections, poor growth, failure to thrive, frequent hospitalization, poor quality of life and premature death [35]. These do occur, especially in developing countries where diagnosis and treatment are challenging. Cardiac diseases though can occur alone, but there is usually a significant association with comorbidities and syndromes, and these biological or genetic risk factors affect the medical outcomes of management. Some of these genetic risk factors include William syndrome, Downs syndrome, Turner, Noonan, Digeorge, CHARGE, PHACE, CATCH 22, *etc* [36].

There is an increased risk of intelligence, language development (expressive and receptive attention), psychosocial maladjustment, motor deficit and other neurological deficit. The severity also depends on the level of exposure to the risk factors. These children are at increased risk of neuro-developmental delays, motor dysfunction and central nervous system abnormalities [37].

Cognitive and social interactions, impaired behavior and core communication skills can occur as morbidities among children with cardiac diseases. During diagnosis of heart diseases, the outcome can be discouraging, especially in late diagnosis, where the disease may not be amenable to treatment or cure without a greater consequence or complication. For instance, multiple valvular diseases in RHD with very poor ejection fraction, severe pulmonary hypertension and Eisenmenger syndrome, dilated cardiomyopathy, severe arrhythmias, cerebral infarction, abscess and stroke in cyanotic heart lesions portend a guarded prognosis [38]. Other conditions do present with a bad prognosis at onset, especially in the duct-dependent lesions after the first few weeks of life. Examples of such lesions are complex congenital heart disease requiring complex surgery *e.g.*, hypoplastic left heart syndrome, transposition of the great artery with intact septum and cardiomyopathies.

## ECONOMIC BURDEN OF PEDIATRIC HEART DISEASES

Disease burden is the impact of health problems as measured by the financial cost, mortality, morbidity or other indicators [39]. While mortality and morbidity data are important in measuring the burden of diseases, there is a gap in determining how the diseases affect human welfare, household income, the society and the country's Gross Domestic Product (GDP). These are what the economic burden of the disease usually addresses. The economic burden of disease is the cost saved by preventing a certain disease in an individual [39]. This concept is not usually addressed in everyday practice but with increasing technology, innovations, and the rising cost of disease management in recent times where there are limited resources. The economic burden of diseases is a veritable tool in the hands of clinicians and policymakers to plan the management of diseases, such that individuals and households are not further impoverished, and the health system is not overburdened [39].

About 15 million children die or are incapacitated annually due to preventable or treated cardiac conditions in resource-poor countries, and these are not given adequate attention because of the ravaging effect of communicable diseases which are targeted because of the perceived low cost [40, 41]. However, the global disease burden of pediatric heart diseases shows that congenital diseases are major causes of childhood mortality and significant lifelong disability, which accounted for 6% of all infants' death and 96% of these deaths occurred in low and middle-income countries [40]. In addition, acquired heart diseases still have significant mortality and morbidity in low and middle-income countries. The global disease burden estimates that there is 15.6 million prevalence of rheumatic heart disease, with 282000 incident cases and 233000 deaths due to rheumatic fever and heart diseases annually, and the disability-adjusted life year burden was estimated to be 1430 (944-2067) cases in 2010 [40]. These data are projections from the high to low-income countries that may have a higher incidence of these diseases due to poverty, ignorance, lack of awareness, poor access to health care, dearth of highly specialized personnel and technology for diagnosis [42, 43].

## Economic Burden

The economic burden of a disease is important in that it estimates the maximal cost reduction if a disease is prevented in an individual. It involves the identification, assessment and valuing of resources that are related to an illness [39]. Pediatric heart diseases are divided into congenital and acquired heart diseases, and care for these diseases requires specialized skills and enormous financial resources. The prevalence of congenital heart diseases seems to be uniform globally with a slight increase in Asian countries ranging from 10 to 12 per 1000 live births which represents about 1.35 million live births in a year [40]. Half of these children with CHD tend to die within one year if no intervention is done, these interventions range from medical treatment to highly specialized surgical interventions [40, 44]. The cost of which is usually overwhelming for poor households in low-income and middle-income countries, where there is low coverage in health insurance, and most of the health financing is out of pocket payment without financial risk protection [44]. In a study in India, it was found that the average total cost of surgery for most congenital heart diseases is about $11,989 ($9696- $15804), and in Nigeria, it ranges from $62030 -$11200 [45, 46]. These countries have low Gross per Capita income when compared to high-income countries. The aim of the cost estimation of illness is to assess critically the cost of disease not in morbidity or mortality but in monetary terms, and estimate its burden to the household, society and the health system. Societal cost is the most encompassing in that it is independent of who bears the cost, and includes the opportunity cost of the disease [39, 47]. The cost of illness is not only the cost paid for treatment or medications, but it also includes indirect costs such as transportation, employment loss, work absenteeism, and opportunity cost which are the alternatives forgone or adjustment in employment or lifestyles, changes adapted due to illness and transportation [41, 48].

**Direct cost:** Refers to the cost of medical treatment, surgery, rehabilitation and medical assistance. It is measured by the micro-costing technique, whereby every resource is identified and the total cost is identified [48].

**Non-direct costs**: Refers to expenses that cover non-medical resources such as transportation and nutrition outside the home.

**Indirect cost**: This refers to the loss of productivity associated with the disease. It is usually measured using the human capital approach or friction cost approach. The loss of productivity is related to the friction period, which is the time required for the patient to be replaced by another employee and to achieve productivity to its former level [48]. The economic cost of cardiac diseases is usually higher in high-income countries compared to low and middle-income countries. This is because of high technology, the availability of specialized care and high-end treatment. However, the impact is usually cushioned because of early referral that mitigates against complications, availability of health insurance with good coverage, social welfare packages and higher gross per capita income as compared to low and middle-income countries [42].

In high-income countries, the illness cost of cardiovascular diseases constitutes a major part of the gross domestic product, and this costs about 169 billion Euro annually with health care accounting for 62%, productivity losses at 21% and informal care at 21% [43]. This cost includes not only the cost of care but also the informal care, opportunity cost of relatives that assist the patient, the loss of productivity due to inability to work, disability and premature death. Most of the costs are borne by the social welfare system or health care insurance but in Low and Middle-Income Countries (LMIC); the costs are usually borne by non-governmental organizations and out-of-pocket expenditures by individuals with a smaller fraction by health insurance [40, 49].

The cost of an acute episode of cardiac disease and the annual cost of care usually is more than the total health expenditure per capita in most LMICs, and these expenditures are usually out-of-pocket expenses. These costs constitute a financial barrier for health care leading to poor utilization of health care services and further treatment for the patients that are on chronic therapy [48]. This mode of health financing for pediatric cardiac services causes a delay in health-seeking behavior, leading to late presentation of heart diseases to health care facilities and financial impoverishment for the individuals, families and society.

It is known that late presentation leads to more costs in cardiac diseases. Complications of heart diseases such as pulmonary hypertension, heart failure, cardiomyopathies, stroke and infective endocarditis also increase the cost of health by increasing the cost of intensive care unit stay, prolonged hospital stay, complex procedures and loss of productivity [40, 43]. Studies in India and the European Union show that the cost of illness was found to be dependent on the anomaly, the procedures and the risk category [46].

## Factors that Contribute to the Increased Economic Burden of Cardiovascular Diseases in Children

Different factors have been noted to contribute to the increased economic burden of Pediatric heart diseases. Some of these factors include:

### *Late Referral and Diagnosis*

Most Pediatric heart diseases are preventable, and for those that are amenable to treatment, early diagnosis and referral to facilities that manage the condition help in mitigating complications such as heart failure and irreversible complications of pulmonary hypertension which tend to lead to prolonged medical management. This is usually due to a lack of echocardiography facilities, ignorance and a dearth of specialized health personnel.

### *Poor Health Financing*

Out of pocket payment is a major health financing mechanism in low and middle-income countries, this method has no financial protection for the household or individuals. In some countries, it contributes to about 70% of health financing methods [43, 47]. Cardiovascular care is capital intensive, and payment for such services is usually catastrophic for the individuals and households affected, such that it drives them further below the poverty line, such that they may not be able to access care, procure some chronic medication, afford surgery and other intervention services. Even when they can access the care they need to forgo or adapt to lifestyle changes.

## Lack of Health Insurance or Social Welfare System

Health insurance affords individual and household financial risk protection during illness. It tends to distribute the risk such that households are not impoverished due to ill health. Lack of health insurance worsens the economic burden due to cardiovascular diseases in children. It also puts a strain on the health system which may be saddled with the responsibility to provide care for the uninsured, especially in emergency cases, without adequate reimbursement.

## The Complexity of the Diseases Process and Intervention

Patients who have a more complex disease process are bound to have prolonged treatment, if it is a structural defect, the intervention tends to be more complex. The increased cost is also related to the preoperative state of the patient. Risk adjustment in congenital heart surgery (RACHS-1) score has been shown to be a predictor of higher surgical cost, prolonged intensive care unit stay and hospital stay in patients with congenital heart diseases, such that patients in RACHS-3 and 4 incur more total health care expenditure than RACHS-1 categories both at the household and health system levels [45, 49]. These high-risk categories also tend to require prolonged informal care leading to increased productivity loss for the caregivers [42, 45].

In addition, some chronic conditions such as chronic heart failure, valvar heart diseases and hypertension require prolonged care into adulthood such that individuals with such diseases tend to be on chronic medications as they age into adulthood, with continuous care, this tends to increase the economic burden of the disease.

## Health System Challenges

Most health systems in low and middle-income countries have a weak health system, where there is a dearth of well-trained specialists, poor facilities and low budgetary allocations to them [39, 41]. This has led to a referral to centers in high-income countries where specialists and resources can be assessed. This has led to an increasing loss of revenue in medical tourism in these countries with huge expenditure for both the household and the society [43].

In some low-income countries, other challenges increase the cost of illness, and some of these challenges include poor governance, weak policies, poor data collection and research, non-availability of adequate medications, corruption, insufficient care delivery system and poor social welfare services. These tend to affect the poorest of the poor more in these countries [43].

However, the health system also contributes to the increased economic burden of cardiac diseases both in the resource-poor and high-income countries in that some health systems tend to use costly new technologies, overuse specialty care, use more expensive new drugs high administrative costs, use high expensive end of life care for terminal pediatric cardiovascular diseases and practice of defensive medicine. These tend to impact negatively the healthcare cost of individuals and society [49].

## *Family Composition and Socioeconomic Status*

The family or relations are usually the ones that provide informal care to children that have heart diseases, these individuals tend to incur both direct, indirect and opportunity costs during illness [41, 43, 47]. The productivity loss is usually more when both parents are gainfully employed. In India, the productivity loss as calculated by man-hours lost following surgery for congenital heart diseases averages about 35 days during a child's hospitalization, and some have to quit jobs for some period or adapt a new job schedule with loss of revenue during child's illness [45]. The perceived economic stress is usually overwhelming and catastrophic among the lower quintiles of the socioeconomic strata of the society, especially in the low income and medium-income countries where about 35% of affected households spend more than 10% of family income on medications and other services [43]. Such that further demand for cardiovascular services and procurement of chronic medications, and may be hindered.

## *Medical Litigation/Malpractice Cost*

Medical litigation has been noted to increase the economic burden of cardiovascular diseases in that suppliers of health care goods tend to oversupply to avoid litigation, such that individuals that demand the health care goods are usually subjected to multiple investigations, prolonged hospital stays and high-cost procedures to avoid any form of litigation instead of using cost-saving methods during investigations, procedures and procurement of medical consumables. This tends to lead to high medical expenditure both for the household and the country. This practice is common in high-income countries where there is effective health insurance and social welfare system and a high level of medical litigation leading to defensive medicine [40]. In addition, the malpractice cost and indemnity insurance being paid by healthcare providers also contribute to the increased healthcare cost, thereby leading to an increased burden to the health system and patients that demand health.

## CONCLUSION

The economic burden of pediatric cardiovascular diseases is quite huge both for the individual, household and society. The impact includes loss in financial resources, productivity, increase disability-adjusted life years, decreased quality of life, catastrophic expenditure and premature death. These burdens are more in the low and middle-income countries where there is no adequate financial risk protection model of health financing, weak health system and high poverty index with the majority of the population living below $1 a day. However, the burden in high-income countries is usually contributed by expensive new technologies, drugs, the practice of defensive medicine and high administrative costs. Efforts should be made to use cost-effective approaches in disease management, strengthen the health system and provision of adequate insurance both for the health system and individuals to mitigate the modifiable factors that increase the economic burden of heart diseases in children.

## CONSENT FOR PUBLICATION

Not applicable.

## CONFLICT OF INTEREST

The authors declare no conflict of interest, financial or otherwise.

## ACKNOWLEDGMENTS

We acknowledge those that work in the records department for retrieving all necessary documents.

## REFERENCES

[1]     Mc Namara K, Alzubaidi H, Jackson JK. Cardiovascular disease as a leading cause of death: how are pharmacists getting involved? Integr Pharm Res Pract 2019; 8: 1-11.
[http://dx.doi.org/10.2147/IPRP.S133088] [PMID: 30788283]

[2]     Kollia N, Tragaki A, Syngelakis AI, Panagiotakos D. Trends of cardiovascular disease mortality in relation to population aging in Greece (1956-2015). Open Cardiovasc Med J 2018; 12(1): 71-9.
[http://dx.doi.org/10.2174/1874192401812010071] [PMID: 30159093]

[3]     Smith SC Jr, Collins A, Ferrari R, *et al.* Our time: a call to save preventable death from cardiovascular disease (heart disease and stroke). J Am Coll Cardiol 2012; 60(22): 2343-8.
[http://dx.doi.org/10.1016/j.jacc.2012.08.962] [PMID: 22995536]

[4]     Sadoh WE, Uzodimma CC, Daniels Q. Congenital heart disease in Nigerian children: a multicenter echocardiographic study. World J Pediatr Congenit Heart Surg 2013; 4(2): 172-6.
[http://dx.doi.org/10.1177/2150135112474026] [PMID: 23799730]

[5]     Miyague NI, Cardoso SM, Meyer F, *et al.* Epidemiological study of congenital heart defects in children and adolescents: analysis of 4,538 cases. Arq Bras Cardiol 2003; 80(3): 269-78.
[http://dx.doi.org/10.1590/S0066-782X2003000300003] [PMID: 12856270]

[6]     Liu X, Liu G, Wang P, *et al.* Prevalence of congenital heart disease and its related risk indicators among 90 796 Chinese infants aged less than 6 months in Tianjin. Int J Epidemiol 2015; 44(3): 884-93.
[http://dx.doi.org/10.1093/ije/dyv107] [PMID: 26071138]

[7]     Chinawa JM, Eze JC, Obi I, *et al.* Synopsis of congenital cardiac disease among children attending University of Nigeria Teaching Hospital Ituku Ozalla, Enugu. BMC Res Notes 2013; 6(1): 475.
[http://dx.doi.org/10.1186/1756-0500-6-475] [PMID: 24252233]

[8]     Denise V, Elisabeth EM, Konings MA. J Am Coll Cardiol 2011; 58: 2241-7.
[http://dx.doi.org/10.1016/j.jacc.2011.08.025] [PMID: 22078432]

[9]     Dolk H, Loane M, Garne E. Congenital heart defects in Europe: prevalence and perinatal mortality, 2000 to 2005. Circulation 2011; 123(8): 841-9.
[http://dx.doi.org/10.1161/CIRCULATIONAHA.110.958405] [PMID: 21321151]

[10]    Bernier PL, Stefanescu A, Samoukovic G, Tchervenkov CI. The challenge of congenital heart disease worldwide: epidemiologic and demographic facts. Semin Thorac Cardiovasc Surg Pediatr Card Surg Annu 2010; 13(1): 26-34.
[http://dx.doi.org/10.1053/j.pcsu.2010.02.005] [PMID: 20307858]

[11]    Mason CA, Kirby RS, Sever LE, Langlois PH. Prevalence is the preferred measure of frequency of birth defects. Births Defects Res A Clin Mol Teratol 2005; 73: 690-2.
[http://dx.doi.org/10.1002/bdra.20211]

[12]    Khairy P, Ionescu-Ittu R, Mackie AS, Abrahamowicz M, Pilote L, Marelli AJ. Changing mortality in congenital heart disease. J Am Coll Cardiol 2010; 56(14): 1149-57.
[http://dx.doi.org/10.1016/j.jacc.2010.03.085] [PMID: 20863956]

[13]    Somerville J. Grown-up congenital heart disease--medical demands look back, look forward 2000. Thorac Cardiovasc Surg 2001; 49(1): 21-6.
[http://dx.doi.org/10.1055/s-2001-9911] [PMID: 11243517]

[14]    Paar JA, Berrios NM, Rose JD, *et al.* Prevalence of rheumatic heart disease in children and young adults in Nicaragua. Am J Cardiol 2010; 105(12): 1809-14.
[http://dx.doi.org/10.1016/j.amjcard.2010.01.364] [PMID: 20538135]

[15]    Saxena A, Desai A, Narvencar K, *et al.* Echocardiographic prevalence of rheumatic heart disease in Indian school children using World Heart Federation criteria - A multi site extension of RHEUMATIC study (the e-RHEUMATIC study). Int J Cardiol 2017; 249: 438-2.
[http://dx.doi.org/10.1016/j.ijcard.2017.09.184] [PMID: 28966041]

[16]    Wilkinson JD, Sleeper LA, Alvarez JA, Bublik N, Lipshultz SE. The pediatric cardiomyopathy registry: 1995–2007. Prog Pediatr Cardiol 2008; 25(1): 31-6.
[http://dx.doi.org/10.1016/j.ppedcard.2007.11.006] [PMID: 19343086]

[17]    Lipshultz SE, Sleeper LA, Towbin JA, *et al.* The incidence of pediatric cardiomyopathy in two regions of the United States. N Engl J Med 2003; 348(17): 1647-55.
[http://dx.doi.org/10.1056/NEJMoa021715] [PMID: 12711739]

[18]    Bublik N, Alvarez JA, Lipshultz SE. Pediatric cardiomyopathy as a chronic disease: A perspective on comprehensive care programs. Prog Pediatr Cardiol 2008; 25(1): 103-11.
[http://dx.doi.org/10.1016/j.ppedcard.2007.11.011] [PMID: 19122765]

[19]    Towbin JA, Lowe AM, Colan SD, *et al.* Incidence, causes, and outcomes of dilated cardiomyopathy in children. JAMA 2006; 296(15): 1867-76.
[http://dx.doi.org/10.1001/jama.296.15.1867] [PMID: 17047217]

[20]    Hänselmann A, Veltmann C, Bauersachs J, Berliner D. Dilated cardiomyopathies and non-compaction cardiomyopathy. Herz 2020; 45(3): 212-20.
[http://dx.doi.org/10.1007/s00059-020-04903-5] [PMID: 32107565]

[21]    Fisher SD, Easley KA, Orav EJ, *et al.* Mild dilated cardiomyopathy and increased left ventricular mass predict mortality: The Prospective P2C2 HIV Multicenter Study. Am Heart J 2005; 150(3): 439-47.
[http://dx.doi.org/10.1016/j.ahj.2005.06.012] [PMID: 16169321]

[22]    Lipshultz SE. Dilated cardiomyopathy in HIV-infected patients. N Engl J Med 1998; 339(16): 1153-5.
[http://dx.doi.org/10.1056/NEJM199810153391609] [PMID: 9770563]

[23]    Alvarez JA, Wilkinson JD, Lipshultz SE. Outcome predictors for pediatric dilated cardiomyopathy: A systematic review. Prog Pediatr Cardiol 2007; 23(1-2): 25-32.
[http://dx.doi.org/10.1016/j.ppedcard.2007.05.009] [PMID: 19701490]

[24]    Andrews RE, Fenton MJ, Ridout DA, Burch M. New-onset heart failure due to heart muscle disease in childhood: a prospective study in the United kingdom and Ireland. Circulation 2008; 117(1): 79-84.
[http://dx.doi.org/10.1161/CIRCULATIONAHA.106.671735] [PMID: 18086928]

[25]    Go AS, Mozaffarian D, Roger VL, *et al.* Heart disease and stroke statistics--2013 update: a report from the American Heart Association. Circulation 2013; 127(1): 6-245.
[http://dx.doi.org/10.1161/CIR.0b013e31828124ad]

[26]    Mendis S, Puska P, Norrving B. Global Atlas on Cardiovascular Disease Prevention and Control (PDF). World Health Organization in collaboration with the World Heart Federation and the World Stroke Organization 2011: 3–18.

[27]    Lipshultz SE, Colan SD, Towbin JA, Wilkinson JD. Introduction for "idiopathic and primary cardiomyopathy in children". Prog Pediatr Cardiol 2007; 23(1-2): 3.
[http://dx.doi.org/10.1016/j.ppedcard.2007.05.007]

[28]    Mampuya WM. Cardiac rehabilitation past, present and future: an overview. Cardiovasc Diagn Ther 2012; 2(1): 38-49.
[PMID: 24282695]

[29]    Kreatsoulas C, Anand SS. The impact of social determinants on cardiovascular disease. Can J Cardiol 2010; 26(Suppl C) (Suppl. C): 8C-13C.
[http://dx.doi.org/10.1016/S0828-282X(10)71075-8] [PMID: 20847985]

[30]    Almesned S, Al-Akhfash A, Al Mesned A. Social impact on families of children with complex congenital heart disease. Ann Saudi Med 2013; 33(2): 140-3.
[http://dx.doi.org/10.5144/0256-4947.2013.140] [PMID: 23563001]

[31]    Allabadi H, Alkaiyat A, Alkhayyat A, *et al.* Depression and anxiety symptoms in cardiac patients: a cross-sectional hospital-based study in a Palestinian population. BMC Public Health 2019; 19(1): 232.
[http://dx.doi.org/10.1186/s12889-019-6561-3] [PMID: 30808333]

[32]    Amini-Rarani M, Vahedi S, Borjali M, Nosratabadi M. Socioeconomic inequality in congenital heart diseases in Iran. Int J Equity Health 2021; 20(1): 251.
[http://dx.doi.org/10.1186/s12939-021-01591-3] [PMID: 34863190]

[33]    Shear MK, Simon N, Wall M, *et al.* Complicated grief and related bereavement issues for DSM-5. Depress Anxiety 2011; 28(2): 103-17.
[http://dx.doi.org/10.1002/da.20780] [PMID: 21284063]

[34]    Hudsmith LE, Thorne SA. Transition of care from paediatric to adult services in cardiology. Arch Dis Child 2007; 92(10): 927-30.
[http://dx.doi.org/10.1136/adc.2006.103812] [PMID: 17895343]

[35]    Craig S, Elyse F, Karen U, Katherine B, Mary M, Heidi C. Best Practices in Managing Transition to Adulthood for Adolescents With Congenital Heart Disease: The Transition Process and Medical and Psychosocial Issues. Circulation 2012; 126: 1143-72.

[36]    Marino BS, Lipkin PH, Newburger JW, *et al.* Neurodevelopmental outcomes in children with congenital heart disease: evaluation and management: a scientific statement from the American Heart Association. Circulation 2012; 126(9): 1143-72.

[http://dx.doi.org/10.1161/CIR.0b013e318265ee8a] [PMID: 22851541]

[37]    Sika-Paotonu D, Beaton A, Raghu A, *et al.* Acute Rheumatic Fever and Rheumatic Heart Disease.Streptococcus pyogenes: Basic Biology to Clinical Manifestations. Oklahoma City, OK: University of Oklahoma Health Sciences Center 2016.

[38]    Sani MU, Karaye KM, Borodo MM. Prevalence and pattern of rheumatic heart disease in the Nigerian savannah: an echocardiographic study. Cardiovasc J Afr 2007; 18(5): 295-9.
[PMID: 17957324]

[39]    Mosadeghrad AM. Factors influencing healthcare service quality. Int J Health Policy Manag 2014; 3(2): 77-89.
[http://dx.doi.org/10.15171/ijhpm.2014.65]

[40]    Musa NL, Hjortdal V, Zheleva B, *et al.* The global burden of paediatric heart disease. Cardiol Young 2017; 27(S6): S3-8.
[http://dx.doi.org/10.1017/S1047951117002530]

[41]    Leal J, Luengo-Fernández R, Gray A, Petersen S, Rayner M. Economic burden of cardiovascular diseases in the enlarged European Union. Eur Heart J 2006; 27(13): 1610-9.
[http://dx.doi.org/10.1093/eurheartj/ehi733] [PMID: 16495286]

[42]    Gheorghe A, Griffiths U, Murphy A, Legido-Quigley H, Lamptey P, Perel P. The economic burden of cardiovascular disease and hypertension in low- and middle-income countries: a systematic review. BMC Public Health 2018; 18(1): 975.
[http://dx.doi.org/10.1186/s12889-018-5806-x] [PMID: 30081871]

[43]    Sadoh WE, Nwaneri DU, Owobu AC. The cost of out-patient management of chronic heart failure in children with congenital heart disease. Niger J Clin Pract 2011; 14(1): 65-9.
[http://dx.doi.org/10.4103/1119-3077.79255] [PMID: 21493995]

[44]    Raj M, Paul M, Sudhakar A, *et al.* Micro-economic impact of congenital heart surgery: results of a prospective study from a limited-resource setting. PLoS One 2015; 10(6): e0131348.
[http://dx.doi.org/10.1371/journal.pone.0131348] [PMID: 26110639]

[45]    Falase B, Sanusi M, Majekodunmi A, Ajose I, Idowu A, Oke D. The cost of open heart surgery in Nigeria. Pan Afr Med J 2013; 2: 61.
[http://dx.doi.org/10.11604/pamj.2013.14.61.2162] [PMID: 23565308]

[46]    Chamorro Velásquez CL, Sandoval Reyes NF, Taborda Restrepo A, *et al.* The economic impact of critical congenital heart disease to the health system and families in Colombia. F1000 Res 2019; 8: 92.
[http://dx.doi.org/10.12688/f1000research.17631.1]

[47]    Connor JA, Kline NE, Mott S, Harris SK, Jenkins KJ. The meaning of cost for families of children with congenital heart disease. J Pediatr Health Care 2010; 24(5): 318-25.
[http://dx.doi.org/10.1016/j.pedhc.2009.09.002] [PMID: 20804952]

[48]    Pandey KR, Meltzer DO. Financial burden and impoverishment due to cardiovascular medications in Low and Middle Income Countries: An Illustration from India. PLoS One 2016; 11(5): e0155293.
[http://dx.doi.org/10.1371/journal.pone.0155293] [PMID: 27159055]

[49]    Willems R, Tack P, François K, Annemans L. Direct medical costs of Pediatric congenital Heart disease surgery in a Belgian University Hospital. World J Pediatr Congenit Heart Surg 2019; 10(1): 28-36.
[http://dx.doi.org/10.1177/2150135118808747] [PMID: 30799714]

# CHAPTER 7

# Meconium Stained Newborn

**Mohammad Moonis Akbar Faridi**[1,*] and **Sumaiya Shamsi**[1]

*[1] Era's Lucknow Medical College, Era University, Lucknow, India*

**Abstract:** Meconium Stained Amniotic Fluid (MSAF) and Meconium Aspiration Syndrome (MAS) in newborn are commonly encountered by obstetricians and neonatologists world over, and more so in developing countries. MAS is a serious condition as it causes severe respiratory morbidity and complications like air leak, pneumothorax, Persistent Pulmonary Hypertension (PPHN), surfactant inactivation and death in many cases. There have been several changes in the management of pregnant mothers and their neonates, as well as in the endotracheal suctioning guidelines for babies born with MSAF ever since the pathogenesis of intra-uterine passage of meconium and meconium aspiration syndrome, and evidence on intervention outcomes became known. This chapter shall review the mechanism of meconium stained amniotic fluid, the pathophysiology of meconium aspiration syndrome and management of the newborn infant in the labor room, NICU and beyond, as per the present consensus. Potential newer therapies and drugs shall also be briefly addressed.

**Keywords:** Amniotic fluid, Chemical pneumonitis, ECMO, Endotracheal suction, Fetal distress, High-frequency ventilation, Inhaled nitric oxide, Meconium stained amniotic fluid, Meconium staining, Meconium aspiration, Meconium aspiration syndrome, Mecometer, Meconiumcrit, Neonatal pneumothorax, Non-vigorous infant, NRP, Persistent pulmonary hypertension, Respiratory distress, Surfactant, Vigorous infant.

## INTRODUCTION

The earliest stool of the newborn is meconium, which may occasionally be passed before birth, in-utero or during the process of being delivered, thereby causing staining of the amniotic fluid. This condition is called Meconium-Stained Amniotic Fluid (MSAF). The MSAF has always been a cause of concern to obstetricians and neonatologists, pertaining to its management and perinatal outcome after Schwartz (1857) first time opined that intra-uterine passage of meconium as a marker of perinatal hypoxia. Right from Aristotle's time, when he

* **Corresponding author Mohammad Moonis Akbar Faridi:** Era's Lucknow Medical College, Era University, Lucknow, India; Tel: 91-88006 96442; Fax: 0522-2407824; E-mails: mmafaridi@yahoo.co.in and drmmafaridi@gmail.com

**Nima Rezaei and Noosha Samieefar (Eds.)**
**All rights reserved-© 2023 Bentham Science Publishers**

associated MSAF with a state of sleepiness and depression in a neonate, to date the subject has been a topic of research and inquisition. The Meconium Aspiration Syndrome (MAS) is perhaps the diffusion of meconium into the fetal airways that poses serious neonatal morbidity and mortality. Debates and controversies have continued to surround the management of MSAF and MAS.

Meconium, derived from the Greek word *mekoni* meaning poppy juice or opium, was believed to keep the baby calm and quiet in the womb. Meconium is the fetal feces that accumulate in the colon throughout gestation. It is thick, blackish-green in color, odorless in smell, and consists of desquamated cells from the intestine and skin, lanugo hair, mucin from the gastrointestinal tract, vernix fat and secretions from the amniotic fluid. It is comprised of: 75% water and 25% solids viz, lipids, cholesterol, mucopolysaccharides, protein, enzymes including pancreatic phospholipase A2, bile acids and salts and some drug metabolites if the mother is taking medicines. Amniotic fluid is clear and colorless and essentially sterile, except for a few vernix particles and some microbiome DNA; the significance of the latter is not known as of now [1, 2]. However, the in-utero passage of meconium imparts color to the amniotic fluid and is alarmingly a telltale sign of fetal hypoxia and acidosis until proven otherwise.

Meconium appears in the fetal intestine around the 10th week of gestation, and gradually increases in amount to about 200 grams at term. Low motilin levels, a hormone that initiates intestinal peristalsis, and the presence of a terminal cap of viscous meconium and a tonic anal sphincter prevent gut peristalsis and passage of meconium during fetal life. The gastrointestinal system matures as gestation progresses. Increasing cholinergic innervations near term gestation and transient parasympathetic stimulation of the gut; transient umbilical cord or fetal head compression after rupturing of membranes and rising motilin levels may account for MSAF in the term and post-term newborn infants in the absence of perinatal asphyxia. The incidence of MSAF is about 10%–15% of all pregnancies worldwide, being higher in the blacks and South Asian ethnicity, and associated with 20% of non-vigorous infants [3]. MAS develops in approximately 10% of babies [4, 5], and contributes to one neonatal death in 2000 infants [6]. The incidence of MSAF rises with advancing gestational age, ranging from 13% for infants 36–39 weeks to 31.5% for infants born after 42 weeks gestation [7]. However, changes in clinical practice to avoid gestation beyond 41 weeks have consequently shown a decline in the prevalence of MSAF and MAS [8]. Poor integrity and maturation of the parasympathetic system and low levels of the hormone in early gestation make MSAF an uncommon event in preterm infants. The reported incidence of MSAF is only 3–6.7% in the preterm population [9].

## ETIOLOGY

Apart from fetal maturation a hypoxic insult to the fetus in the form of fetoplacental insufficiency, nuchal cord, cord compression, abruptio placentae or metabolic acidosis and intra-uterine infection by E. Coli, Group B streptococci and Listeria, can also cause increased intestinal peristalsis and relaxation of anal sphincter leading to passage of meconium in-utero (Table **1**).

**Table 1. Etiology of meconium-stained amniotic fluid.**

| Antenatal Period | Intra Natal Period |
|---|---|
| Placenta and umbilical cord structure and function abnormalities. | Physiological gut maturation and peristalsis. |
| Placental low glycogen stores. | Sudden pressure on the forehead and umbilical cord on the spontaneous rupture of membranes. |
| Placental senescence: full-term gestation, gestational diabetes, smoking and drug abuse. | Cephalo-pelvic disproportion. |
| Intra-uterine growth retardation | Prolong labor. |
| Abruptio placentae. | Fetal heart arrhythmia, Fetal heart decelerations on Cardiotocography CTG. |
| Nuchal cord, hyper-coiled cord and low umbilical coiling index. | Uterine atony or tetany. |
| Pre–eclampsia and chorioamnionitis. | Umbilical cord avulsion. |
| Intra-uterine infection: Listeria, E. coli and Group B Streptococci. | Perinatal asphyxia with acidosis. |

Note: the underlying pathology for MASF remains perinatal asphyxia until proven otherwise.

Meconium Staining is a state when the umbilical cord, skin, and nails of a newborn infant are stained yellow at birth. Meconium Aspiration (MA) is a condition when meconium is present below the vocal cords. When a neonate aspirates meconium during intrauterine gasping or initial breaths at birth, it is described as primary meconium aspiration. The infant also ingests MSAF during delivery which may cause gastritis. Secondary meconium aspiration results after birth when the infant may vomit MSAF and aspirate. Meconium aspiration can be diagnosed by direct visualization of the meconium below the vocal cords by laryngoscope, by aspiration of meconium through an endotracheal tube, or after taking a chest skiagram. Meconium may be present in the fore –waters or hind-waters; the former has more pathological significance. The presence of meconium in the forewaters has similar significance in breech delivery as in vertex presentation.

The color and consistency of the MSAF both have attracted researchers in predicting the fetal outcome, associating perinatal asphyxia, or planning interventions and management. Green-colored amniotic fluid indicates an acute event, either a hypoxic insult or a 'normal physiological maturation' while yellow amniotic fluid results from a past event, and symbolizes chronic hypoxia. MSAF is referred to as thin, thick, and pea-soup or mild and severe based on subjective assessment of the concentration of meconium in the amniotic fluid. However, to add objectivity, several methods have been devised for the quantitative estimation of meconium in amniotic liquor. Meconiumcrit [10] is the solid component of meconium in the amniotic fluid expressed as volume percent based on the principle of hematocrit calculation. A meconiumcrit of 10% or less imparts green color to the amniotic fluid, and more than 30% meconiumcrit renders blackish-green color to the amniotic fluid. Spectrophotometry is another method to estimate the meconium content in the amniotic fluid. Both these methods require expertise and instruments, and thus cannot be used in clinical practice at the periphery (Fig. **1**).

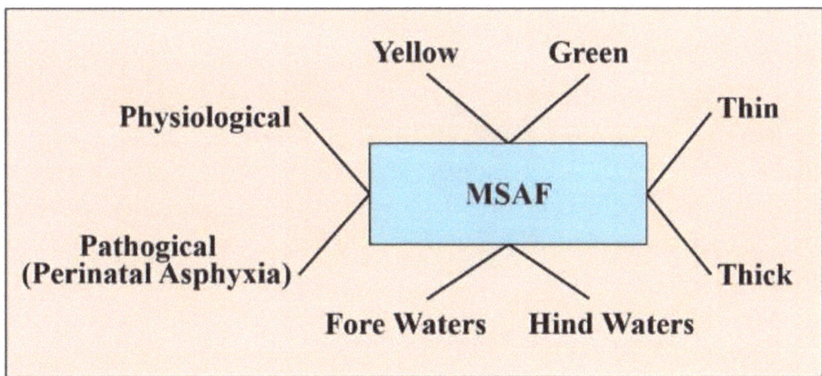


**Fig. (1).** Attributes of Meconium Stained Amniotic Fluid.

'Mecometer', designed by Korean scientists [11], is a standard color scale based on optical density. The absorbance of the standard scale and MSAF samples were measured at 420nm, and a linear correlation between the meconium content and optical density was established, thus making it simpler and easy to use the tool in routine practice.

## Etiology and Risk Factors for MSAF

The exact etiology of the in-utero passage of meconium remains unclear [12]. However, one thing established is that MSAF may be a physiological event. Perinatal asphyxia, especially with metabolic acidosis is frequently associated with MSAF. Advanced gestational age at delivery, feto-maternal stress factors like hypoxia or intra-uterine bacterial infection, uncontrolled gestational diabetes, cord compression or fetal head impaction after rupturing of membranes or cephalo-pelvic disproportion, hypo or hypercoiling of umbilical cord vessels and fetal heart rate abnormalities have all been shown an association with the meconium staining of the amniotic fluid in various studies. All factors pertaining to placental insufficiency, maternal hypertension, pre-eclampsia, oligo-hydramnios and maternal drug abuse can predispose to meconium passage in-utero. Infants born to women living with Human Immunodeficiency Virus (HIV) have a higher risk of MSAF and MAS [13].

The aspiration of MSAF poses a greater risk for the development of respiratory distress in infants than with clear amniotic fluid. This warrants a careful and protocol-based identification of the maternal risk factors and antepartum fetal monitoring to timely anticipate the need for fetal and neonatal resuscitation and management of respiratory distress in meconium settings.

## MECONIUM ASPIRATION SYNDROME

MAS is a clinical entity that develops in an infant born with MSAF envisaging meconium aspiration, clinical signs of respiratory distress, and an X-ray of chest consistent with the meconium aspiration. The MAS is considered a massive airway disease characterized by tachypnea, chest retractions, decreased SpO2, respiratory alkalosis followed by mixed acidosis and increasing oxygen requirement. The incidence of MAS varies from 5% to 16%, and is significantly more in asphyxiated infants [14].

### Pathophysiology of MAS

The pathophysiology of MAS is intricate and incompletely understood despite the substantial literature available. The complex composition of meconium has made it difficult to identify a single agent explaining the pathogenesis of respiratory morbidity which includes in-utero hypoxia, metabolic acidosis and fetal cardiac arrhythmias; airway obstruction, surfactant inactivation, intra-pulmonary hypertension, chemical pneumonitis, inflammation of pulmonary parenchyma, secondary bacterial infection and other toxic effects. Several factors contribute to the development of MAS (Fig. **2**).

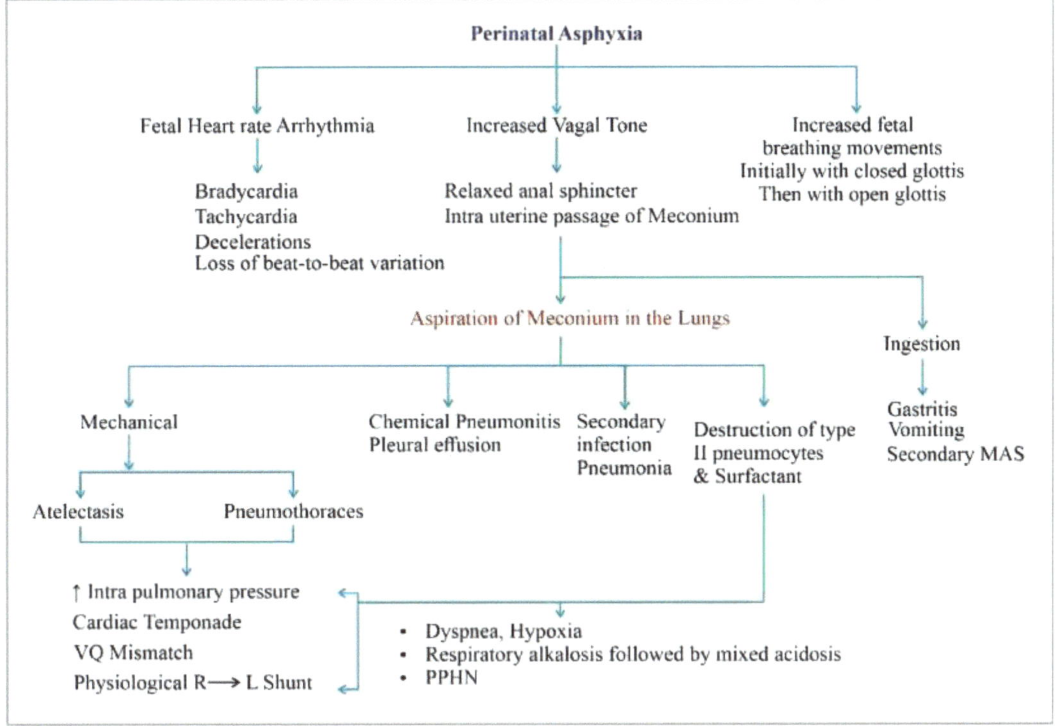



**Fig. (2).** Pathophysiology of MAS.

## *Fetal Hypoxia*

*In utero* breathing efforts of the fetus, a part of the antenatal ultrasonographic assessment of Bio-Physical Profile (BPP), are characterized by short inspiratory and long expiratory phases with the closed glottis. Amniotic fluid reaches up to the pharynx during the active inspiratory phase but does not enter into the trachea as the glottis remains closed. It returns to the amniotic sac during the expiratory phase. However, when perinatal hypoxia sets in the vagal reflex, it activates gut ischemia due to the fetal diving reflex, anal sphincter tone decreases, and the passage of meconium occurs. Hypoxia leads to metabolic acidosis. The fetal breathing efforts turn into gasping, fetal heart decompensates leading to early and late decelerations and poor cardiac output, the fetal diving reflex is lost, the glottis opens, and MSAF is aspirated in the trachea and bronchi. The meconium reaches terminal bronchioles when the baby initiates breathing at birth. The MSAF is twice as common with a BPP score of ≤6 as compared to a BPP score of ≥8 [15], supporting chronic stress and perinatal hypoxia theory. Erythropoietin levels also rise in babies born through MSAF indicating chronic hypoxia contributing to meconium passage [16]. The rise in erythropoietin levels enhances the production of nucleated RBCs in fetal circulation. The rise in erythroid precursors can be taken as a surrogate marker of chronic fetal hypoxia [17].

## Mechanical Obstruction of Airways

The solid meconium particles cause physical obstruction in the airways. A *large amount* of meconium may completely block the terminal bronchioles. As a result, atelectasis occurs beyond the obstruction site rendering the collapsed alveoli incapable of participating in the perfusion-diffusion of gases (V/Q mismatch). The atelectatic pulmonary lobule acts as a physiologic right-to-left shunt that further worsens neonatal hypoxia. A small amount of meconium partially obstructs the distal bronchioles, and frequently causes a ball-valve phenomenon. The air enters the alveoli during inspiration which is an active process but cannot come out during exhalation due to the passive nature of the latter. The size of the distal alveoli goes on increasing with subsequent breaths. Distended alveoli ultimately burst, and cause pneumothorax, pneumopericardium, and even cardiac tamponade. Traditionally mechanical blockage of the airways has been implicated in the main pathophysiologic mechanism.

## Surfactant Inactivation

Surfactant is synthesized, and secreted by type II alveolar epithelial cells which differentiate between 24 and 34 weeks of gestation. It is made up of 70%- 80% phospholipids, approximately 10% protein (SP-A, SP-B, SP-C and SP-D) and 10% neutral lipids, mainly cholesterol [18]. Surfactant reduces surface tension at the air-liquid interface of the alveolus and prevents its collapse during end-expiration. Recent studies have suggested that surfactant also has a role in the innate host defense against inhaled pathogens [19]. Meconium damages type II pneumocytes decreases secretion of the surfactant and inhibits its surface tension-lowering properties. This leads to a significant reduction in lung compliance and functional residual capacity, and an increase in expiratory lung resistance [20]. Treatment with large doses of natural surfactant improves lung compliance, work of breathing and ventilation, and thus explains its use in the management of MAS in newborn infants.

## Inflammation and Chemical Pneumonitis

Why some neonates born with MSAF develop MAS and others do not has been an interesting question. The assumption of chemical pneumonitis being caused by meconium has been suggested after finding leucocyte infiltration in the rabbit lungs in experimental meconium aspiration [21]. Meconium-induced pulmonary parenchymal inflammation is supported by the fact that the former exhibits pro-inflammatory properties such as Interleukin (IL)-1, Tumor Necrosis Factor (TNF),

IL-8 and Phospholipase- A2 [22 - 24]. The raised concentration of C-Reactive Protein (CRP) [25] and Procalcitonin (PCT) in the non-infectious infants born with MSAF further supports the inflammation theory [26]. Chemical pneumonitis sets in 6-8 hours after aspiration of MSAF followed by secondary bacterial infection worsening the condition of the newborn infant.

## Persistent Pulmonary Hypertension

Persistent Pulmonary Hypertension of the Newborn (PPHN) is a syndrome characterized by sustained elevation of Pulmonary Vascular Resistance (PVR), and is often associated with normal or low Systemic Vascular Resistance (SVR). It leads to extra-pulmonary shunting from right to left across persistent fetal channels (Patent Ductus Arteriosus (PDA) and Patent Foramen Ovale (PFO)) leading to labile hypoxemia. It is often secondary to an unsuccessful pulmonary transition at birth. Significant PPHN occurs in 20-40% of infants who suffer from MAS. PPHN in infants with MAS may be caused by (a) pulmonary vasoconstriction secondary to hypoxia, hypercarbia and acidosis, (b) hypertrophy of the post-acinar capillaries as a result of chronic intrauterine hypoxia, and (c) pulmonary vasoconstriction due to pulmonary inflammation. Activation of inflammatory mediators like thromboxane A2, angiotensin II and cytokines possibly contributes to pulmonary hypertension. Levels of leukotrienes, platelet-activating factor, thromboxanes and endothelin -1 ET-1 are elevated [27].

## Secondary Infection

Meconium is a rich culture medium for bacterial growth *in vitro*. Autopsy in MAS-affected neonates has shown features of bacterial pneumonia on histopathology [28]. Studies have also shown an increased incidence of chorioamnionitis and positive amniotic fluid cultures in babies with MSAF. Whether the bacterial infection is a consequence or a cause of MSAF is debatable [29]. Acute phase reactants like CRP and PCT may rise without bacterial infection in infants with MSAF.

## Clinical Features

Wide variability in the clinical features of MAS is seen. From mild respiratory distress requiring minimal or no oxygen to severe distress causing respiratory failure even with the use of the best oxygenation modalities, and complicated by sepsis, a neonate can have a storming course.

Babies born with thick MSAF, low Apgar score at 1 minute, fetal bradycardia and fetal cardiac decelerations and intrapartum maternal fever develop severe respiratory morbidity and PPHN, and carry a higher risk of mortality [30]. Death due to MAS varies from 19.4%-32% in the Indian Sub-continent [31, 32] to <5% in the developed countries [33, 34].

Commonly neonates are born with greenish-yellow staining of the amniotic fluid, vernix, nails and umbilical cord with or without immediate respiratory distress depending on the amount, thickness and duration of in-utero passage of meconium and several other factors associated with the meconium passage. In general, skin and nails become stained after 2 to 6 hours of exposure, respectively. Being common in post-term neonates, signs of post-maturity, peeling of the skin, over-grown nails, decreased vernix and weight loss are also seen. A large number of infants born with thin MSAF and vigorous at birth remain normal, feed well, and behave like peers of the same gestational age and birth weight. Few of them may develop tachypnea with a respiratory rate of 60-80 per minute without chest retractions, maintain SpO2 in room air and settle within 24 hours. They, however, need close monitoring. Some people define this state as subclinical MAS. The respiratory distress may appear soon after birth if the infant is non-vigorous (No/feeble cry, flaccid muscle tone and heart rate <100 per minute), and has aspirated MSAF before or during delivery, otherwise symptoms appear 4-6 hours after birth when meconium migrates from proximal to distal airways or chemical pneumonitis develops. Hence, a period of careful monitoring of vitals in meconium-stained infants for at least 24 hours is warranted.

Features of respiratory distress include tachypnea, retractions, grunting, nasal flaring and or cyanosis. Antero-Posterior diameter of the chest may increase giving a barrel-shaped appearance because of over-inflation. On auscultation, rales and rhonchi can be heard, and a systolic murmur of tricuspid regurgitation due to PPHN may be audible on careful auscultation. Severely affected infants have increasing oxygen requirements and inotropic support, and may need mechanical ventilation, Extra Corporeal Membrane Oxygenation (ECMO), etc. The presence of pneumothoraces, shock, hypoxia and lactic acidosis further complicates the disease. About 20% to 30% of neonates may have neurologic and /or respiratory depression at birth. The PaO2/FiO2 ratio <200 can predict mortality with 94.1% and 96.6% sensitivity and specificity, respectively among infants suffering from MAS [35].

The infant may also ingest meconium in-utero or during labor. Meconium-induced gastritis causes vomiting and retching, and feeds intolerance in the first 24-48 hours of birth. Gastric lavage in the labor room or afterward does not make any difference in the causation of gastritis and secondary MAS [36].

Cleary and Wiswell [37] have proposed severity criteria to define MAS depending on oxygen requirement: (a) mild MAS is a disease that requires less than 40%

oxygen for less than 48 hours, (b) moderate MAS is a disease that requires more than 40% oxygen for more than 48 hours with no air leak, and (c) severe MAS is a disease that requires assisted ventilation for more than 48 hours, and is often associated with PPHN. The symptoms and signs of MAS get mixed up with those of hypoxic-ischemic encephalopathy as most of these infants have already suffered from perinatal asphyxia. Infants can have seizures, altered sensorium and metabolic derangements like hypoglycemia, hypocalcemia and hypothermia. The immediate prognosis is good if there is no hypoxic damage to the brain.

The development of MAS poses serious long-term pulmonary sequelae that include airway obstruction, hyperinflation, elevated closing volumes and airway hyper-reactivity [38]. Persistent pulmonary insufficiency has been seen in children till 8 years of age [39]. The possibility of neurodevelopmental disabilities in MAS-treated infants is still investigational, although the associated hypoxic insult with sequelae is not an uncommon phenomenon amongst survivors.

**Diagnosis**

The diagnosis of MAS is clinical. The presence of respiratory manifestations in neonates born with MSAF, with suggestive x-ray features in the absence of other plausible causes is considered MAS. The chest x-ray may be near normal or show pneumothoraces. There can be asymmetric coarse patchy pulmonary opacities due to sub-segmental atelectasis, increased lung volumes and flattened diaphragm due to hyper-inflated lungs secondary to distal small airway obstruction and gas trapping in 20-40% cases and multifocal consolidation due to chemical pneumonitis.

Ultrasonography (USG) is another reliable, accurate and non-radiation exposure tool to diagnose MAS.USG features include pulmonary consolidation with air bronchogram, pleural line anomalies and disappearance of A-line, alveolar-interstitial syndrome or B-line in the non-consolidation area, atelectasis and pleural effusion. The first three features are pathognomonic of MAS, and are almost always found. Atelectasis and pleural effusion are found in less than 15% of patients [40].

Arterial blood gas analysis shows hypoxemia and hypercarbia; initial metabolic alkalosis, due to hyperventilation, turns to metabolic or mixed acidosis. A higher amount of $FiO_2$ is required to maintain $SpO_2$ between 92%-94%. 2D ECHO is the gold standard to confirm PPHN and monitor the efficacy of therapeutic interventions. It gives a view of hemodynamics, the direction of the shunt, and systemic blood pressure measurement with tricuspid regurgitation velocity.

Differential Diagnosis of MAS includes other causes of respiratory distress in the newborn infant which occur in 4%–9% of cases born with MSAF. These are Transient Tachypnea of the Newborn (TTNB), delayed transition from fetal circulation, sepsis and congenital heart diseases.

## Management

The objective of the management of MSAF is the prevention of MAS, and to do timely intervention to reduce its incidence and severity. Better antepartum monitoring based on clinical parameters and cardiotocography, removing the infant from the inimical intrauterine environment by enhancing delivery, normal or assisted or Lower (uterine) Segment Caesarean Section (LSCS), involvement of an expert neonatal resuscitation team at birth and proper neonatal care beyond the labor room decrease the incidence, complications, and severity of MAS. There is a paradigm shift in the airway management of newborn infants at birth from universal tracheal suction of meconium [41] to no endotracheal suction. Extensive research has been carried out in the last five decades regarding the pharmacological and supportive treatment of MAS.

### *Neonatal Management in the Delivery Room*

Receive the infant in the pre-warmed linen immediately after birth, sever cord and assess cry, muscle tone and heart rate while moving towards the warmer in the labor room.

### *Vigorous Infant*

A vigorous infant is crying spontaneously, limbs are flexed and actively moving, and heart rate is >10 at 6 seconds (HR >100/min). The recent International Liaison Committee on Resuscitation (ILCOR) guidelines 2020 [42] recommend that vigorous newborn infants with MSAF do not require routine intubation and tracheal suctioning. Steps of routine care should be initiated with the baby being with the mother, and gentle clearing of secretions from the mouth if necessary. Respiration, heart rate, and color of the infant are noted. An infant with spontaneous breathing, heart rate >100 per min and pink lips and tongue is regarded to have the best transition from the intra-uterine sojourn to extra-uterine life. Infants should be provided skin-to-skin touch with the mother, and initiate breastfeeding within an hour. Keep the infant under strict monitoring either with the mother, if she is comfortable or in the NICU. Respiratory rate, heart rate, blood pressure and $SpO_2$ should be measured at least 4 hourly. The infant is evaluated for using accessory muscles in the form of flaring of alae nasi, subcostal and inter-costal retractions, grunt and cyanosis.

## *Non-vigorous Infant*

If the infant is depressed and flaccid, does not cry, or has feeble gasping respiration, and heart rate is <100 per min then he should be immediately put under a warmer, the position is made with the neck slightly extended. According to 2015 NRP guidelines, emphasis should be placed on supportive interventions-oxygenation and ventilation - as needed which may include intubation and suction if airway obstruction is present, and endotracheal suction may be done directly by 3# endotracheal tube applying negative pressure while withdrawing the tube. One or two attempts may be made till no more meconium is aspirated. However, current evidence doubts its efficacy [43, 44]. After suction, the infant should be dried and mopped, and stimulated by rubbing the back or stocking the soles. The initial steps should not take more than 30 sec. Now evaluate heart rate, respiration and color. Give bag and mask ventilation if the heart rate is <100 per min or the infant is not breathing. Follow the rest of the initial steps for neonatal resuscitation.

## *Gastric Lavage*

The infant may ingest MSAF before delivery in the intrauterine period or during labor. Meconium is acidic in nature, pH 7.1-7.2, and may be vomited out as a result of gastritis. This may cause feed intolerance. In many centers, gastric lavage is performed in the labor room or after admission to the NICU with normal saline to prevent feed intolerance and secondary MAS. However, recent randomized controlled trials have shown that gastric lavage does not offer any benefit, and is not required [36, 45].

### *Management Beyond the Delivery Room*

The non-vigorous infant should be managed in the NICU. Frequent monitoring of vital signs with the help of a non-invasive monitor is very useful. CHART Pulse (C=color; H=heart rate; A=apnea, respiratory rate; R=capillary refill time; T=temperature; P=blood pressure) is a good acronym for remembering the clinical evaluation of the baby presenting with MAS. Intake/output charting is important. The infant's urine output of>1 mL/Kg/hr. is acceptable. Downes scoring (Table **2**) is based on simple clinical parameters, and is useful in monitoring the respiratory status of the infant [46] A Downes score of >7 indicates impending respiratory failure.

Baseline investigations include CBC, CRP, blood culture, blood sugar, blood urea, serum electrolytes, serum calcium and arterial blood gas analysis. Since frequent blood gas samples may be required to guide further management, an indwelling arterial catheter is preferred. Pre-ductal and post-ductal oxygen saturation difference of > 5-10% in the right upper limb and leg is significant. Lactate levels rise in the cord blood, indicate significant perinatal asphyxia, and may predict the need for mechanical ventilation [47].

**Table 2. Downes score.**

| Feature | Score 0 | Score 1 | Score 2 |
|---|---|---|---|
| Cyanosis | None | In room air | In 40% $FiO_2$ |
| Retractions | None | Mild | Severe |
| Grunting | None | Audible with stethoscope | Audible without stethoscope |
| Air entry | Normal | Decreased | Barely audible |
| Respiratory | <60 | 60-80 | >80 or apnea |

Score <4 no respiratory distress, 4-7 Clinical respiratory distress, >7 impending respiratory failure.

Maintenance of temperature with the infant being placed in a neutral thermal environment, correction of hypovolemia, and circulatory support with normal saline or packed red blood cells should be done in patients with marginal oxygenation; the target is to keep hematocrit above 40%. The patient may need inotropic support with cardiotonic agents such as dopamine, dobutamine and noradrenaline. Anticipation and prompt treatment of hypoglycemia, acidosis, hypocalcemia and polycythemia are crucial in determining the outcome.

## Supportive Therapy and General Measures

### *Respiratory Support*

Management of hypoxemia is of paramount importance as worsening hypoxia may cause severe pulmonary vasoconstriction, and contribute to the development of PPHN which carries a higher risk of mortality in MAS. Hypoxia in an infant who has suffered from perinatal asphyxia may further damage the brain. Fine titration of oxygen therapy is important for intact survival. The requirement for respiratory support depends on the severity of MAS. Some infants require only humidified oxygen by a hood or nasal prongs. About 10% of infants maintain oxygen saturation on continuous positive airway pressure, while about 40%of patients need mechanical ventilation. The target oxygen saturation is 90% to 95%. Baseline ABG shows respiratory alkalosis due to tachypnea and washing of carbon dioxide and reduced ionic calcium. Later on, when work of breathing increases the infant develops mixed acidosis, hypercarbia and hypoxia. Cyanosis develops relatively late compared to older infants due to the abundance of fetal hemoglobin in the neonates.

## Mechanical Ventilation

The complex pathophysiology of MAS coexisting with the areas of hyperinflation and atelectasis makes optimal ventilatory management a challenge. The aim is to improve oxygenation, and minimize barotrauma, volutrauma and thermotrauma in the lungs. High oxygen requirement (FiO$_2$ >0.8), PaO$_2$ <50mmHg, PaCO$_2$ >60 mmHg, respiratory acidosis (pH <7.25), PPHN or circulatory failure warrants intubation and mechanical ventilation [48]. The appropriate mode of ventilation though debatable and Synchronized Intermittent Mandatory Ventilation (SIMV) is the most commonly used mode by convention. Target blood gas and ventilator settings depend upon the presence or absence of PPHN and associated predominant lung abnormality. A trial of bubble nasal Continuous Positive Airway Pressure (CPAP) has shown a reduced need for mechanical ventilation in a recent study [49].

In cases with marked regional or global atelectasis, high-Peak Inspiratory Pressure (PIP) (up to a maximum of 30cm of water) and high Positive-End Expiratory Pressure (PEEP; 4–7 cm) with longer inspiratory time help in the recruitment of alveoli. If there is obvious gas trapping, PEEP should be decreased (3–4 cm) with optimal expiratory time (0.5–0.7) and rapid ventilator rates [50].

In the presence of PPHN higher ventilator rates (50–70), and higher FiO$_2$ (80%–100%) with an oxygen saturation target of 95% or above should be considered to maintain PaO$_2$ between 70 and 100 mmHg and PaCO$_2$ between 35 and 45 mmHg along with volume expansion, vasopressors and other supportive measures [48]. Hyperventilation may induce alkalosis, and lead to the risk of cerebral vasoconstriction which may induce neurologic injury and sensorineural hearing loss. Other modalities like inhaled nitric oxide and high-frequency ventilation should be considered early in such situations.

## High-Frequency Ventilation

High-Frequency Ventilation (HFV) is a new technique of ventilation that uses respiratory rates that greatly exceed the rate of normal breathing. The ability of High-Frequency Oscillatory Ventilation (HFOV) to maintain oxygenation and ventilation while using minimal tidal volumes allows for minimizing barotrauma and volutrauma, and thus reduces the morbidity associated with ventilator management. HFV has been shown to be beneficial over conventional ventilation in MAS which is often complicated with air leak syndromes.

About 20%–30% of all infants requiring intubation and ventilation with MAS are treated with high-frequency ventilation [51]. HFOV is even better in cases complicated with significant atelectasis. Infants with severe PPHN responded better to inhale iNO with HFOV than with conventional ventilation in many studies. Also, the ECMO requirement was much less with this mode in such babies [50].

## Surfactant Therapy

The effect of meconium in causing surfactant deficiency and inhibiting its surface tension-lowering properties has been reported. In-vitro studies have shown that when a surfactant is low, even diluted meconium can be detrimental in raising the surface tension in the alveoli to the extent that it becomes incompatible with normal physiological functioning. The effect of surfactant administration on different aspects of MAS has been studied. There are two ways in which surfactant therapy has been tried- bolus therapy and surfactant lavage. Bolus surfactant therapy decreases the severity of the MAS and the requirement for ECMO. However, it does not alter the duration of ventilation, hospital stay, oxygen use, air leak syndromes or mortality [52].

Meconium causes alveolar epithelial damage thereby leading to surfactant dysfunction. Surfactant lavage therapy may remove the meconium and thereby the surfactant inhibitors in it. This shall augment the surfactant response and effect. Research combining both therapies by administering lavage with dilute surfactant followed by a bolus dose has suggested improving gas exchange and pulmonary mechanics [53]. However, the superiority of none of the two surfactant modes of therapy has been established, so far. More research is needed to confirm the treatment effect, define the optimal doses and method of surfactant administration, and compare lavage with bolus administration. The Canadian Pediatric Society [54] recommends exogenous surfactant for all intubated infants with MAS requiring $FiO_2 \geq 50\%$, and prefer natural surfactant when compared to artificial ones. Airway obstruction, air leaks and hemorrhagic pulmonary edema are a few major complications of surfactant therapy.

## Corticosteroid Therapy

Inflammation plays a key role in the pathophysiology of MAS. This has led the researchers to look for the possible benefits of steroids on pulmonary and systemic inflammation. Conclusive evidence could not be brought to date. A Cochrane meta-analysis showed no effect of steroids in MAS on the need for mechanical ventilation, duration of hospital stay or decrease in mortality, instead, it demonstrated an increase in the requirement of oxygen [55].

A recent Indian study with inhaled steroids has shown the reduced duration of oxygen therapy, as well as hospital stay in cases of MAS [56]. Few recent trials using corticosteroids have also shown the shortened duration of stay and oxygen dependence with improved radiological clearance in steroid-treated patients of MAS [57, 58]. In view of the limited experience, steroid therapy is not currently recommended in MAS.

## *Antibiotics*

The role of routine antibiotics in the management of MAS is controversial, although MSAF culture shows an increased incidence of bacterial growth. Studies have shown that routine antibiotic prophylaxis is not beneficial without other risk factors for sepsis [59]. A meta-analysis of three RCTs has concluded that the use of antibiotics for MAS did not result in a significant reduction in mortality, sepsis or duration of hospital stay [60].

Presently there is no recommendation for antibiotics in the treatment of MAS, and further studies are needed to support or refute their role. If there is strong clinical evidence of chorioamnionitis in the mother or sepsis screen warrants the risk of bacterial infection, then third-generation cephalosporin with an aminoglycoside can be used.

## *Inhaled Nitric oxide*

Pulmonary vasoconstriction leading to increased pulmonary vascular resistance and causing PPHN is a common complication leading to death in MAS. Inhaled nitric oxide iNO is a selective pulmonary vasodilator. It causes vasodilatation, improves oxygenation in the ventilated areas of the lung, and decreases ventilation-perfusion mismatch (VQ mismatch). iNO does not affect systemic vascular resistance while improving pulmonary flow. Hence, the right-to-left shunt is reduced. The use of iNO reduces mortality and ECMO in the term and near term due to MAS. Combining HFV along with iNO has shown even better outcomes in decreasing intra-pulmonary shunting and augmenting oxygen delivery to the pulmonary circulation.

The cost of setting iNO in developing countries becomes a limiting factor. When PPHN does not respond to iNO then sildenafil, which is a phosphodiesterase inhibitor or milrinone dipyramidole, has been tried [61]. Studies with agents like super-oxide dismutase, prostacyclin, magnesium sulfate and bosentan, an endothelial antagonist, have also been tried in limited numbers.

## *Extracorporeal Membrane Oxygenation*

PPHN is a difficult entity and remains frequently nonresponsive to iNO and other respiratory support maneuvers. ECMO is based on the principle of oxygenating the patient's blood outside the corpse; the patient's deoxygenated blood is drained *via* a venous cannula, carbon dioxide ($CO_2$) is removed, and $O_2$ is added through an "extracorporeal" devise. The 'oxygenated' blood is then returned to the systemic circulation *via* another vein (VV ECMO) or artery (VA ECMO). MAS is the commonest indication for ECMO in neonates. The selection criteria for ECMO include: 1) gestation age more than 34 weeks, 2) birthweight more than 2000 g, 3) no serious coagulopathy or active bleeding,4) no major intracranial bleeding, 5) duration of mechanical ventilation less than 10to14days and reversible lung disease, 6) failure of optimal medical management, and 7) infants with high predicted risk mortality.

The accepted criteria to start ECMO is persistent hypoxemia (Oxygenation Index, OI>40), in spite of aggressive management with mechanical ventilation and iNO. With the advent of newer therapies, the number of infants requiring ECMO has reduced. In developed countries, 95%of infants with MAS survive [62].

## *Future Therapy*

At present all treatment modalities of MAS are mainly supportive. Recent evidence of the interplay of various inflammatory mediators in the causation of MAS and oxidative damage and free radical injury to the pulmonary parenchyma has led to experiments with antioxidants like N-Acetylcysteine (NAC) in experimental animals with MAS. NAC suppresses IL-8 and IL-1β formation along with neutrophil migration. It may also reduce the viscosity of meconium by breaking disulfide bonds between protein molecules [63]. Research has advocated that a combination of NAC with surfactants shows enhanced therapeutic benefits than either treatment alone [64, 65].

A study on the mechanism of cell death in meconium has led to the role of the renin-angiotensin system in apoptosis. It was seen that pre-treatment of rabbits with captopril, followed by meconium instillation intratracheally reduced apoptosis in the lung epithelium [66].

The administration of cyclooxygenase II inhibitor parecoxib in meconium-treated rabbits reduces the expression of myeloperoxidase and COX-II receptors and attenuates histopathologic damage and meconium-induced acute lung injury with significant improvement in respiratory functions [67].

Rescue therapy with intratracheal albumin also improves lung function by binding and blocking active substances like free fatty acids and bile acids in meconium [68]. A protease inhibitor cocktail prevents cell detachment induced by meconium, suggesting a possible role of fetal pancreatic digestive enzymes in the treatment of MAS [69]. Liquid ventilation with perfluorocarbons has been found beneficial in improving survival in animal models of MAS, offering research potential for its use in humans [70]. All these therapies are in the experimental stage, with only animal studies available so far, and await further human trials.

## CONCLUSION

Newborn infant passes thick blackish-green sticky stools in the first 3-4 days of life. It is called meconium. Sometimes it may be evacuated in the fetal period staining the amniotic fluid yellow (old) or green (fresh) depending upon the duration. MSAF is considered a marker of perinatal asphyxia, characterized by hypoxia and metabolic acidosis until proven otherwise. Physiological maturation of the intestinal peristalsis in the fetus of full-term gestation and transient pressure on the forehead or umbilical cord after rupture of the membranes may cause hypercarbia, without hypoxia or acidosis, leading to the passage of meconium in-utero. Endotracheal [ET] suctioning of the meconium at birth is not indicated in vigorous infants. The benefit of endotracheal ET suction in non-vigorous infants is controversial. Gastric lavage neither reduces feed intolerance nor the incidence of secondary MAS. Infants may aspirate MSAF during delivery or at birth. Meconium aspiration can be diagnosed by direct visualization of the meconium below the vocal cord or by imaging techniques such as x-ray and USG chest, Meconium exerts mechanical and chemical effects on the pulmonary parenchyma causing atelectasis, pneumothoraces and pneumonitis. All infants do not develop MAS after meconium aspiration. MAS is a clinical condition when an infant born with MSAF develops respiratory distress and a chest x-ray/USG shows features suggestive of meconium aspiration. MAS carries a higher risk of mortality due to pneumothorax, pneumomediastinum, pulmonary hemorrhage, secondary infection and PPHN. Infants with MAS should be admitted to the NICU. Monitoring of vital parameters, SpO2 and intake output should be done regularly. Respiratory distress can be evaluated frequently by Downe's scoring. Physiological and metabolic homeostasis must be ensured. There is no role of prophylactic antibiotics in MAS. Oxygen therapy is the cornerstone of the management of MAS. Supportive measures such as care in the thermoneutral environment, adequate hydration, breastfeeding/expressed breast milk feeding and timely management of hypoglycemia, hypocalcemia and acidosis improve survival. Administration of surfactant and broad-spectrum antibiotics in the presence of bacterial infection is useful in the treatment of MAS but steroid therapy is not helpful. MAS causes long-term morbidity in the form of hyperactive airway disease, airway obstruction, hyperinflation, elevated closing volumes, and persistent pulmonary insufficiency in children till 8 years of age.

## ABBREVIATIONS

**ABG**     Arterial Blood Gas

**BPP**     Biophysical Profile

| | |
|---|---|
| **CBC** | Complete Blood Count |
| **CHART** | Color, Heart rate, Apnea, capillary Refill time, Temperature. |
| **CPAP** | Continuous Positive Airway Pressure |
| **CTG** | Cardiotocography |
| **CRP** | C- Reactive Protein |
| **ECMO** | Extra Corporeal Membrane Oxygenation |
| **ET** | Endotracheal |
| **FiO2** | Fraction of Inspired Oxygen |
| **HFOV** | High Frequency Oscillatory Ventilation |
| **HFV** | High-Frequency Ventilation |
| **HIV** | Human Immunodeficiency Virus |
| **MA** | Meconium Aspiration |
| **MAS** | Meconium Aspiration Syndrome |
| **MSAF** | Meconium Stained Amniotic Fluid |
| **NICU** | Neonatal Intensive Care Unit |
| **NRP** | Neonatal Resuscitation Program |
| **PaCo2** | Partial Pressure of Carbon Dioxide in Arterial Blood. |
| **PaO2** | Partial Pressure of Oxygen in Arterial Blood |
| **PDA** | Patent Ductus Arteriosus |
| **PFO** | Patent Foramen Ovale |
| **PPHN** | Persistent Pulmonary Hypertension |
| **PVR** | Pulmonary Vascular Resistance |
| **SVR** | Systemic Vascular Resistance |
| **USG** | Ultrasonography |

## CONSENT FOR PUBLICATION

Not applicable.

## CONFLICT OF INTEREST

The authors declare no conflict of interest, financial or otherwise.

## ACKNOWLEDGMENTS

I am first and foremost thankful to God almighty for making me write this chapter in these challenging times when the COVID-19 pandemic has severely halted every stream of life.

I am highly thankful to my colleague, also the co-author of the chapter, for her valuable contribution to writing and drafting this chapter.

## REFERENCES

[1]    Stinson L, Hallingström M, Barman M, *et al.* Comparison of bacterial DNA profiles in mid-trimester amniotic fluid samples from preterm and term deliveries. Front Microbiol 2020; 11: 415.
[http://dx.doi.org/10.3389/fmicb.2020.00415]

[2]    de Goffau MC, Lager S, Sovio U, *et al.* Human placenta has no microbiome but can contain potential pathogens. Nature 2019; 572(7769): 329-34.
[http://dx.doi.org/10.1038/s41586-019-1451-5] [PMID: 31367035]

[3]    Wiswell TE. Appropriate management of the non-vigorous meconium-stained neonate: An unanswered question. Pediatr 2018; 142: 6.

[4]    Narang A, Nair PM, Bhakoo ON, Vashisht K. Management of meconium stained amniotic fluid: a team approach. Indian Pediatr 1993; 30(1): 9-13.
[PMID: 8406722]

[5]    Bhat RY, Rao A. Meconium-stained amniotic fluid and meconium aspiration syndrome: a prospective study. Ann Trop Paediatr 2008; 28(3): 199-203.
[http://dx.doi.org/10.1179/146532808X335642] [PMID: 18727848]

[6]    Rokade J, Mule V, Solanke G. To study the perinatal outcome in meconium stained amniotic fluid. Inter J Scientific Res Publications 2016; 6: 7.

[7]    Steer PJ, Eigbe E, Lissauer TJ, Beard RW. Interrelationships Among Abnormal Cardiotocograms in Labor, Meconium Staining of the Amniotic Fluid, Arterial Cord Blood pH, and Apgar Scores. Obstet Anesthes Dig 1990; 10(1): 10.
[http://dx.doi.org/10.1097/00132582-199004000-00013]

[8]    Yoder BA, Kirsch EA, Barth WH Jr, Gordon MC. Changing obstetric practices associated with decreasing incidence of meconium aspiration syndrome. Obstet Gynecol 2002; 99(5, Part 1): 731-9.
[http://dx.doi.org/10.1097/00006250-200205000-00011] [PMID: 11978280]

[9]    Henry JA, Baker RW, Yanowitz TD. The in utero passage of meconium by very low birth weight infants: a marker for adverse outcomes. J Perinatol 2006; 26(2): 125-9.
[http://dx.doi.org/10.1038/sj.jp.7211435] [PMID: 16407963]

[10]   Trimmer KJ, Gilstrap LC III. "Meconiumcrit" and birth asphyxia. Am J Obstet Gynecol 1991; 165(4): 1010-3.
[http://dx.doi.org/10.1016/0002-9378(91)90460-9] [PMID: 1951504]

[11]   Park SK, Shin SH. Newly developed mecometer method for objective assessment of meconium content. J Korean Med Sci 2002; 17(1): 15-7.
[http://dx.doi.org/10.3346/jkms.2002.17.1.15] [PMID: 11850582]

[12]   Ghidini A, Spong CY. Severe meconium aspiration syndrome is not caused by aspiration of meconium. Am J Obstet Gynecol 2001; 185(4): 931-8.
[http://dx.doi.org/10.1067/mob.2001.116828] [PMID: 11641681]

[13]   Gupta SK, Haerr P, David R, Rastogi A, Pyati S. Meconium aspiration syndrome in infants of HIV-positive women: a case-control study. J Perinat Med 2016; 44(4): 469-75.
[http://dx.doi.org/10.1515/jpm-2014-0377] [PMID: 25999326]

[14]   Yurdakök M. Meconium aspiration syndrome: do we know? Turk J Pediatr 2011; 53(2): 121-9.
[PMID: 21853647]

[15]   Manning FA, Harman CR, Morrison I, Menticoglou S. Fetal assessment based on fetal biophysical profile scoring. Am J Obstet Gynecol 1990; 162(2): 398-402.
[http://dx.doi.org/10.1016/0002-9378(90)90395-N] [PMID: 2309823]

[16] Richey SD, Ramin SM, Bawdon RE, *et al.* Markers of acute and chronic asphyxia in infants with meconium-stained amniotic fluid. Am J Obstet Gynecol 1995; 172(4): 1212-5.
[http://dx.doi.org/10.1016/0002-9378(95)91481-1] [PMID: 7726258]

[17] Garg P, Saxena S. Comparison of hematological parameters among newborns with meconium stained amniotic fluid and clear amniotic fluid. Int J Contemp Pediatrics 2019; 6(6): 2480.
[http://dx.doi.org/10.18203/2349-3291.ijcp20194720]

[18] Nkadi PO, Merritt TA, Pillers DAM. An overview of pulmonary surfactant in the neonate: Genetics, metabolism, and the role of surfactant in health and disease. Mol Genet Metab 2009; 97(2): 95-101.
[http://dx.doi.org/10.1016/j.ymgme.2009.01.015] [PMID: 19299177]

[19] Malloy JL, Veldhuizen RAW, Thibodeaux BA, O'Callaghan RJ, Wright JR. *Pseudomonas aeruginosa* protease IV degrades surfactant proteins and inhibits surfactant host defense and biophysical functions. Am J Physiol Lung Cell Mol Physiol 2005; 288(2): L409-18.
[http://dx.doi.org/10.1152/ajplung.00322.2004] [PMID: 15516485]

[20] Moses D, Holm BA, Spitale P, Liu M, Enhorning G. Inhibition of pulmonary surfactant function by meconium. Am J Obstet Gynecol 1991; 164(2): 477-81.
[http://dx.doi.org/10.1016/S0002-9378(11)80003-7] [PMID: 1992687]

[21] Tyler DC, Murphy J, Cheney FW. Mechanical and chemical damage to lung tissue caused by meconium aspiration. Pediatrics 1978; 62(4): 454-9.
[http://dx.doi.org/10.1542/peds.62.4.454] [PMID: 714576]

[22] Vidyasagar D, Zagariya A. Studies of meconium-induced lung injury: inflammatory cytokine expression and apoptosis. J Perinatol 2008; 28(S3) (Suppl. 3): S102-7.
[http://dx.doi.org/10.1038/jp.2008.153] [PMID: 19057598]

[23] Zagariya A, Sierzputovska M, Navale S, Vidyasagar D. Role of meconium and hypoxia in meconium aspiration-induced lung injury in neonatal rabbits. Mediators Inflamm 2010; 2010: 1-6.
[http://dx.doi.org/10.1155/2010/204831] [PMID: 21234319]

[24] Romero R, Yoon BH, Chaemsaithong P, *et al.* Secreted phospholipase A $_2$ is increased in meconium-stained amniotic fluid of term gestations: potential implications for the genesis of meconium aspiration syndrome. J Matern Fetal Neonatal Med 2014; 27(10): 975-83.
[http://dx.doi.org/10.3109/14767058.2013.847918] [PMID: 24063538]

[25] Hofer N, Müller W, Resch B. CCLM.2011.048. Epub 1515; 2010(Dec): 3.

[26] K M, Faridi M, Singh N, Batra P. Procalcitonin as Predictor of Bacterial Infection in Meconium Aspiration Syndrome. Am J Perinatol 2018; 35(8): 769-73.
[http://dx.doi.org/10.1055/s-0037-1615793] [PMID: 29287292]

[27] Soukka H, Jalonen J, Kero P, Kääpä P. Endothelin-1, atrial natriuretic peptide and pathophysiology of pulmonary hypertension in porcine meconium aspiration. Acta Paediatr 1998; 87(4): 424-8.
[http://dx.doi.org/10.1111/j.1651-2227.1998.tb01472.x] [PMID: 9628300]

[28] Yeh TF. Core Concepts: Meconium Aspiration Syndrome: Pathogenesis and Current Management. Neoreviews 2010; 11(9): e503-12.
[http://dx.doi.org/10.1542/neo.11-9-e503]

[29] Hutton EK, Thorpe J. Consequences of meconium stained amniotic fluid: What does the evidence tell us? Early Hum Dev 2014; 90(7): 333-9.
[http://dx.doi.org/10.1016/j.earlhumdev.2014.04.005] [PMID: 24794305]

[30] Oliveira CPL, Flôr-de-Lima F, Rocha GMD, Machado AP, Guimarães Pereira Areias MHF. Meconium aspiration syndrome: risk factors and predictors of severity. J Matern Fetal Neonatal Med 2019; 32(9): 1492-8.
[http://dx.doi.org/10.1080/14767058.2017.1410700] [PMID: 29219011]

[31] Shaikh M, Irfan Waheed KA, Javaid S, Gul R, Hashmi MA, Fatima ST. Detrimental Complications Of

Meconium Aspiration Syndrome And Their Impact On Outcome. J Ayub Med Coll Abbottabad 2016; 28(3): 506-9.
[PMID: 28712223]

[32]   Louis D, Sundaram V, Mukhopadhyay K, Dutta S, Kumar P. Predictors of mortality in neonates with meconium aspiration syndrome. Indian Pediatr 2014; 51(8): 637-40.
[http://dx.doi.org/10.1007/s13312-014-0466-0] [PMID: 25128996]

[33]   Espinheira MC, Grilo M, Rocha G, Guedes B, Guimarães H. Meconium aspiration syndrome - the experience of a tertiary center. Rev Port Pneumol 2011; 17(2): 71-6.
[http://dx.doi.org/10.1016/S0873-2159(11)70017-4] [PMID: 21477569]

[34]   Edwards E, Lakshminrusimha S, Ehret D, Horbar J. NICU Admissions for Meconium Aspiration Syndrome before and after a National Resuscitation Program Suctioning Guideline Change. Children (Basel) 2019; 6(5): 68.
[http://dx.doi.org/10.3390/children6050068] [PMID: 31067816]

[35]   Narayanan A, Batra P, Faridi M, Harit D. PaO2/FiO2 Ratio as Predictor of Mortality in Neonates with Meconium Aspiration Syndrome. Am J Perinatol 2019; 36(6): 609-14.
[http://dx.doi.org/10.1055/s-0038-1672171] [PMID: 30282105]

[36]   Gidaganti S, Faridi MMA, Narang M, Batra P. Effect of Gastric Lavage on Meconium Aspiration Syndrome and Feed Intolerance in Vigorous Infants Born with Meconium Stained Amniotic Fluid — A Randomized Control Trial. Indian Pediatr 2018; 55(3): 206-10.
[http://dx.doi.org/10.1007/s13312-018-1318-0] [PMID: 29629694]

[37]   Cleary GM, Wiswell TE. Meconium-stained amniotic fluid and the meconium aspiration syndrome. An update. Pediatr Clin North Am 1998; 45(3): 511-29.
[http://dx.doi.org/10.1016/S0031-3955(05)70025-0] [PMID: 9653434]

[38]   Swaminathan S, Quinn J, Stabile MW, Bader D, Platzker ACG, Keens TG. Long-term pulmonary sequelae of meconium aspiration syndrome. J Pediatr 1989; 114(3): 356-61.
[http://dx.doi.org/10.1016/S0022-3476(89)80551-7] [PMID: 2921679]

[39]   Macfarlane PI, Heaf DP. Pulmonary function in children after neonatal meconium aspiration syndrome. Arch Dis Child 1988; 63(4): 368-72.
[http://dx.doi.org/10.1136/adc.63.4.368] [PMID: 3365005]

[40]   Liu J, Cao HY, Fu W. Lung ultrasonography to diagnose meconium aspiration syndrome of the newborn. J Int Med Res 2016; 44(6): 1534-42.
[http://dx.doi.org/10.1177/0300060516663954] [PMID: 27807253]

[41]   Gregory GA, Gooding CA, Phibbs RH, Tooley WH. Meconium aspiration in infants—a prospective study. J Pediatr 1974; 85(6): 848-52.
[http://dx.doi.org/10.1016/S0022-3476(74)80358-6] [PMID: 4472964]

[42]   Aziz K, Lee HC, Escobedo MB, Hoover AV, Kamath-Rayne BD, Kapadia VS, *et al.* Part 5: Neonatal Resuscitation: 2020 American Heart Association Guidelines for Cardiopulmonary Resuscitation and Emergency Cardiovascular Care Circulation 2020 Oct 20;142 (16_suppl_2).
[PMID: 26473001]

[43]   Nangia S, Sunder S, Biswas R, Saili A. Endotracheal suction in term non vigorous meconium stained neonates—A pilot study. Resuscitation 2016; 105: 79-84.
[http://dx.doi.org/10.1016/j.resuscitation.2016.05.015] [PMID: 27255954]

[44]   Chettri S, Adhisivam B, Bhat BV. Endotracheal Suction for Nonvigorous Neonates Born through Meconium Stained Amniotic Fluid: A Randomized Controlled Trial. J Pediatr 2015; 166(5): 1208-1213.e1.
[http://dx.doi.org/10.1016/j.jpeds.2014.12.076] [PMID: 25661412]

[45]   Yadav SK, Venkatnarayan K, Adhikari KM, Sinha R, Mathai SS. Gastric lavage in babies born through meconium stained amniotic fluid in prevention of early feed intolerance: A randomized

controlled trial. J Neonatal Perinatal Med 2018; 11(4): 393-7.
[http://dx.doi.org/10.3233/NPM-17154] [PMID: 30149474]

[46] Downes JJ, Vidyasagar D, Morrow GM, Boggs TR. Respiratory distress syndrome of newborn infants. I. New clinical scoring system (RDS score) with acid--base and blood-gas correlations. Clin Pediatr (Phila) 1970; 9(6): 325-31.
[http://dx.doi.org/10.1177/000992287000900607] [PMID: 5419441]

[47] Mazouri A, Fallah R, Saboute M, Taherifard P, Dehghan M. The prognostic value of the level of lactate in umbilical cord blood in predicting complications of neonates with meconium aspiration syndrome. J Matern Fetal Neonatal Med 2021; 34(7): 1-7.
[http://dx.doi.org/10.1080/14767058.2019.1623195] [PMID: 31340690]

[48] Goldsmith JP. Continuous positive airway pressure and conventional mechanical ventilation in the treatment of meconium aspiration syndrome. J Perinatol 2008; 28(S3) (Suppl. 3): S49-55.
[http://dx.doi.org/10.1038/jp.2008.156] [PMID: 19057611]

[49] Pandita A, Murki S, Oleti TP, *et al.* Effect of Nasal Continuous Positive Airway Pressure on Infants With Meconium Aspiration Syndrome. JAMA Pediatr 2018; 172(2): 161-5.
[http://dx.doi.org/10.1001/jamapediatrics.2017.3873] [PMID: 29204652]

[50] Dargaville PA. Respiratory support in meconium aspiration syndrome: a practical guide. Int J Pediatr 2012; 2012: 1-9.
[http://dx.doi.org/10.1155/2012/965159] [PMID: 22518190]

[51] Tingay DG, Mills JF, Morley CJ, Pellicano A, Dargaville PA. Australian and New Zealand Neonatal Network. Trends in use and outcome of newborn infants treated with high frequency ventilation in Australia and New Zealand, 1996-2003. J Paediatr Child Health 2007; 43(3): 160-6.

[52] Dargaville PA, Copnell B, Mills JF, *et al.* Randomized controlled trial of lung lavage with dilute surfactant for meconium aspiration syndrome. J Pediatr 2011; 158(3): 383-389.e2.
[http://dx.doi.org/10.1016/j.jpeds.2010.08.044] [PMID: 20947097]

[53] Henn R, Fiori RM, Fiori HH, *et al.* Surfactant with and without bronchoalveolar lavage in an experimental model of meconium aspiration syndrome. J Perinat Med 2016; 44(6): 685-9.
[http://dx.doi.org/10.1515/jpm-2014-0287] [PMID: 25719289]

[54] Recommendations for neonatal surfactant therapy. Paediatr Child Health 2005; 10(2): 109-16.
[PMID: 19668609]

[55] Ward MC, Sinn JKH. Steroid therapy for meconium aspiration syndrome in newborn infants. Cochrane Libr 2003; 2003(4): CD003485.
[http://dx.doi.org/10.1002/14651858.CD003485] [PMID: 14583981]

[56] Garg N, Choudhary M, Sharma D, Dabi D, Choudhary JS, Choudhary SK. The role of early inhaled budesonide therapy in meconium aspiration in term newborns: a randomized control study. J Matern Fetal Neonatal Med 2016; 29(1): 36-40.
[http://dx.doi.org/10.3109/14767058.2014.985202] [PMID: 25373430]

[57] Basu S, Kumar A, Bhatia BD, Satya K, Singh TB. Role of steroids on the clinical course and outcome of meconium aspiration syndrome-a randomized controlled trial. J Trop Pediatr 2007; 53(5): 331-7.
[http://dx.doi.org/10.1093/tropej/fmm035] [PMID: 17535827]

[58] Tripathi S, Saili A. The effect of steroids on the clinical course and outcome of neonates with meconium aspiration syndrome. J Trop Pediatr 2006; 53(1): 8-12.
[http://dx.doi.org/10.1093/tropej/fml018] [PMID: 16705003]

[59] Goel A, Nangia S, Saili A, Garg A, Sharma S, Randhawa VS. Role of prophylactic antibiotics in neonates born through meconium-stained amniotic fluid (MSAF)—a randomized controlled trial. Eur J Pediatr 2015; 174(2): 237-43.
[http://dx.doi.org/10.1007/s00431-014-2385-4] [PMID: 25084971]

[60] Natarajan CK, Sankar MJ, Jain K, Agarwal R, Paul VK. Surfactant therapy and antibiotics in neonates

with meconium aspiration syndrome: a systematic review and meta-analysis. J Perinatol 2016; 36(S1) (Suppl. 1): S49-54.
[http://dx.doi.org/10.1038/jp.2016.32] [PMID: 27109092]

[61]   Swarnam K, Soraisham AS, Sivanandan S. Advances in the management of meconium aspiration syndrome. Int J Pediatr 2012; 2012: 1-7.
[http://dx.doi.org/10.1155/2012/359571] [PMID: 22164183]

[62]   Kinsella JP, Abman SH. Inhaled nitric oxide and high frequency oscillatory ventilation in persistent pulmonary hypertension of the newborn. Eur J Pediatr 1998; 157(S1) (Suppl. 1): S28-30.
[http://dx.doi.org/10.1007/PL00014288] [PMID: 9462904]

[63]   Kopincová J, Mokrá D, Mikolka P, Kolomazník M, Čalkovská A. N-acetylcysteine advancement of surfactant therapy in experimental meconium aspiration syndrome: possible mechanisms. Physiol Res 2014; 63 (Suppl. 4): S629-42.
[http://dx.doi.org/10.33549/physiolres.932938] [PMID: 25669694]

[64]   Ivanov VA. Meconium aspiration syndrome treatment – New approaches using old drugs. Med Hypotheses 2006; 66(4): 808-10.
[http://dx.doi.org/10.1016/j.mehy.2005.09.046] [PMID: 16364559]

[65]   Carson BS, Losey RW, Bowes WA Jr, Simmons MA. Combined obstetric and pediatric approach to prevent meconium aspiration syndrome. Am J Obstet Gynecol 1976; 126(6): 712-5.
[http://dx.doi.org/10.1016/0002-9378(76)90525-1] [PMID: 984149]

[66]   Uhal BD, Abdul-Hafez A. Angiotensin II in apoptotic lung injury: potential role in meconium aspiration syndrome. J Perinatol 2008; 28(S3) (Suppl. 3): S108-12.
[http://dx.doi.org/10.1038/jp.2008.149] [PMID: 19057599]

[67]   Li AM, Zhang LN, Li WZ. Amelioration of meconium-induced acute lung injury by parecoxib in a rabbit model. Int J Clin Exp Med 2015; 8(5): 6804-12.
[PMID: 26221218]

[68]   Saugstad OD, Tølløfsrud PA, Lindenskov P, Drevon CA. Toxic effects of different meconium fractions on lung function: new therapeutic strategies for meconium aspiration syndrome? J Perinatol 2008; 28(S3) (Suppl. 3): S113-5.
[http://dx.doi.org/10.1038/jp.2008.151] [PMID: 19057600]

[69]   Ivanov VA, Gewolb IH, Uhal BD. A new look at the pathogenesis of the meconium aspiration syndrome: a role for fetal pancreatic proteolytic enzymes in epithelial cell detachment. Pediatr Res 2010; 68(3): 221-4.
[http://dx.doi.org/10.1203/PDR.0b013e3181ebd4c3] [PMID: 20551860]

[70]   Jeng MJ, Soong WJ, Lee YS, *et al.* Effects of therapeutic bronchoalveolar lavage and partial liquid ventilation on meconium-aspirated newborn piglets. Crit Care Med 2006; 34(4): 1099-105.
[http://dx.doi.org/10.1097/01.CCM.0000205662.60832.35] [PMID: 16484898]

**CHAPTER 8**

# Transient Tachypnea of the Newborn

**Fahri Ovali**[1,*]

[1] *Istanbul Medeniyet University, Faculty of Medicine, Department of Pediatrics, Division of Neonatology, Neonatal Intensive Care Unit, Göztepe Education and Traning Hospital, Kadıköy, Istanbul, Turkey*

**Abstract:** Transient Tachypnea of the Newborn (TTN) is the most common respiratory morbidity in term infants. In fetal life, the lungs are filled with fetal alveolar fluid, which is secreted by the alveolar epithelium through chloride channels. In late gestation and by the onset of labor, chloride-secreting channels switch to sodium-absorbing channels, and alveolar fluid is cleared away, leaving space for air after birth. Disorders that compromise the absorption of fetal lung fluid would end up in respiratory distress, tachypnea and hypoxemia. Elective cesarean section is the major risk factor for TTN, as well as other risk factors. Clinical features and chest radiograms are sufficient for the diagnosis. The disease is usually benign and self-limiting, but in some cases, respiratory support may be needed along with supportive treatment. The prognosis is usually good but with an increased risk of asthma in childhood.

**Keywords:** Alveolar epithelium, Amiloride, Asthma, Aquaporin, Beta-adrenergics, Cesarean section, Chloride channels, Cyanosis, Fetal alveolar fluid, Glucocorticoid, late preterm, Lung ultrasound, Mechanical ventilation, Oxygen, Preterm, Respiratory distress, Sodium channels, Surfactant, Tachypnea, Transient tachypnea, Vascular markings.

## INTRODUCTION

Transient Tachypnea of the Newborn (TTN) was first described by Avery *et al.* in 1966, and has been one of the most common causes of neonatal respiratory distress. Synonymous names include wet lung, respiratory distress type 2, and benign respiratory distress. Since most of the infants recover uneventfully, pathological findings are difficult to describe. Due to the same reason, the true incidence of the disease is not known, but it is estimated that the incidence is about 3.6 to 5.7 per 1000 term infants [1, 2], and almost 4% in late preterm infants [3]. In infants delivered by cesarean section before the onset of labor, respiratory

---

* **Corresponding author Fahri Ovali:** Istanbul Medeniyet University, Faculty of Medicine, Department of Pediatrics, Division of Neonatology, Neonatal Intensive Care Unit, Göztepe Education and Traning Hospital, Kadıköy, Istanbul, Turkey; Tel: +90 5324116715; Fax: +902166022805; E-mail: fahri.ovali@medeniyet.edu.tr

**Nima Rezaei and Noosha Samieefar (Eds.)**

symptoms occur in 35.5 infants per 1000, whereas in infants delivered by cesarean section with labor, the rate is 12.2 per 1000. This rate is 5.3 per 1000 births in infants delivered through the vaginal route [4]. Some mild cases of respiratory distress syndrome as well as infants with pulmonary maladaptation may actually be TTN. On the other hand, some persistent cases may actually be respiratory distress syndrome or may be called "malignant" tachypnea of the newborn.

## Dynamics of Fetal Lung Fluid

During fetal life, lungs are filled with Fetal Lung Fluid (FLF), which maintains alveolar distention and development. Although lungs receive only 10% of total cardiac output, this is sufficient for the production of FLF. Fetal lung fluid is produced by type I alveolar cells, fills in the alveolar space, and moves towards the trachea by fetal chest movements. Some of FLF is swallowed through the esophagus, while some of it joins the amniotic fluid. Since intratracheal pressure is almost 2 mm Hg higher than the amniotic fluid pressure, flow is maintained by the pressure gradient. Research in fetal lambs have revealed that FLF is produced 50 ml/kg per day in mid-trimester, increasing to 120 ml/kg per day in late-gestation [4]. The amount of fluid increases from 4-6 ml/kg body weight at mid-gestation to about 30-50 ml/kg near term in fetal lambs [5]. This increase is associated with increased pulmonary vasculature and increased epithelial surface [6]. A few days before vaginal delivery, the fluid begins to decrease to approximately 15-18 ml/kg [7]. Fetal lung fluid contains 157 meq/L chloride, and since fetal alveolar eptihelium is inpermeable to proteins, its protein and bicarbonate content are very low.

The activity of ions and water through the lung epithelium is analyzed in 3 phases:

1. Fetal phase: Although the protein content of the fetal lung interstitium and the osmotic gradient is high, alveolar epithelium actively secretes chloride to the airways, followed by obligatory water secretion. In spite of chloride secretion, sodium channels are inactive, and sodium absorption is very low. Chloride enters the epithelial cell through the basement membrane with sodium and potassium. Thereafter, with the help of the Na-K-ATPase enzyme at the basolateral membrane, sodium is exchanged with potassium, and it moves to the extracellular space. (3 sodium ions are exchanged for 2 potassium ions), increasing the chloride content of intracellular space. This reaction uses energy. Increased chloride within the cell crosses the apical membrane through Cystic Fibrosis Transmembrane Regulator (CTFR) and other chloride channels passively into the alveoli. Sodium is transferred into the alveoli through

paracellular routes. Water moves through the epithelial cells, and couples with chloride through water channels such as Aquaporin 5. Aquaporin 5 is expressed heavily on type 1 cell surfaces, and the majority of water transport occurs through these channels [8]. Type I cells are permeable to water, and secretes chloride to the alveoli also [9] (Fig. **1**). Low pH activates chloride channels, and increases FLF [10].

2. Transition phase: This stage involves the reversal in the direction of ions and water movement. It is expected that immediately before birth, the epithelium absorbs water from the alveoli and alveoli becomes ready to be filled with air after birth. This two-step process is completed in 2-6 hours by an interplay of change in sodium, potassium and chloride absorption, and secretion by Na-K-ATPase through amiloride-sensitive Epithelial Sodium Channels (ENaC) on the epithelial cell surface. The number of these channels is very low in preterm compared to term infants [11]. The first step is passive movement of sodium from lumen across the apical membrane into the cell through Na channels. The second step is active extrusion of sodium from the cell across the basolateral membrane into the serosal space. In the first step, by the intracellular transport of sodium, membrane potential begins to change, and chloride starts to move into the cell through chloride channels. A concomitant increase in Na-K-ATPase facilitates sodium absorption, followed by intracellular movement of water. Secretion of this fluid may be inhibited by bumetanide, which implies Na-K-2Cl co-transport [5]. In cases of oligohydramnios, the movement of FLF to the amniotic fluid is increased due to the increased pressure gradient, which results in decreased intraalveolar pressure and lung hypoplasia.

Amiloride blocks sodium transport on the luminal surface of the epithelium, whereas ouabain blocks Na-K-ATPase activity on the basolateral surface. The stress associated with preterm delivery does not affect sodium absorption; therefore, lung edema is frequently observed in preterm infants [9]. Glucocorticoids increase the expression of Na-K-ATPase, epithelial sodium channels and aquaporins as well as alpha, beta and gamma subunits of ENaC, which results in increased number and decreased breakdown of membrane channels [12].

Cation channels on the apical surface are the rate-limiting step, responsible for more than 90% of the resistance to the transcellular sodium transport [13]. In vaginally delivered infants, ENaC levels fall dramatically within 30 hours after birth. In preterm infants and in infants delivered through cesarean section, this fall is much slower. In other words, slow rates of epithelium sodium transport due to ENaC levels contribute to the development of TTN. The expression of sodium channels is regulated by the "microenvironment" which includes glucocorticoids, oxygen, beta-adrenergics and surfactant [14 - 17].

3   Postnatal phase: Pulmonary circulation increases after birth, triggering the absorption of FLF through several mechanisms. Lung epithelium switches from a predominantly chloride secreting membrane to a predominantly sodium absorbing membrane. With the start of active labor and increase in catecholamine secretion, the production of FLF decreases, coupled with an increase in its absorption. About two thirds of FLF is absorbed through these mechanisms, and the remainder one third is cleared away by respiratory movements. In elective cesarean sections where active labor does not begin, this mechanism does not work, and the risk of TTN is increased.

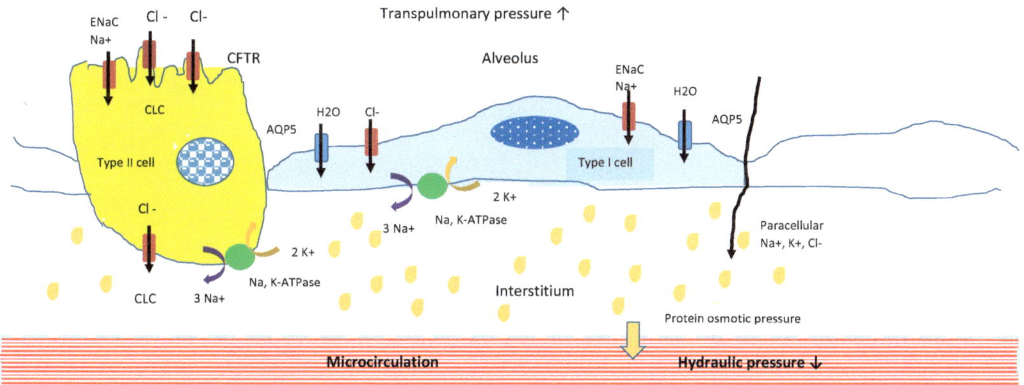


**Fig. (1).** With the onset of labor, sodium enters type I and type II cells through the apical surface *via* ENaC channels. Chloride uses the CFTR and Chloride Channels (CLC) to balance sodium. Increased sodium in the cell stimulates Na-K-ATPase at the basolateral membrane which promotes extrusion of 3 molecules of sodium from the cell and entrance of 2 molecules of potassium into the cell. This ion transport creates an osmotic gradient which transfers water into the intersititium by aquaporins (AQP5). The onset of respiration decreases the capillary hydrostatic pressure in the pulmonary circulation. Intersititial water is cleared by the pulmonary circulation and lymphatics.

Catecholamines stimulate the absorption of sodium, followed by the transport of water. Absorbed water is cleared from the lung by pulmonary circulation and lymphatics. Thyroid hormones, hydrocortisone, terbutalin and aminophyllin increase the absorption of water [18, 19]. Maturation of catecholamine receptors is increased towards term, which explains why preterm infants are more prone to TTN. In asphyxiated infants, acidification of intraalveolar fluid activates chloride channels and inhibits aquaporins, which result in decreased absorbtion of FLF and increased respiratory distress. Increased concentration of oxygen after birth also contributes to the shift of chloride secretion to sodium absorption [20]. Antenatal glucocorticoids and beta-adrenergic agonists increase the expression of RNA of ENaC subunits and aquaporins. However, the administration of adrenergic agents after birth is not effective in clearing the FLF [21].

Glucocorticoids stimulate transcription ENaC and induce sodium reabsorption in late gestation [12]. They increase the number of channels by decreasing their degradation and increasing the activity of existing channels. Glucocorticoids also enhance the responsiveness of lungs to beta-adrenergic agents and thyroid hormones [12, 22]. On the other hand, beta-agonists increase the activity of sodium channels in the lung through a cAMP-PKA mediated route.

Drainage of the FLF after birth is towards lung lymphatic, lung circulation, pleural space, mediastinum and upper airways. Lung lymphatics can clear only 15% of FLF [23]. With the onset of respiration, left atrium pressure and pulmonary circulation increase and most of the FLF is cleared by the pulmonary circulation. For a long time, it was believed that squeezing of the thoracic wall during vaginal labor contributed to the clearance of the FLF *via* trachea; but current evidence suggests that this mechanism is responsible for only a small portion of FLF clearance [19]. Compared to infants born through the vaginal route, thoracic volume of the infants born through cesarean section is 40% less.

After birth, alveolar fluid is not completely cleared away; a tiny layer of fluid remains on the epithelial surface, which serves as a barrier against various mechanical and chemical irritants [24]. Accumulation of fluid in the peribronchiolar lymphatics and intersititium leads to partial collapse of the bronchioles and air trapping. Continued perfusion of poorly ventilated alveoli leads to ventilation-perfusion mismatch,hypoxemia and hypercapnia.

## ETIOLOGY

Disturbances in the clearance of FLF would leave the fluid in the alveoli, where air should pour in. Risk factors include cesarean delivery, macrosomia, maternal diabetes or asthma, prolonged delivery especially after administration of magnesium sulphate to the mother, perinatal asphyxia, excessive fluid load to the mother and cardiogenic edema, twins and male gender [25].

Since the protein content of the FLF is low, its absorption is easy. In cases of asphyxia, change in capillary permeability or aspiration of amniotic fluid may increase the protein content of the FLF, hence slowing down its absorption. Excessive hypotonic fluid resuscitation to the mother during the delivery process may decrease the oncotic pressure and osmotic gradient, which results in attenuation of reabsorption. In cases of placental transfusion which increases the central venous pressure, hydrostatic pressure within the pulmonary capillaries may decrease the reabsorption process.

Genetic background of transient tachypnea of the newborn is controversial. Mild or moderate surfactant deficiency may cause TTN. However, in a study of surfactant gene polymorphisms, heterozygosity in the SP-B121ins2 gene and variations in the intron4 gene were not significantly different than those seen in healthy controls [26]. ENaC gene mutations are associated with pseudohypoaldosteronisms, but its association with TTN is unclear [27]. Some studies suggest that polymorphisms in the beta-adrenergic receptor genes may blunt the response to adrenergic stimuli, and would predispose the infant to TTN in the newborn period and to asthma later in life [28]. However, since many factors may influence surfactant protein structure, and are associated with disor-

ders of epithelial sodium channels, there is insufficient evidence regarding the genetic background of TTN.

The role of Nitric Oxide (NO) in the pathogenesis of TTN is also controversial. Asymmetric Dimethylarginine (ADMA) is an endogenous NO synthase inhibitor, and increased concentrations of ADMA may reduce NO synthesis, leading to pulmonary vascular resistance and fluid retention. ADMA levels are elevated in newborns with TTN [29]. Risk factors for TTN are summarized in Table **1**.

## CLINICAL FEATURES

Diagnosis of TTN is based on clinical and radiological findings, and most of the time, is a diagnosis of exclusion. Most prominent symptom is tachypnea, which starts within the first 1-2 hours after birth, and may be as high as 100-120 breaths per minute. Nasal flaring, grunting, intercostal retractions and cyanosis may ensue. Antero-posterior diameter of the chest may have increased (*i.e.* barrel chest) pushing down the liver and spleen towards the abdomen, making them palpable. Breath sounds are clear, without rales or ronchi. There is no "normal" length of time for tachypnea after birth; this may be arbitrarily between 2 -12 hours; but 6 hours is a reasonable limit since after this time, tachypnea may interfere with the nutrition of the infant [30]. In 75% of cases, these symptoms disappear by 48 hours, and the infant recovers completely. Shorter periods of tachypnea are referred as "transitional delay" or "adaptive delay". If at 6 hours of life, the respiratory symptoms are still prominent, oxygen requirement is more than 40%, and the infant has not recovered yet, s/he should be admitted to the neonatal intensive care unit. However, in some cases, it may last more than 72 hours. In such instances, other causes of tachypnea should be investigated [5]. Peak respiratory rate of 90 per minute or higher at 36 hours of life strongly suggests prolonged tachypnea [31].

The infant should be monitored by a pulse oximeter (One problem is that pulse oximeters appear to be influenced by skin colour) . Arterial blood gases are generally within normal limits, and respiratory or metabolic acidosis is very rare. Even if present, hypoxemia responds to less than 40% oxygen administration.

Rarely, some infants develop hypoxemia requiring high concentrations of oxygen (> 60%), and may need respiratory support including mechanical ventilation. If tachypnea persists beyond 5-6 days, an echocardiography should be obtained to rule out congenital heart disease.

**Table 1. Risk factors for transient tachypnea of the newborn.**

| |
|---|
| Preterm or late preterm birth |
| Cesarean section |
| Multiple births |
| Breech presentation |
| Nulliparity |
| Prolonged labor |
| Maternal diabetes mellitus |
| Hypotonic fluid administration to the mother |
| Macrosomia |
| Maternal asthma |
| Maternal obesity |
| Maternal drug use (narcotics) |
| Maternal epilepsy |
| Perinatal asphyxia |
| Male gender |
| Fetal hypothyroxinemia |

## LABORATORY FINDINGS

Complete blood count with differential is required to exclude infection and polycytemia. Sepsis markers such as C-Reactive Protein (CRP) and procalcitonin may be obtained if there is a strong suspicion of sepsis.

Chest radiography reveals areas of overaeration with perihilar radial vascular markings, cardiomegaly, widening of intercostal spaces, flattening of diaphragmatic contours and edema of interlobar septums (Fig. **2**). Perihilar markings are the result of engorgement of periarterial lymphatic channels which are filled with FLF cleared from the alveoli. However, in respiratory distress syndrome, there is reticulo-granular appearance and air bronchograms, all of which render the differential diagnosis easier. Radiological findings may begin to improve by 24 hours, but may last 3-7 days in some cases.

Lung ultrasound may be used in the diagnosis of TTN. In an infant with TTN, pleural line and pleural sliding are seen normally. In the lower lung fields, compact B lines may be evident whereas in the upper lung fields, compact B lines are less pronounced; this is known as "double lung point". Lung consolidation excludes TTN [32, 33] (Fig. **3**).

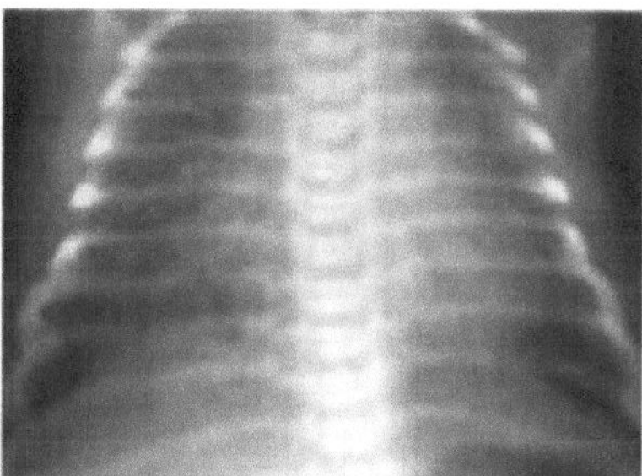

**Fig. (2).** Chest radiography in transient tachypnea of the newborn. The lungs are well-aerated but vascular markings are prominent at the hilum.

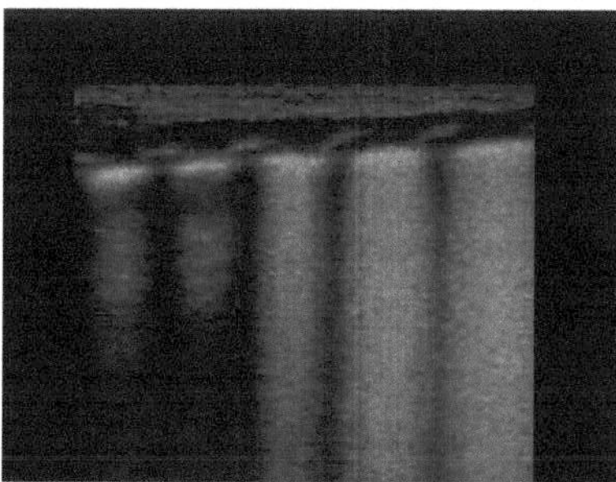

**Fig. (3).** Lung ultrasonography in the transient tachypnea of the newborn. Compact B lines are prominent in the lower lung fields whereas less compact B lines are seen in the upper lung fields (double lung point).

## DIFFERENTIAL DIAGNOSIS

Although the symptoms and clinical findings may be similar to those of respiratory distress syndrome, lung radiography features make the diagnosis easier. In cases of severe hypercarbia, another diagnosis should be contemplated. Tachypnea may be the result of a central irritation, frequently as a result of perinatal asphyxia. However, in such cases, history of asphyxia during delivery and relevant laboratory results may lead to correct diagnosis. In cases of sepsis, results of cultures and other ancillary laboratory findings may help the diagnosis. Other diseases that should be excluded include pneumonia, congenital heart diseases, aspiration syndromes, metabolic disorders, polycytemia and other neurological disorders. Tachypnea due to metabolic acidosis can be ruled out by measurement of capillary blood gas. Causes of tachypnea in the newborn infant are summarized in Table **2**.

**Table 2. Causes of tachypnea in the term newborn infant.**

| |
|---|
| Transient tachypnea of the newborn |
| Pneumonia |
| Aspiration syndromes (meconium, blood, amniotic fluid) |
| Congenital malformations (congenital diaphragmatic hernia, cystic adenomatoid malformations) |
| Central nervous system irritation (Perinatal asphyxia or intracranial hemorrhage) |
| Pulmonary hypertension |
| Pulmonary edema (anomalous venous drainage, left-to-right shunts, *i.e.* patent ductus arteriosus) |
| Air leaks |
| Metabolic acidosis |
| Respiratory distress syndrome |

## MANAGEMENT

TTN is a self-limiting condition, and in most cases, supportive treatment is sufficient. Oxygenation is the primary goal, and not more than 40% of $FiO_2$ is needed to keep the oxygen saturation above 90%, generally provided by hood or nasal cannula. Cardiopulmonary monitorization, maintaing neutral thermal environment, providing nutrition, blood glucose and fluid management and observing for possible signs of an infection are required. Mechanical ventilation is not generally needed. Monitorization of oxygen saturation with pulse oxymeter blood gas analysis would suffice in most cases. Restricted fluids administration is recommended, and shortens the duration of respiratory support in these infants [34, 35]. Fluid therapy should be adjusted according to the needs of the infant, and should not exceed 50-60 ml/kg in the first few days of life. Caution should be taken while feeding the infant. Routine antibiotics are not recommended; if there is a strong suspicion of infection, antibiotics may be administered until the cultures are proven negative by 48 hours. If the respiratory rate is more than 60-80 breaths per minute, oral feeding should be withheld, and the infant should be started on IV fluids, and fed with an orogastric tube. If however, the respiratory rate is more than 80 breaths per minute, enteral feeding should be stopped. Re-feeding should be started in a gentle manner by advancing volume in small increments.

In persistent cases, a single dose of furosemide has been used to help clear the alveoli, but this approach is not evidence-based, and is not recommended. Inhaled racemic epinephrine, inhaled beta-agonists and inhaled corticosteroids are also not recommended during the management of TTN [36-41]. Tachypnea rarely persists to 7 days.

## PREVENTION

Although TTN is a benign condition, it may be frustrating to the family and physicians since it may require transfer of the infant to a neonatal intensive care unit, separation from the mother, multiple diagnostic studies, delay in discharge, prolonged hospitalization and increased healthcare costs [5]. Elective cesarean operations should not be performed before 39 weeks of completed gestation, and vaginal delivery should be advocated unless a medical indication exists for operative delivery. In cases of elective cesarean section in late preterm infants, administration of antenatal steroids may decrease neonatal morbidities, and should be contemplated and discussed with the mother [42]. The American College of Obstetrics and Gynecology (ACOG) provides criteria for establishing fetal lung maturity before elective cesarean section. Spinal anesthesia may be preferred instead of general anesthesia for cesarean section [43].

## PROGNOSIS

Transient tachypnea of the newborn is a benign disease, and most patients recover within 48 hours. Tachypnea does not recur. Infants born to mothers who have asthma are at higher risk for the development of TTN, and infants who have TTN have an increased risk of asthma diagnosed at preschool. This association is stronger in male infants [44, 45].

## CONCLUSION

Transient tachypnea of the newborn is the most common respiratory disease in term infants and results from the delayed absorption of fetal lung fluid during and after labor. Although it is a benign and self-limiting disease, care should be taken to exclude other causes of respiratory distress and the family should be counseled accordingly. Rarely, some patients may need respiratory support. Avoidance of elective cesarean section is the mainstay of prevention.

## CONSENT FOR PUBLICATION

Not applicable.

## CONFLICT OF INTEREST

The authors declare no conflict of interest, financial or otherwise.

## ACKNOWLEDGEMENT

Declared none.

# REFERENCES

[1]     Field DJ, Milner AD, Hopkin IE, Madeley RJ. Changing patterns in neonatal respiratory diseases. Pediatr Pulmonol 1987; 3(4): 231-5.
[http://dx.doi.org/10.1002/ppul.1950030407] [PMID: 3658528]

[2]     Morrison JJ, Rennie JM, Milton PJ. Neonatal respiratory morbidity and mode of delivery at term: influence of timing of elective caesarean section. BJOG 1995; 102(2): 101-6.
[http://dx.doi.org/10.1111/j.1471-0528.1995.tb09060.x] [PMID: 7756199]

[3]     Jain L. Respiratory morbidity in late-preterm infants: prevention is better than cure! Am J Perinatol 2008; 25(2): 075-8.
[http://dx.doi.org/10.1055/s-2007-1022471] [PMID: 18214813]

[4]     Cassin S, Gause G, Perks AM. The effects of bumetanide and furosemide on lung liquid secretion in fetal sheep. Exp Biol Med (Maywood) 1986; 181(3): 427-31.
[http://dx.doi.org/10.3181/00379727-181-42276] [PMID: 3945652]

[5]     Guglani L, Lakshminrusimha S, Ryan RM. Transient tachypnea of the newborn. Pediatrics in review 2008; 29(11): e59-65.

[6]     Lines A, Hooper SB, Harding R. Lung liquid production rates and volumes do not decrease before labor in healthy fetal sheep. J Appl Physiol 1997; 82(3): 927-32.
[http://dx.doi.org/10.1152/jappl.1997.82.3.927] [PMID: 9074984]

[7]     Kıtterman J. Ballard PL,Clements JA, Mescher EJ, Tooley WH. *Tracheal fluid in fetal lambs: spontaneous decrease before birth.* J Appl Physiol 1979; 47: 985-9.
[http://dx.doi.org/10.1152/jappl.1979.47.5.985] [PMID: 41832]

[8]     Li Y, Marcoux MO, Gineste M, Vanpee M, Zelenina M, Casper C. Expression of water and ion transporters in tracheal aspirates from neonates with respiratory distress. Acta Paediatr 2009; 98(11): 1729-37.
[http://dx.doi.org/10.1111/j.1651-2227.2009.01496.x] [PMID: 19719801]

[9]     Keene SD. Lung fluid balance during development and in neonatal lung disease.The newborn lung Neonatology questions and controversies. 3rd edition ed.., Philadelphia: Saunders-elsevier 2019.

[10]    Blaisdell CJ, Edmonds RD, Wang XT, Guggino S, Zeitlin PL. pH-regulated chloride secretion in fetal lung epithelia. Am J Physiol Lung Cell Mol Physiol 2000; 278(6): L1248-55.
[http://dx.doi.org/10.1152/ajplung.2000.278.6.L1248] [PMID: 10835331]

[11]    Helve O, Janér C, Pitkänen O, Andersson S. Expression of the epithelial sodium channel in airway epithelium of newborn infants depends on gestational age. Pediatrics 2007; 120(6): 1311-6.
[http://dx.doi.org/10.1542/peds.2007-0100] [PMID: 18055681]

[12]    Venkatesh VC, Katzberg HD. Glucocorticoid regulation of epithelial sodium channel genes in human fetal lung. Am J Physiol 1997; 273(1 Pt 1): L227-33.
[PMID: 9252560]

[13]    Chen XJ. Mechanisms and regulation of ion transport in adult mammalian alveolar type II pneumocytes. American Journal of Physiology-Cell Physiology 1991; 261: c727-38.

[14]    Chen XJ, Eaton DC, Jain L. β-Adrenergic regulation of amiloride-sensitive lung sodium channels. Am J Physiol Lung Cell Mol Physiol 2002; 282(4): L609-20.
[http://dx.doi.org/10.1152/ajplung.00356.2001] [PMID: 11880285]

[15]    Renard S, Voilley N, Bassilana F, Lazdunski M, Barbry P. Localization and regulation by steroids of the?? and? subunits of the amiloride-sensitive Na+ channel in colon, lung and kidney. Pflugers Arch 1995; 430(3): 299-307.
[http://dx.doi.org/10.1007/BF00373903] [PMID: 7491252]

[16]    Garty H, Benos DJ. Characteristics and regulatory mechanisms of the amiloride-blockable Na+ channel. Physiol Rev 1988; 68(2): 309-73.

[http://dx.doi.org/10.1152/physrev.1988.68.2.309] [PMID: 2451832]

[17] Guidot DM, Modelska K, Lois M, *et al.* Ethanol ingestion *via* glutathione depletion impairs alveolar epithelial barrier function in rats. Am J Physiol Lung Cell Mol Physiol 2000; 279(1): L127-35.
[http://dx.doi.org/10.1152/ajplung.2000.279.1.L127] [PMID: 10893211]

[18] Barker PM, Walters DV, Markiewicz M, Strang LB. Development of the lung liquid reabsorptive mechanism in fetal sheep: synergism of triiodothyronine and hydrocortisone. J Physiol 1991; 433(1): 435-49.
[http://dx.doi.org/10.1113/jphysiol.1991.sp018436] [PMID: 1841951]

[19] Chapman DL, Carlton DP, Nielson DW, Cummings JJ, Poulain FR, Bland RD. Changes in lung lipid during spontaneous labor in fetal sheep. J Appl Physiol 1994; 76(2): 523-30.
[http://dx.doi.org/10.1152/jappl.1994.76.2.523] [PMID: 8175558]

[20] Ramminger SJ, Baines DL, Olver RE, Wilson SM. The effects of $P_{O2}$ upon transepithelial ion transport in fetal rat distal lung epithelial cells. J Physiol 2000; 524(2): 539-47.
[http://dx.doi.org/10.1111/j.1469-7793.2000.t01-1-00539.x] [PMID: 10766932]

[21] Finley N, Norlin A, Baines DL, Folkesson HG. Alveolar epithelial fluid clearance is mediated by endogenous catecholamines at birth in guinea pigs. J Clin Invest 1998; 101(5): 972-81.
[http://dx.doi.org/10.1172/JCI1478] [PMID: 9486967]

[22] Jobe AH, Ikegami M, Padbury J, *et al.* Combined effects of fetal beta agonist stimulation and glucocorticoids on lung function of preterm lambs. Neonatology 1997; 72(5): 305-13.
[http://dx.doi.org/10.1159/000244497] [PMID: 9395841]

[23] Bland RD, Hansen TN, Haberkern CM, *et al.* Lung fluid balance in lambs before and after birth. J Appl Physiol 1982; 53(4): 992-1004.
[http://dx.doi.org/10.1152/jappl.1982.53.4.992] [PMID: 7153132]

[24] Jain L, Eaton DC. Physiology of fetal lung fluid clearance and the effect of labor. Seminars in Perinatology 2006; 30(1): 34-43.

[25] Crowley MA. Neonatal respiratory disorders.Fanaroff and martin's neonatal-perinatal medicine Diseases of the fetus and infant. 11th ed. St louis: Elsevier 2020; pp. 1203-30.

[26] Tutdibi E, Hospes B, Landmann E, *et al.* Transient tachypnea of the newborn (TTN): a role for polymorphisms of surfactant protein B (SP-B) encoding gene? Klin Padiatr 2003; 215(5): 248-52.
[http://dx.doi.org/10.1055/s-2003-42670] [PMID: 14520584]

[27] Edelheit O, Hanukoglu I, Gizewska M, *et al.* Novel mutations in epithelial sodium channel (ENaC) subunit genes and phenotypic expression of multisystem pseudohypoaldosteronism. Clin Endocrinol (Oxf) 2005; 62(5): 547-53.
[http://dx.doi.org/10.1111/j.1365-2265.2005.02255.x] [PMID: 15853823]

[28] Aslan E, Tutdibi E, Martens S, Han Y, Monz D, Gortner L. Transient tachypnea of the newborn (TTN): A role for polymorphisms in the β-adrenergic receptor (ADRB) encoding genes? Acta Paediatr 2008; 97(10): 1346-50.
[http://dx.doi.org/10.1111/j.1651-2227.2008.00888.x] [PMID: 18540901]

[29] Isik DU, Bas AY, Demirel N, *et al.* Increased asymmetric dimethylarginine levels in severe transient tachypnea of the newborn. J Perinatol 2016; 36(6): 459-62.
[http://dx.doi.org/10.1038/jp.2016.9] [PMID: 26866680]

[30] Hagen E, Chu A, Lew C. Transient tachypnea of the newborn. Neoreviews 2017; 18(3): e141-8.
[http://dx.doi.org/10.1542/neo.18-3-e141]

[31] Gowen CW Jr, Lawson EE, Gingras J, Boucher RC, Gatzy JT, Knowles MR. Electrical potential difference and ion transport across nasal epithelium of term neonates: Correlation with mode of delivery, transient tachypnea of the newborn, and respiratory rate. J Pediatr 1988; 113(1): 121-7.
[http://dx.doi.org/10.1016/S0022-3476(88)80545-6] [PMID: 3385520]

[32]　Palacio M, Bonet-carne E, Cobo T, Perez-moreno A, Sabrià J. Prediction of neonatal respiratory morbidity by quantitative ultrasound lung texture analysis: A multicenter study. American Journal of Obstetrics and Gynecology 2017; 217(2): 196.e1-196.e14.

[33]　Sharma D, Farahbakhsh N. Role of chest ultrasound in neonatal lung disease: a review of current evidences. J Matern Fetal Neonatal Med 2019; 32(2): 310-6.
[http://dx.doi.org/10.1080/14767058.2017.1376317] [PMID: 28870125]

[34]　Stroustrup A, Trasande L. Randomized controlled trial of restrictive fluid management in transient tachypnea of the newborn. The Journal of Pediatrics 2012; 160: 38-43.

[35]　Dehdashtian M, Aramesh MR, Melekian A, Aletayeb MH, Ghaemmaghami A. Restricted versus standard maintenance fluid volume in management of transient tachypnea of newborn: a clinical trial. Iran J Pediatr 2014; 24(5): 575-80.
[PMID: 25793064]

[36]　Kassab M, Khriesat WM, Bawadi H, Anabrees J. Furosemide for transient tachypnoea of the newborn. Cochrane database of systematic reviews 2013; (6): CD003064.

[37]　Kao B, Stewart de Ramirez SA, Belfort MB, Hansen A. Inhaled epinephrine for the treatment of transient tachypnea of the newborn. J Perinatol 2008; 28(3): 205-10.
[http://dx.doi.org/10.1038/sj.jp.7211917] [PMID: 18200024]

[38]　Armangil D, Yurdakök M, Korkmaz A, Yiğit Ş, Tekinalp G. Inhaled beta-2 agonist salbutamol for the treatment of transient tachypnea of the newborn. The Journal of Pediatrics 2011; 159: 398-403.
[http://dx.doi.org/10.1016/j.jpeds.2011.02.028]

[39]　Moresco L, Bruschettini M, Cohen A. Salbutamol for transient tachypnea of the newborn. Cochrane Database Syst Rev 2016; (5): CD011878.

[40]　Du X. Epinephrine for transient tachypnea of the newborn. Cochrane database of systematic reviews 2016; (5): CD011877.

[41]　Vaisbourd Y, Abu-Raya B, Zangen S, et al. Inhaled corticosteroids in transient tachypnea of the newborn: A randomized, placebo-controlled study. Pediatr Pulmonol 2017; 52(8): 1043-50.
[http://dx.doi.org/10.1002/ppul.23756] [PMID: 28672098]

[42]　Smith GC. Antenatal betamethasone for women at risk for late preterm delivery. N Engl J Med 2016; 375(5): 486.
[PMID: 27518672]

[43]　Ozden Omaygenc D, Dogu T, Omaygenc MO, et al. Type of anesthesia affects neonatal wellbeing and frequency of transient tachypnea in elective cesarean sections. J Matern Fetal Neonatal Med 2015; 28(5): 568-72.
[http://dx.doi.org/10.3109/14767058.2014.926328] [PMID: 24844161]

[44]　Liem JJ, Huq SI, Ekuma O, Becker AB, Kozyrskyj AL. Transient tachypnea of the newborn may be an early clinical manifestation of wheezing symptoms. J Pediatr 2007; 151(1): 29-33.
[http://dx.doi.org/10.1016/j.jpeds.2007.02.021] [PMID: 17586187]

[45]　Schatz M, Zeiger RS, Hoffman CP, Saunders BS, Harden KM, Forsythe AB. Increased transient tachypnea of the newborn in infants of asthmatic mothers. Am J Dis Child 1991; 145(2): 156-8.
[PMID: 1994679]

CHAPTER 9

# Fetal Tumors: Diagnosis and Management

**Forough Jabbari[1], Parnian Jabbari[2,3], Nazanin Taraghikhah[2,3], Behnaz Moradi[4,5] and Nima Rezaei[2,5,6,*]**

[1] *Department of Gynecology, Yas Women's Hospital, Tehran University of Medical Sciences, Tehran, Iran*

[2] *Network of Immunity in Infection, Malignancy and Autoimmunity (NIIMA), Universal Scientific Education and Research Network (USERN), Tehran, Iran*

[3] *Department of Radiology, Yas Women's Hospital, Tehran University of Medical Sciences, Tehran, Iran*

[4] *Department of Radiology, Advanced Diagnostic and Interventional Radiology Research Center (ADIR), Medical Imaging Center, Imam Khomeini Hospital Complex, Tehran University of Medical Sciences, Tehran, Iran*

[5] *Research Center for Immunodeficiencies, Children's Medical Center, Tehran University of Medical Sciences, Tehran, Iran*

[6] *Department of Immunology, School of Medicine, Tehran University of Medical Sciences, Tehran, Iran*

**Abstract:** Tumors can be formed in any organ throughout life. The fetal period is no exception to this fact, and it is important to diagnose these tumors as soon as possible to provide timely care to patients. If management is halted, tumors can cause complications in delivery, child development and even death. In this chapter, we discuss the diagnosis and management of several common fetal tumors. We also overview possible future directions in the management of tumors found during the fetal period.

**Keywords:** Broncho-Pulmonary Sequestration, Cancer, Congenital Cystic Adenomatoid Malformation, Diagnostic imaging, Fetal development, Fetal tumors, Glioma, Gynecology, Heart rhabdomyoma, Intracranial tumors, Interstitial Lung Tumors, Kidney tumors, Liver tumors, Management, Obstetrics, Ovarian masses, Pelvic tumors, Perinatal care, Pleuro-Pulmonary Blastoma, Pregnancy, Teratoma.

* **Corresponding author Nima Rezaei:** Research Center for Immunodeficiencies, Children's Medical Center Hospital, Dr. Qarib St, Keshavarz Blvd, Tehran 14194, Iran; Tel: +9821-6692-9234; Fax: +9821-6692-9235; E-mail: rezaei_nima@tums.ac.ir

## INTRODUCTION

Cancers occur at any age and can involve any tissue in the body. Even though the risk of cancers increases with aging as a result of the accumulation of carcinogenic mutations and decreased host immune response to cancer cells, some cancers have a predilection for young individuals [1, 2], such as Leukemia, Neuroblastoma and Wilm's tumor [3]. Rarely, cancers occur before birth, during the fetal period, and their prevalence is estimated to be around 2 to 14 in 100,000 live births [4 - 6]. However, the exact prevalence of fetal cancers cannot be determined as they can remain undiagnosed or be misdiagnosed during pregnancy. These tumors can remain asymptomatic, or can manifest as polyhydramnios or even intrauterine fetal demise, which in many cases are not further investigated. Most fetal masses are benign, however, about 40% of them are malignant based on postnatal investigations [4]. As is the case for other malignancies, timely diagnosis of fetal cancers is important in that decisions regarding prenatal treatment and route of delivery, as well as postnatal care must be made as soon as possible.

Fetal cancers are challenging in many respects. Firstly, their diagnosis is mostly incidental, and usually, an accurate diagnosis is not possible until after delivery, when a histopathologic examination can be performed [7]. Another challenge is the lack of precise guidelines for the management of fetal cancers. Our knowledge regarding the management of fetal cancers is confined to a few case reports. On the other hand, many of the diagnostic tools for the detection of cancers are prohibited during pregnancy [8]. Furthermore, there is no consensus on the management of fetal malignancies.

In this chapter, we describe the most common malignancies of the prenatal period and diagnostic tools for their detection. Current management and possible future directions in the treatment of these cancers are also discussed.

## THE MOST COMMON PRENATAL TUMORS

Many of the tumors that are common in the prenatal period are not malignant. However, we mention all common fetal tumors, regardless of being malignant. Table **1** summarizes some of the most common fetal tumors and malignancies.

**Table 1. Common tumors found during fetal period.**

| Tumor | Incidence | Presentation/ complications. |
|---|---|---|
| Sacrococcygeal Teratoma | ~1 in 40000 live births [9] | Dystocia, fetal hydrops and arrest of delivery. |
| Heart tumors | ~1 in 1000 pregnancies [10] | Arrhythmias and reduced contractility. |

*(Table 1) cont.....*

| Tumor | Incidence | Presentation/ complications. |
|---|---|---|
| Brain tumors | ~1 in 500000 live births [11] | Polyhydramnios and decreased fetal movement. |
| Neuroblastoma | ~1 in 100000 live births [12] | Mass (mostly adrenal). |
| Wilm's tumor | ~1 in 63000 live births [13] | Polyhydramnios and fetal hydrops. |

To date, there is no consensus regarding the classification of prenatal tumors. However, an acceptable classification based on the location of these tumors was proposed by Meinzer [14]. He classified locations in which the tumors arise into four major categories, including 1) head and brain, 2) face and neck, 3) thorax and 4) abdomen and retroperitoneum, as well as four minor locations being 1) extremities, 2) genitalia, 3) sacrococcygeal region and 4) skin. We follow a similar classification for the tumors reviewed.

**Intracranial Tumors**

The prevalence of intracranial tumors varies between 0.34 to 3.4 per one million live births, due to different temporal classifications [11, 15]. However, their incidence has increased in the past two decades [16]. These tumors either remain asymptomatic, or present with non-specific manifestations such as hydrocephalus, macrocephaly or intracranial mass. Ultrasound (US) is the first-line diagnostic tool in the detection of intracranial lesions. Further imaging investigation using Computed Tomography (CT) and Magnetic Resonance Imaging (MRI) can unveil more details regarding the lesion. Intracranial lesions other than tumors, such as vascular malformations or hemorrhage must be considered as well [17]. A definite diagnosis is mostly halted until after birth following a histopathologic study. Unlike many other fetal cancers, tumors of the Central Nervous System (CNS) are sporadic, and not associated with other abnormalities such as aneuploidy [18]. These tumors are associated with poor prognosis and mostly lead to death either prenatally or shortly after birth [18]. The survival rate for tumors of the CNS is reported to be approximately 28% [19].

*Teratoma*

Teratomas are the most common tumors of the CNS diagnosed perinatally [20], and account for 27%-62% of prenatal CNS tumors in different series [11, 18, 19, 21]. Even though they are benign in nature, they have the worst outcome of intracranial tumors and have an overall survival of as low as 10% [20, 22]. Their prognosis is greatly affected by tumor size, and gestational age at diagnosis and larger tumors, and those diagnosed at an earlier gestational age have worse prognoses. On imaging, teratomas present as heterogeneous masses mostly due to cysts resulting from necrotic lesions, and to a lesser extent due to hemorrhage within the mass. Cystic lesions can help differentiate teratomas from other intracranial masses with a heterogeneous presentation [20]. Teratomas are commonly observed in cerebral hemispheres followed by third and lateral ventricles [19, 23]. They are often large, and can replace the entire normal brain tissue [20].

## *Glioma*

Gliomas are the second most common prenatal CNS tumors, and account for approximately 25% of these tumors [24]. They are mostly low-grade during the fetal period (*i.e.* astrocytoma). However, the CNS can give rise to high-grade gliomas such as glioblastoma multiforme prenatally. These tumors are mostly located in the cerebral hemispheres, and they can distort the brain structure by displacing ventricles, which can lead to hydrocephalus and expansion of the cranium. Similar to teratomas, they appear as large, heterogeneous masses, however, their heterogeneity is mainly due to intratumoral hemorrhage. The outcome of the tumor depends on various factors such as the size of the tumor and its histology [25].

## *Other Intracranial Tumors*

Other intracranial tumors include craniopharyngioma, ependymomas, primitive neuroectodermal tumors, choroid plexus papillomas, and medulloblastoma, to name a few. The most common of these are craniopharyngiomas which are benign epithelial tumors arising from remnants of Rathke's pouch and account for up to 11% of congenital brain tumors [20]. They are mostly detected in the third trimester as midline heterogeneous masses with cysts and foci of calcifications [26].

## Thoracic Tumors

Many of the intrathoracic lesions during the fetal period are cystic lesions; however, solid or microcystic lesions are also common. Therefore, it is important to always consider malignancies when faced with a cystic lesion in the thoracic cavity during prenatal assessments. The prevalence of these tumors is different in various series. In a series of 84 fetal tumors detected among 4895 fetal malformations, thoracic tumors were the most common tumors, with heart tumors accounting for the majority of cases, and they can complicate about 0.2% of pregnancies, and cause fetal heart failure [27 - 29]. Most of these tumors are benign, and occur earlier in the course of pregnancy, in contrast to the malignant tumors that present in the late-second to the third trimester [30]. Even though many tumors can be present in the thoracic cavity, such as neuroblastomas, in this section, we focus on the tumors whose most common origins are the lungs and the heart.

## Congenital Cystic Adenomatoid Malformation (CCAM)

CCAMs are benign lung tumors resulting from overgrowth of terminal bronchioles accompanied by a reduced number of alveoli [31]. They are relatively rare with an approximate prevalence of 1:25,000 live births with a predilection towards the male gender [32, 33]. CCAMs can be detected *via* US as early as the second trimester. Appearance of CCAMs can vary from mostly solid masses and unilobar to purely cystic masses, frequently observed in the left lobe (Fig. **1**) [31]. These lesions can be differentiated from malignant lesions as they begin to regress in the third trimester [34]. The prognosis for fetal CCAMs varies from 9% to 49% in different series.

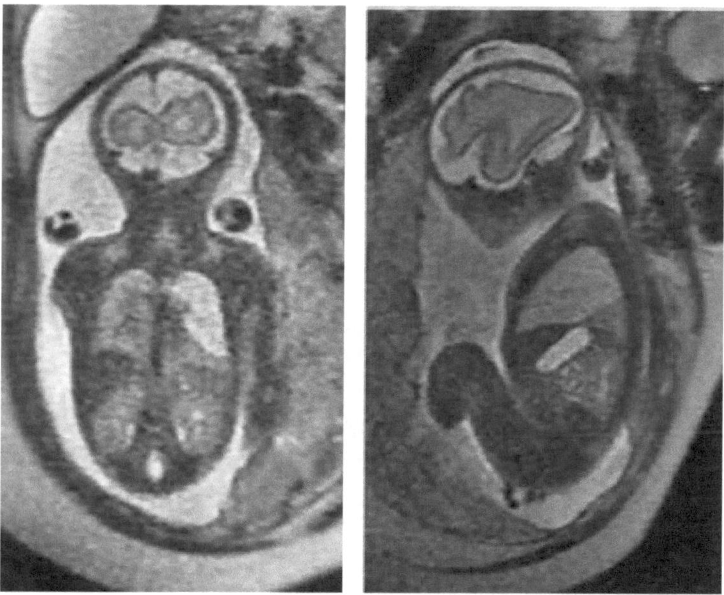

**Fig. (1).**  High T2 signal mass in left hemithorax without systemic artery found in the third trimester, suggestive of CCAM. Post-natal evaluation confirms the diagnosis of CCAM type 3.

## Broncho-Pulmonary Sequestration (BPS)

BPS is a rare, benign, nonfunctioning mass of the lung isolated from the tracheobronchial tree. These lesions can be either intralobar or extralobar, the latter usually placed in the abdominal cavity, and are associated with diaphragmatic hernias [35]. The incidence of BPS is estimated to be 1 in 15000 births with a male predilection [36]. These tumors can be detected in the prenatal US, as early as early second trimester, presenting as hyper-echogenic solid masses, mostly found in lower left lobes. Lesions diagnosed before week 26 of gestation are associated with a poorer prognosis, and may lead to mediastinal shift, polyhydramnios, hydrops and fetal demise [37, 38]. PBS is reported to be associated with other anomalies, especially those of the thorax such as tracheoesophageal fistula, esophageal duplication and diverticula, as well as esophageal and bronchogenic cysts [39 - 42].

### *Pleuro-Pulmonary Blastoma (PPB)*

Even though rare when compared to other fetal lung abnormalities, these tumors are the most common malignancies of the lung in the fetal period [43]. Thus far, around 500 cases of PPB have been reported, and the prevalence of these tumors is estimated at around 1: 250,000 live births [44], many of which are associated with other malignancies [43]. On imaging, these tumors can be difficult to distinguish from other lung abnormalities, especially airway malformations. In the US, these lesions appear as either pure cystic, mostly solid or a mix of two, which is the basis for their classification as type I, type III, and type II, respectively [45]. The overall prognosis for type I tumors is better than those of type II and III tumors. Type I tumors have long-term survival and cure rates of 83%, compared to the 42% for type II and III tumors [46]. Type II tumors involving pleura are reported to have a worse prognosis [47].

### *Interstitial Lung Tumors (ILTs)*

ILTs can be described as foci of septa widening in the lung interstitium accompanied by immature growth of airspaces [48] adjacent to the normally developed lung parenchyma. During the prenatal period, they can appear as well-demarcated homogeneous solid or microcystic lesions *via* US. These tumors are exceedingly rare, however, due to challenges in distinguishing these tumors from other fetal lung masses, especially PPB, their exact prevalence is not known. Based on the reported cases, these tumors have a slight male predilection. In most cases, these tumors are not associated with complications in pregnancy, however, they can cause fetal hydrops [49].

### *Heart Rhabdomyoma*

Heart rhabdomyomas are the most common tumors of the heart during the fetal period, and account for up to 60% of fetal heart tumors with an estimated prevalence of 1: 20,000 births [50, 51]. Around 50% to 90% of these tumors are associated with Tuberous Sclerosis (TS) [51]. These tumors can grow intramurally, inside the ventricular cavity or extra-cardiacally. However, mostly present in the interventricular septum or the right ventricle [52]. They may be incidental findings during routine third-trimester ultrasonographic assessment (Fig. **2**) [53], however, they can cause pregnancy complications such as fetal heart failure, dysrhythmias and fetal hydrops [51]. Fetal color-coded echocardiography has high sensitivity and specificity in the detection of heart tumors, including rhabdomyomas. The prognosis of the fetus and child is highly dependent on cardiac complications of the tumor, and co-existing tuberous sclerosis, which can be detected prenatally by genetic studies.

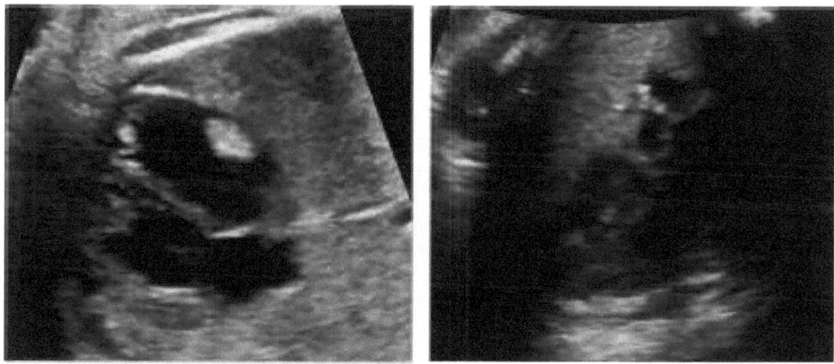

**Fig. (2).** Fetal echocardiography revealing multiple rhabdomyomas in a 32 weeks' gestational age.

## *Pericardial Teratomas*

Pericardial teratomas are the second most prevalent tumors of the heart, and account for 20% of fetal heart tumors [28]. Similar to other cardiac tumors, these tumors are also discovered during the third-trimester US appearing as a heterogeneous mass. Even though these tumors can be well managed through excision, their prognosis depends on the complications they cause, including pericardial effusion and tamponade, heart failure, and fetal hydrops [54].

## *Other Thoracic Tumors*

Some tumors such as infantile hemangiomas which are the most common benign tumors of infancy, can rarely originate in the lungs [49]. However, hemangiomas and lymphangiomas can also be detected in the axillae and mediastinum. Fibrosarcomas are tumors that usually involve extremities. However, they can rarely be observed in the lungs and heart, which are hard to distinguish them from hemangiomas based on US findings. Heart fibromas account for 12% of fetal cardiac tumors which usually appear as round, pedunculated masses in US. These tumors can be hard to distinguish from heart rhabdomyomas, however, calcifications which are sometimes observed in fibromas can help with differentiating them [50].

## **Intra-Abdominal and Pelvic Tumors**

In a study by Kamil *et al.* [29], the abdomen and pelvis were the third and fourth most common origins of fetal tumors, and accounted for approximately 20% and 10% of these tumors, respectively. In a study by Amari *et al.* [55], the most common intra-abdominal and pelvic tumors were those of the urinary tract accounting for approximately 60% of cases, followed by genital tract and gastrointestinal tumors. The majority of these tumors are cystic lesions found incidentally in the late second-trimester to early third-trimester during routine prenatal evaluation. Tumors arising in the abdomen usually have a good prognosis, and some of these tumors undergo spontaneous remission [55]. However, tumors involving the pelvis are associated with high rates of complications or mortality [29]. These tumors are associated with aneuploidy in some cases, which warrants prenatal genetic evaluation [55].

## Kidney Tumors

Kidney tumors account for approximately 5% of all prenatal tumors [56]. Many of these tumors appear as homogeneous or heterogeneous hypo-echogenic solid masses well demarcated with a hyper-echogenic rim [57]. Due to the high similarity in US appearance, distinguishing these tumors may need investigation with MRI. The definite diagnosis is mostly postponed until after birth when biopsy and histopathologic examination is more feasible, however, due to the advancement of prenatal interventions, prenatal renal biopsies can be performed, facilitating timely management [58].

Even though Wilms' tumor is the most recognized renal tumor of childhood, these tumors are not frequently detected during the antenatal period. Congenital Mesoblastic Nephromas (CMNs) are the most common tumors arising from the kidney or renal fossa. These tumors have a male predilection, and are more commonly observed in the right kidney [59]. These tumors can be found in the third-trimester during routine antenatal US as an enlarging homogenous mass. In most cases, CMNs are associated with complications, mostly polyhydramnios rather than oligohydramnios [60].

Nephroblastoma (Wilms' tumors) rarely occur prenatally with a prevalence of 1:10,000 births, and accounts for approximately 0.16% of all renal tumors [59]. The prognosis of these tumors depends on their histology and stage, as well as genetic mutations. However, their overall prognosis for lower stages is favorable [58].

## Hepatic Tumors

Most tumors found in the liver during the fetal period are metastatic. Infantile hepatic hemangiomas are the most common primary hepatic tumors, followed by mesenchymal hamartomas and hepatoblastomas [61]. Although mostly diagnosed postnatally, they can be diagnosed antenatally through US as well as demarcated single or multiple hepatic masses, mostly found in the right hepatic lobe, however, can extend to extrahepatic regions. These tumors have favorable prognosis with an approximately 70% and 60% survival for single and multiple masses, respectively.

Mesenchymal hamartomas are cystic, solid or a mix of both, however, they are mostly present as cystic masses in US. Close monitoring of the masses is warranted due to the rapid growth rate of the tumors. These tumors have a favorable prognosis with an overall survival rate of 64% among fetuses [62]. Mesenchymal hamartomas can be associated with placental mesenchymal dysplasia which worsens the prognosis of the fetus [63].

Hepatoblastomas are the third most common hepatic tumors of the fetal period and the most common hepatic malignancy of childhood [64]. These tumors are categorized into four stages that greatly affect the prognosis. However, the overall survival for these tumors is approximately 25%, and those with stage 4 are associated with the worst prognosis [62]. These tumors grow fast which helps with distinguishing them from hepatic hemangiomas, however, this warrants close monitoring for complications of the tumor and timely management. Large hepatoblastomas can cause compression of the inferior vena cava, consumptive coagulopathy, anemia and in severe cases can lead to hydrops and fetal demise [65]. These tumors are associated with other fetal anomalies and lower birth weights which must be investigated during antenatal evaluation [63].

Despite favorable prognosis, hepatic tumors can lead to complications including hydramnios, rupture of the liver and hemorrhage during delivery, fetal hydrops, respiratory distress, heart failure and fetal demise. Hepatic hemangiomas can also lead to thrombocytopenia and disseminated intravascular coagulation [62].

## *Pelvic Tumors*

### *Sacrococcygeal Teratoma*

Fetal Sacrococcygeal Teratomas (FSTs) are rare tumors with an approximate prevalence of 1:14,000 births and a prevalence for the female sex [66]. These tumors highly vary in characteristics. They can be cystic or solid with high levels of vascularization (Fig. **3**). These tumors are divided into four classes, with class I tumors growing externally, and class IV tumors growing intra-abdominally. They can grow rapidly to volumes that not only complicate delivery, but also jeopardize fetal life due to complications such as polyhydramnios, heart failure and hydrops, and fetal hemorrhage which is the leading cause of fetal mortality [67]. Therefore, even though these tumors are benign in nature, they can be associated with high rates of fetal mortality and morbidity [68]. In the prenatal US, these tumors have various presentations, and can present as cystic or solid echogenic masses or a combination of both. Similar to many other fetal tumors, these tumors are associated with other fetal abnormalities including hydronephrosis and hip dysplasia, as well as genetic abnormalities such as Trisomy 13 [69, 70], which warrants antenatal evaluation for genetic abnormalities.

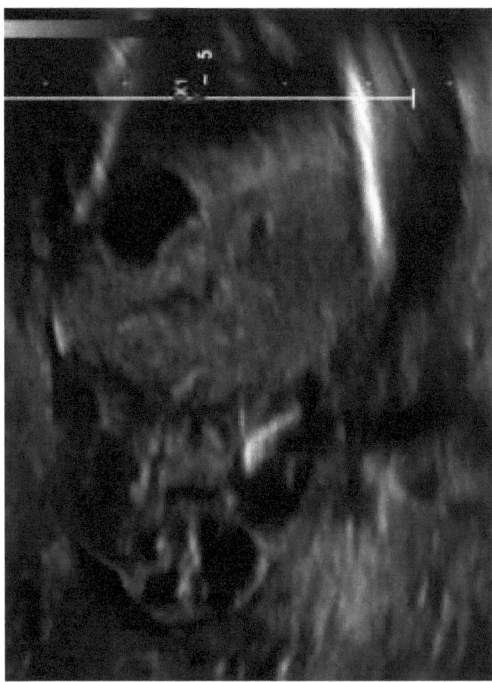

**Fig. (3).** A caudal complex mass composed of solid and cystic components found in second trimester suggestive of sacrococcygygeal teratoma.

## *Ovarian Masses*

Ovarian cysts are the most common masses found during prenatal US evaluation [71]. The prevalence of these tumors is estimated to be around 1:2500 live births [72]. Many factors have been proposed for the etiology of these cysts including maternal pre-existing conditions such as diabetes, or fetal hormonal causes such as congenital adrenal hyperplasia or hypothyroidism, along with genetic abnormalities [73 - 75]. These tumors are mostly found incidentally during antenatal US evaluation in third trimester as unilateral masses. The characteristics of these masses depend on the type of ovarian cysts: uncomplicated cysts appear as unilocular, thin-walled, anechogenic masses. On the other hand, complicated cysts appear as thick-walled cysts with septa and hyper-echogenic components. Even though the US characteristics of the ovarian cysts can suggest a long list of differential diagnoses including other intra-abdominal tumors, the presence of a daughter cyst sign manifested by the presence of a cystic lesion adjacent to the wall of a cyst, provides about 80% sensitivity and 100% specificity [76]. The prognosis of these tumors is generally good, however, in cases of extremely large cysts, complications such as respiratory distress or heart failure may occur which warrant invasive interventions.

## Other Significant Tumors and Malignancies

### *Neuroblastoma*

Neuroblastoma (NB) is the most common malignant, solid tumor in infancy [12]. These tumors are mostly found in adrenal glands, however, they can also be found in other locations such as the thoracic cavity and the rest of the abdomen. The prevalence of these tumors has been reported to be as high as 1:10,000 live births. The appearance of these tumors in the antenatal US may vary from purely cystic masses to hyper-echogenic, heterogeneous masses (Fig. **4**) [77]. The prognosis of these tumors depends on many factors, including the genetic profile of the tumor and age at diagnosis. Those tumors diagnosed before one year of age have a better prognosis, with some tumors going through spontaneous remission [78].

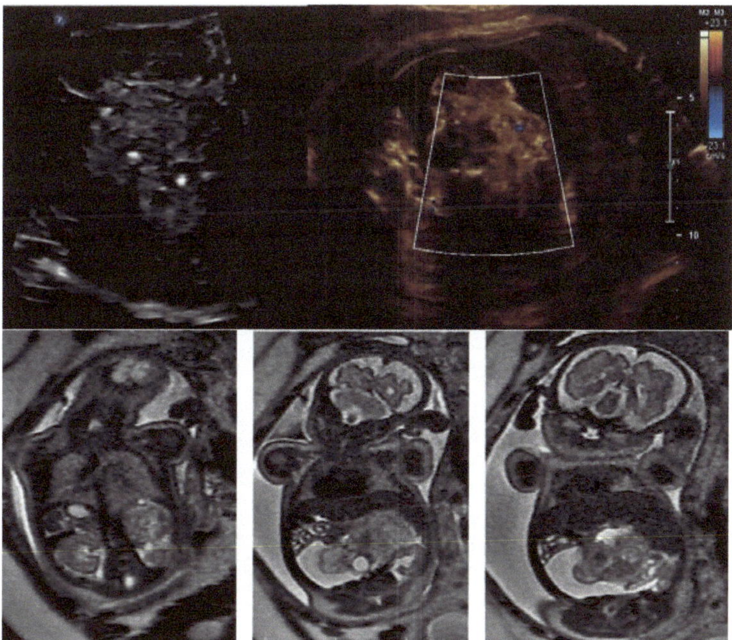

**Fig. (4).** Large intra-abdominal mass with calcification found in third trimester during routine prenatal evaluation (upper panel). MRI shows calcification and high level of vascularization in a mass originated from the right adrenal gland displacing the right kidney inferiorly suggestive of neuroblastoma (lower panel).

## PRENATAL DIAGNOSTIC TOOLS

### Imaging Modalities

Imaging modalities can be used throughout the pregnancy to evaluate the normal development or abnormalities that might occur. Therefore, it is of utmost importance to implement tools that are safe for both mother and the fetus. Therefore, imaging modalities associated with a risk of ionizing radiation such as plain radiography with X-ray, CT scan, and nuclear and Positron Emission Tomography (PET) scanning must be avoided, as much as possible during pregnancy. On the other hand, US and MRI provide safe and accurate diagnostic tools. Each of these imaging modalities has its cons and pros which will be discussed.

### Ultrasonography

Integration of US with obstetrics dates back to the 1950s. Currently, US is the first imaging tool used in prenatal evaluation of the fetus, and is used for detection of a variety of fetal abnormalities. This is because of feasibility, affordability, low risk, providing real-time images and availability of US in nearly every obstetric setting. This modality has progressed over time in terms of the quality of the imaging thanks to advanced technologies such as 3D/4D imaging, color and Doppler US. Therefore, this imaging technique is becoming more reliable in the detection of abnormalities. Furthermore, advances in imaging technologies allow for earlier detection of fetal tumors which is a cornerstone of timely management and decision-making. Even though US provides a narrow field of view and the images obtained are operator dependent and of low contrast, its advantages outweigh these disadvantages [79].

Fetal tumors are usually incidental findings that are found mostly in the third trimester [29, 80]. The sensitivity and specificity of US in the detection and diagnosis of these tumors vary based on the site of the tumor and its presentation. Even though US findings of fetal tumors are not helpful in providing a definite diagnosis, some features of the tumors appearing in US imaging can strongly point toward a specific diagnosis [6].

Once the presence of a tumor in the fetus is suspected or confirmed, US is the modality of choice for follow-up of the tumor, if termination of pregnancy is not performed in the first place. However, US findings may warrant reassessment with more accurate imaging modalities such as MRI [81].

## Magnetic Resonance Imaging

Even though MRI is not associated with the risk of ionizing radiation, the use of MRI for prenatal fetal assessments is limited due to a number of factors. In contrast to US, MRI is not widely available, and is costlier compared to US [82]. Another factor that limited the widespread use of MRI was the high level of artifacts associated with maternal and fetal movements, which would warrant maternal and fetal sedation. However, this is no longer an issue thanks to the development of ultrafast MRI technics which can obtain high-quality images at a rate of one section per second [18].

Despite the fact that many of the factors mentioned are currently resolved, the use of MRI for the assessment of fetal abnormalities is reserved for cases where more details of a lesion are needed in order to reveal its nature. However, MRI is not merely used for better assessment of the lesion itself, there are instances where MRI is used to investigate the presence of other abnormalities, such as the cases of heart rhabdomyoma that warrant MRI of the CNS in order to investigate the presence of CNS lesions associated with tuberous sclerosis. The MRI findings, in combination with US findings, provide more accurate characteristics which narrow the list of differential diagnoses [83].

## Prenatal Tissue Sampling

Even though biopsy sampling of the tumors detected prenatally is mostly postponed until after birth, current techniques allow for the sampling of fetal tumors antenatally. Before, fetal tissue sampling was mostly performed to evaluate metabolic and hereditary conditions through direct examination of skin, liver, and muscle tissues, however, biopsy sampling can also be performed on tumor tissue. This allows for histopathologic examination of the tumors which results in definite diagnosis prenatally. Advances in both imaging and sampling techniques allow for more accurate sampling, which is also associated with a lower risk of damaging fetal tissues. The most commonly used techniques include US, MRI and fetoscopy, which allow for diagnosis, and at times, treatment of prenatal tumors. These techniques allow for the sampling of many fetal organs including, but not limited to brain, kidneys, liver, lung, oropharyngeal tumors and bone marrow [84 - 89].

## Genetic Studies

Even though genetic studies have been used for more than 30 years for the diagnosis of various congenital disorders, namely chromosomal abnormalities and metabolic disorders, their use in prenatal diagnosis of malignancies is limited, despite advances in prenatal genetic diagnostic methods [84]. Most of the currently implemented genetic diagnostic tests in prenatal evaluation of cancers are concerned with malignancies occurring in later stages of life, rather than during the prenatal period, such as prenatal assessment of BRCA-1 gene for prediction of development of breast cancer in the fetus in future [90]. Some of these genetic diagnostics are performed as part of Assisted Reproductive Technology (ART), and some are performed during the fetal period, along with the assessment of other genetic abnormalities [84].

Genetic studies for the assessment of fetal malignancies during pregnancy can be performed *via* tumor sampling. In some disorders, such as neuroblastoma, whose prognosis varies based on several genetic mutations, prenatal genetic studies can be helpful [91]. However, minimally aggressive genetic diagnostic tests, such as cell-free DNA, cannot be implemented for the diagnosis of fetal malignancies.

## MANAGEMENT

Timely diagnosis and close follow-up of fetuses with prenatally diagnosed tumors and malignancies is crucial for making decisions regarding the management of the pregnancy and planning postnatal care [80]. The location and size of the tumor and its histology are some of the main factors affecting the course of the tumor progression, with the latter dramatically affecting the middle. Another factor that affects the possibility of tumor resection is the vascularity of the tumor, which can be easily determined through prenatal imaging [80, 92 - 94]. These factors determine whether to provide treatment for the fetal tumor before or after birth. In this section, we will review the current management for categories of tumors discussed earlier.

### Head and Neck Tumors

As mentioned earlier, the majority of intracranial tumors are detected in the late second to early third trimester of pregnancy. It is important to determine the nature of the lesions with more sensitive imaging tools such as Doppler ultrasounds and MRI to differentiate tumors from less invasive lesions such as arteriovenous malformations. The nature of the tumor determines the treatment approach. Rapidly progressive lesions must be closely monitored as they can lead to significant macrocephaly, leading to pregnancy complications occurring mainly during labor such as obstructed delivery or intracranial hemorrhage.

Purely cystic lesions or tumors with large cystic components have the potential to complicate delivery due to huge macrocephaly. These can be managed prenatally with cephalocentesis [95, 96]. However, the procedure carries a high risk of fetal demise due to rapid intracranial decompression. Ventricular drainage can also be used for intracranial decompression. Other interventions for brain tumors which are mainly reserved for after birth include surgical resection of the tumors and chemotherapy. Unlike brain tumors occurring in later stages of life, radiotherapy is not recommended for brain tumors diagnosed in infants due to the high risk of developmental retardation, development of future neoplasms as well as neuro-endocrine abnormalities [97]. Gross total resection improves the outcome of patients, and even though it can be achieved through an endoscopic approach for small ventricular tumors, large parenchymal tumors mostly require open craniotomy for resection [98].

The chemotherapy regimen and whether it should be performed before or after surgery are determined by the histopathology of the tumor, its size, and its vascularity. Induction multi-drug combination therapy is used for induction following surgery. Neoadjuvant therapy for large tumors or those with high levels of vascularity can improve the possibility of gross total resection [99].

For fetuses diagnosed with neck tumors, it is important to determine whether the mass is obstructing the fetal trachea or fetal swallowing (Fig. **5**). MRI can help better determine tracheal obstruction. However, there are cases in that certainty cannot be achieved even with MRI for which fetoscopic laryngo-tracheoscopy can determine patency of the airway [34], and can also be used to secure the airway through fetoscopic intubation [100]. Fetuses with tracheal obstruction must be planned to be delivered *via* Ex-Utero Intrapartum Treatment (EXIT)-a procedure in centers with experts for managing fetal airway obstruction from multiple surgical teams, including obstetricians as well as ear-nose-throat specialists [98, 101]. In such cases, the airway must be secured either through endotracheal intubation or through tracheostomy while the fetus still depends on maternal circulation for oxygenation. However, these procedures may not result in the survival of the fetus in cases of large masses obstructing the airway [102]. Other head and neck tumors that do not require prompt airway obstruction can be managed postnatally to debulk the tumor [103].

**Thoracic Tumors**

When a lesion of the fetal lung is suspected, the first step towards its management is to determine whether the lesion is benign, such as in the case of CCAM, or malignant. Very large masses, especially those causing a mediastinal shift or pleural effusion, can be managed prenatally with less invasive procedures. For CCAMs proliferating at a significant pace, transplacental steroids can slow the progression of the mass, and prevent the development of hydrops. However, if CCAMs become associated with hydrops, thoracic-amniotic shunts can resolve the hydrops [104, 105].

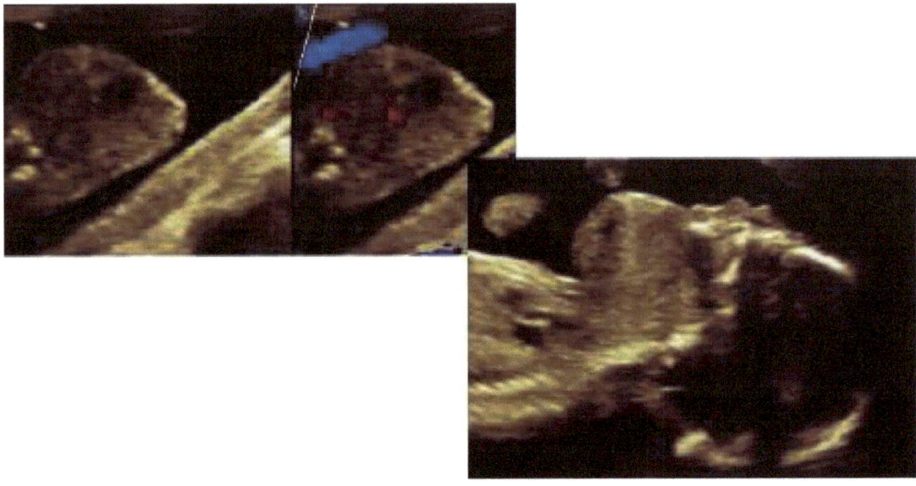

**Fig. (5).** A large, mostly-solid, anterior neck mass with high levels of vascularity and calcifications found at 19 weeks suggestive of neck teratoma. The mass resulted in fetal neck hyperextension and airway compression necessitating early termination of pregnancy.

Benign lesions, such as BPS, can be managed with conservative or medical treatment such as furosemide and digoxin [106], and more severe cases can be managed through placing thoracoamniotic shunt, alcohol septal ablation or surgical resection [35, 107, 108]. Management of the solid and malignant tumors of the lungs, such as PPB, depends on their stage and histopathology. Primary stage I PPB can be treated with resection alone, however, adjuvant chemotherapy is recommended for primary stage II and stage III PPBs. Recurrent tumors must go through consolidation chemotherapy and autologous stem cell rescue therapy [48]. Resection of the tumor is performed *via* lobectomy which can be performed either antenatally or postnatally [109].

Management of cardiac tumors depends on the number of lesions, their location, their size and whether they obstruct the outflow of cardiac chambers. Rapidly growing tumors or cardiac masses obstructing ventricular inflow/outflow or causing pericardial effusion, such as pericardial teratomas, can result in hydrops, and must be resected promptly [54]. In cases where cardiac mass causes tamponade, immediate intervention is required [110]. Such cases can either go through fetal tumor resection or be temporarily managed by thoracoamniotic shunting until tumor is resected postnatally [111]. Pericardial hemangiomas can be managed postnatally through pericardiocentesis or thoracotomy with a pericardial window, however, if these procedures fail to treat the effusion, tumor resection under cardiopulmonary bypass can be performed [112, 113]. For pericardial hemangiomas invading major nerves and vessels, conservative management may be preferred over resection due to high surgery risk [114]. In such cases, radiotherapy and chemotherapy with steroids, interferons and cyclophosphamide can help manage the tumor [114]. Other cardiac masses that are small or asymptomatic can be closely monitored throughout the pregnancy and managed postnatally. In such cases, the tumor can either be merely monitored in appropriate intervals, go through pericardiocentesis, or be resected antenatally through EXIT surgery [110, 115].

## Intra-Abdominal Tumors

CMNs are benign renal tumors that can be successfully resected postnatally [116]. Nephroblastomas, if not complicating pregnancy due to decreased fetal swallowing potentially leading to hydrops and fetal demise, can be managed postnatally with surgical resection and chemotherapy [13]. Neuroblastoma, which in virtually all fetal cases presents as suprarenal masses, can be managed postnatally as it does not complicate pregnancy. After birth, genetic studies can be performed to determine the prognosis of the mass. Based on the results of the genetic studies, conservative management can be chosen as many of the tumors found during infancy regress spontaneously. In cases where conservative management is not an option, surgical resection followed by chemotherapy and immunotherapy can be performed [117]. Hepatic hemangiomas can complicate pregnancy through microangiopathic hemolysis and consumptive coagulopathy leading to thrombocytopenia and anemia, which in severe cases can lead to heart failure, hydrops, and fetal death. Small hemangiomas can be managed conservatively as they can regress occasionally. The first step toward the management of larger or complicated hepatic hemangiomas is a medical treatment with steroids [118]. Hepatic hemangiomas persistent to medical treatment can be managed surgically [119]. Hepatoblastomas can be managed postnatally with neoadjuvant chemotherapy and surgical resection [120, 121].

## Pelvic Tumors

Sacrococcygeal teratomas, even though benign in nature, have outcomes that are inversely correlated with tumor size. These tumors can complicate pregnancy due to obstructed labor or compression of vital organs which can lead to prematurity [122]. On the other hand, the vascularity of these tumors not only has the potential to impose risks on fetal survival due to cardiac complications, but also affects the treatment plan. Highly vascularized or rapidly growing teratomas can be managed prenatally with less invasive methods such as laser and radiofrequency ablation, sclerotherapy, coiling, and embolization of the tumor, which can decrease the level of tumor vascularity and improve cardiac function [123]. However, these interventions are associated with a risk of preterm delivery and damage to adjacent structures such as skin, bone, and nerves [123]. Other tumors can be managed either prenatally or postnatally through surgical resection of the tumor. Survival rates for tumors managed with surgical resection are better than those managed with less invasive methods, however, surgical resection is also associated with complications such as the risk of Premature Rupture of Membranes (PROM), rectal fistulas, and preterm birth as well as the maternal risk of uterine scarring for tumors managed prenatally [124].

## Ovarian Masses

Ovarian cysts are common findings in routine prenatal US. These cysts vary in size and characteristics, which determine their clinical manifestation. Small cysts are usually asymptomatic, and can regress spontaneously. However, large cysts can complicate pregnancy in different ways, such as obstructed labor and dystocia, intracystic hemorrhage, compression on adjacent structures, and most importantly ovarian torsion [125, 126]. A torsioned cyst is characterized by rapid growth of the cyst, and its acquisition of features of complicated cysts. Immediate surgical care must be provided for ovarian torsion. On the other hand, complicated cysts must be managed surgically, while surgical treatment for simple cysts is controversial [127].

## PERINATAL CARE AND CONSULTATION

Providing accurate consultation to the parents is one of the most important steps toward making decisions for pregnancies, as the final decision must be made by the parents. Parents must be aware of the level of certainty offered by each paraclinical study. For instance, parents must be aware that fetal brain MRI performed to assess the presence of TS lesions in fetuses with heart rhabdomyomas may not show these lesions in spite of their presence [128]. They must also be aware of the risks each intervention imposes on both mother and the fetus. For instance, resection of neck tumors may lead to cervical nerve damage. On the other hand, EXIT surgery for the management of neck tumors obstructing the airway might increase the risk of maternal bleeding due to uterine atony resulting from the use of tocolytics [129].

## FUTURE PERSPECTIVES

Even though each case of prenatally diagnosed tumor must be managed individually based on the special conditions of the fetus and mother, such cases are mostly managed either through termination of pregnancy, conservative management, prenatal resection of the tumor or postnatal resection of the tumor with or without chemotherapy. Currently, medical treatment of fetal tumors is mostly limited to the use of maternal steroids. Chemotherapeutic agents impose high risks on both mother and the fetus. Even though immunotherapy has proven efficacy in many cancers [130], its use to provide treatment for prenatally diagnosed malignancies is not properly investigated.

It is well recognized that immunoglobulin G (IgG) can cross the placenta [131]. On the other hand, T cells can pass through the placenta [132]. Gene-modified T cells, such as chimeric antigen receptor T cells (CAR T cells) and monoclonal antibodies (mAbs) can be used to treat prenatally diagnosed malignancy. These modalities provide targeted therapy that can be safe both to the mother and the fetus.

## CONCLUSION

Based on the wide spectrum of fetal malignancies and their vague presentations, it is important that prenatal care providers be familiar with their features in order to provide timely management. Acquaintance with statistics regarding the nature of the tumors based on their location and imaging presentations is necessary for providing consultation, as well as decision-making regarding the termination of pregnancy or other treatments. Advances in biological treatments, however, are making a shift toward less aggressive treatments in many cases of prenatal tumors.

## CONSENT FOR PUBLICATION

Not applicable.

## CONFLICT OF INTEREST

The authors declare no conflict of interest, financial or otherwise.

## ACKNOWLEDGEMENT

Declared none.

## REFERENCES

[1]     White MC, Holman DM, Boehm JE, Peipins LA, Grossman M, Jane Henley S. Age and cancer risk: a potentially modifiable relationship. Am J Prev Med 2014; 46(3) (Suppl. 1): S7-S15.
        [http://dx.doi.org/10.1016/j.amepre.2013.10.029] [PMID: 24512933]

[2]     Isaevska E, Manasievska M, Alessi D, *et al.* Cancer incidence rates and trends among children and adolescents in Piedmont, 1967–2011. PLoS One 2017; 12(7): e0181805.
        [http://dx.doi.org/10.1371/journal.pone.0181805] [PMID: 28742150]

[3]     Pham A, Wong K, Chang EL. Quality of life in pediatric brain tumor patients treated with proton therapy: a review of the literature. Expert Rev Qual Life Cancer Care 2016; 1(4): 329-38.
        [http://dx.doi.org/10.1080/23809000.2016.1196106]

[4]     Isaacs H Jr. Perinatal (congenital and neonatal) neoplasms: a report of 110 cases. Pediatr Pathol 1985; 3(2-4): 165-216.

[http://dx.doi.org/10.3109/15513818509078782] [PMID: 3879355]

[5]　Parkes SE, Muir KR, Southern L, Cameron AH, Darbyshire PJ, Stevens MCG. Neonatal tumours: A thirty-year population-based study. Med Pediatr Oncol 1994; 22(5): 309-17.
[http://dx.doi.org/10.1002/mpo.2950220503] [PMID: 8127254]

[6]　Cho JY, Lee YH. Fetal tumors: prenatal ultrasonographic findings and clinical characteristics. Ultrasonography 2014; 33(4): 240-51.
[http://dx.doi.org/10.14366/usg.14019] [PMID: 25116458]

[7]　Sebire NJ, Jauniaux E. Fetal and placental malignancies: prenatal diagnosis and management. Ultrasound Obstet Gynecol 2009; 33(2): 235-44.
[http://dx.doi.org/10.1002/uog.6246] [PMID: 19009536]

[8]　Lowe S. Diagnostic imaging in pregnancy: Making informed decisions. Obstet Med 2019; 12(3): 116-22.
[http://dx.doi.org/10.1177/1753495X19838658] [PMID: 31523267]

[9]　Mistri PK, Patua B, Alam H, Ray S, Bhattacharyya SK. Large sacrococcygeal teratoma hindering vaginal delivery attempted at home. Rev Obstet Gynecol 2012; 5(2): 65-8.
[PMID: 22866184]

[10]　Tao TY, Yahyavi-Firouz-Abadi N, Singh GK, Bhalla S. Pediatric cardiac tumors: clinical and imaging features. Radiographics 2014; 34(4): 1031-46.
[http://dx.doi.org/10.1148/rg.344135163] [PMID: 25019440]

[11]　Manoranjan B, Provias JP. Congenital brain tumors: diagnostic pitfalls and therapeutic interventions. J Child Neurol 2011; 26(5): 599-614.
[http://dx.doi.org/10.1177/0883073810394848] [PMID: 21464236]

[12]　Werner H, Daltro P, Davaus T, Araujo Júnior E. Fetal neuroblastoma: ultrasonography and magnetic resonance imaging findings in the prenatal and postnatal IV-S stage. Obstet Gynecol Sci 2016; 59(5): 407-10.
[http://dx.doi.org/10.5468/ogs.2016.59.5.407] [PMID: 27668206]

[13]　Leclair MD, El-Ghoneimi A, Audry G, Ravasse P, Moscovici J, Heloury Y. The outcome of prenatally diagnosed renal tumors. J Urol 2005; 173(1): 186-9.
[http://dx.doi.org/10.1097/01.ju.0000147300.53837.8f] [PMID: 15592071]

[14]　Meizner I. Perinatal oncology–the role of prenatal ultrasound diagnosis. Wiley Online Library 2000.
[http://dx.doi.org/10.1046/j.1469-0705.2000.00297.x]

[15]　Stiller CA, Bunch KJ. Brain and spinal tumours in children aged under two years: incidence and survival in Britain, 1971-85. Br J Cancer Suppl 1992; 18: S50-3.
[PMID: 1503926]

[16]　Chien YH, Tsao PN, Lee WT, Peng SF, Tsou Yau K-I. Congenital intracranial teratoma. Pediatr Neurol 2000; 22(1): 72-4.
[http://dx.doi.org/10.1016/S0887-8994(99)00103-4] [PMID: 10669211]

[17]　Morof DF, Levine D, Stringer KF, Grable I, Folkerth R. Congenital glioblastoma multiforme: prenatal diagnosis on the basis of sonography and magnetic resonance imaging. J Ultrasound Med 2001; 20(12): 1369-75.
[http://dx.doi.org/10.7863/jum.2001.20.12.1369] [PMID: 11762550]

[18]　Milani HJ, Araujo Júnior E, Cavalheiro S, *et al.* Fetal brain tumors: Prenatal diagnosis by ultrasound and magnetic resonance imaging. World J Radiol 2015; 7(1): 17-21.
[http://dx.doi.org/10.4329/wjr.v7.i1.17] [PMID: 25628801]

[19]　Isaacs H Jr. II. Perinatal brain tumors: a review of 250 cases. Pediatr Neurol 2002; 27(5): 333-42.
[http://dx.doi.org/10.1016/S0887-8994(02)00459-9] [PMID: 12504200]

[20]   Hirsig LE, Rajderkar DA. Fetal intracranial neoplasm–not always a teratoma!. Journal of Radiology and Imaging 2016; 1(2): 14-7.
[http://dx.doi.org/10.14312/2399-8172.2016-4]

[21]   Cassart M, Bosson N, Garel C, Eurin D, Avni F. Fetal intracranial tumors: a review of 27 cases. Eur Radiol 2008; 18(10): 2060-6.
[http://dx.doi.org/10.1007/s00330-008-0999-5] [PMID: 18458906]

[22]   Saada J, Enza-Razavi F, Delahaye S, Martinovic J, MacAleese J, Benachi A. Early second-trimester diagnosis of intracranial teratoma. Ultrasound Obstet Gynecol 2009; 33(1): 109-11.
[http://dx.doi.org/10.1002/uog.6231] [PMID: 18991328]

[23]   Isaacs H. Fetal brain tumors: a review of 154 cases. Am J Perinatol 2009; 26(6): 453-66.
[http://dx.doi.org/10.1055/s-0029-1214245] [PMID: 19396744]

[24]   Geraghty AV, Knott PD, Hanna HM. Prenatal diagnosis of fetal glioblastoma multiforme. Prenat Diagn 1989; 9(9): 613-6.
[http://dx.doi.org/10.1002/pd.1970090903] [PMID: 2552427]

[25]   Isaacs H Jr. Perinatal (fetal and neonatal) astrocytoma: a review. Childs Nerv Syst 2016; 32(11): 2085-96.
[http://dx.doi.org/10.1007/s00381-016-3215-y] [PMID: 27568373]

[26]   Joó JG, Rigó J Jr, Sápi Z, Timár B. Foetal craniopharyngioma diagnosed by prenatal ultrasonography and confirmed by histopathological examination. Prenat Diagn 2009; 29(2): 160-3.
[http://dx.doi.org/10.1002/pd.2202] [PMID: 19180629]

[27]   Wacker-Gussmann A, Strasburger JF, Cuneo BF, Wiggins DL, Gotteiner NL, Wakai RT. Fetal arrhythmias associated with cardiac rhabdomyomas. Heart Rhythm 2014; 11(4): 677-83.
[http://dx.doi.org/10.1016/j.hrthm.2013.12.018] [PMID: 24333285]

[28]   Bonnamy L, Perrotin F, Megier P, Haddad G, Body G, Lansac J. Fetal intracardiac tumor(s): prenatal diagnosis and management. Eur J Obstet Gynecol Reprod Biol 2001; 99(1): 112-7.
[http://dx.doi.org/10.1016/S0301-2115(01)00337-2] [PMID: 11604198]

[29]   Kamil D, Tepelmann J, Berg C, *et al.* Spectrum and outcome of prenatally diagnosed fetal tumors. Ultrasound Obstet Gynecol 2008; 31(3): 296-302.
[http://dx.doi.org/10.1002/uog.5260] [PMID: 18307207]

[30]   Phillips J, Blask A, DiPoto Brahmbhatt A, *et al.* Fetal lung interstitial tumor: Prenatal presentation of a rare fetal malignancy. J Neonatal Perinatal Med 2020; 12(4): 473-7.
[http://dx.doi.org/10.3233/NPM-180059] [PMID: 31256075]

[31]   Di Prima FAF, Bellia A, Inclimona G, Grasso F, Teresa M, Cassaro MN. Antenatally diagnosed congenital cystic adenomatoid malformations (CCAM): Research Review. J Prenat Med 2012; 6(2): 22-30.
[PMID: 22905308]

[32]   Laberge JM, Flageole H, Pugash D, *et al.* Outcome of the prenatally diagnosed congenital cystic adenomatoid lung malformation: a Canadian experience. Fetal Diagn Ther 2001; 16(3): 178-86.
[http://dx.doi.org/10.1159/000053905] [PMID: 11316935]

[33]   Langston C, Ed. New concepts in the pathology of congenital lung malformations. Seminars in pediatric surgery 2003.

[34]   Macardle CA, Ehrenberg-Buchner S, Smith EA, *et al.* Surveillance of fetal lung lesions using the congenital pulmonary airway malformation volume ratio: natural history and outcomes. Prenat Diagn 2016; 36(3): 282-9.
[http://dx.doi.org/10.1002/pd.4761] [PMID: 26713859]

[35]   Bermúdez C, Pérez-Wulff J, Bufalino G, Sosa C, Gómez L, Quintero RA. Percutaneous ultrasound-guided sclerotherapy for complicated fetal intralobar bronchopulmonary sequestration. Ultrasound

Obstet Gynecol 2007; 29(5): 586-9.
[http://dx.doi.org/10.1002/uog.3944] [PMID: 17444552]

[36]　Savic B, Birtel FJ, Tholen W, Funke HD, Knoche R. Lung sequestration: report of seven cases and review of 540 published cases. Thorax 1979; 34(1): 96-101.
[http://dx.doi.org/10.1136/thx.34.1.96] [PMID: 442005]

[37]　Welty JL, Belthoff JR, Egbert J, Schwabl H. Relationships between yolk androgens and nest density, laying date, and laying order in Western Burrowing Owls ( *Athene cunicularia hypugaea* ). Can J Zool 2012; 90(2): 182-92.
[http://dx.doi.org/10.1139/z11-125]

[38]　Kitano Y, Adzick NS. New developments in fetal lung surgery. Curr Opin Pulm Med 1999; 5(6): 383-9.
[http://dx.doi.org/10.1097/00063198-199911000-00011] [PMID: 10570741]

[39]　Slotnick RN, McGahan J, Milio L, Schwartz M, Ablin D. Antenatal diagnosis and treatment of fetal bronchopulmonary sequestration. Fetal Diagn Ther 1990; 5(1): 33-9.
[http://dx.doi.org/10.1159/000263532] [PMID: 2101010]

[40]　Siza C. Equine Leptospirosis Seroprevealence in the Central and Bluegrass Regions of Kentucky from 1993-2015. 2016.

[41]　Demos NJ, Teresi A. Congenital lung malformations. J Thorac Cardiovasc Surg 1975; 70(2): 260-4.
[http://dx.doi.org/10.1016/S0022-5223(19)40349-8] [PMID: 1152510]

[42]　Gele R. Congenital bronchopulmonary malformation. N Engl J Med 1968; 278: 1413-9.
[PMID: 5652625]

[43]　Priest JR, Williams GM, Hill DA, Dehner LP, Jaffé A. Pulmonary cysts in early childhood and the risk of malignancy. Pediatr Pulmonol 2009; 44(1): 14-30.
[http://dx.doi.org/10.1002/ppul.20917] [PMID: 19061226]

[44]　Nasr A, Himidan S, Pastor AC, Taylor G, Kim PCW. Is congenital cystic adenomatoid malformation a premalignant lesion for pleuropulmonary blastoma? J Pediatr Surg 2010; 45(6): 1086-9.
[http://dx.doi.org/10.1016/j.jpedsurg.2010.02.067] [PMID: 20620300]

[45]　Miniati DN, Chintagumpala M, Langston C, *et al.* Prenatal presentation and outcome of children with pleuropulmonary blastoma. J Pediatr Surg 2006; 41(1): 66-71.
[http://dx.doi.org/10.1016/j.jpedsurg.2005.10.074] [PMID: 16410110]

[46]　Zhang N, Zeng Q, Ma X, *et al.* Diagnosis and treatment of pleuropulmonary blastoma in children: A single-center report of 41 cases. J Pediatr Surg 2020; 55(7): 1351-5.
[http://dx.doi.org/10.1016/j.jpedsurg.2019.06.009] [PMID: 31277979]

[47]　Indolfi P, Casale F, Carli M, *et al.* Pleuropulmonary blastoma. Cancer 2000; 89(6): 1396-401.
[http://dx.doi.org/10.1002/1097-0142(20000915)89:6<1396::AID-CNCR25>3.0.CO;2-2]　[PMID: 11002236]

[48]　Dishop MK, McKay EM, Kreiger PA, *et al.* Fetal lung interstitial tumor (FLIT): A proposed newly recognized lung tumor of infancy to be differentiated from cystic pleuropulmonary blastoma and other developmental pulmonary lesions. Am J Surg Pathol 2010; 34(12): 1762-72.
[http://dx.doi.org/10.1097/PAS.0b013e3181faf212] [PMID: 21107081]

[49]　Lichtenberger JP III, Biko DM, Carter BW, Pavio MA, Huppmann AR, Chung EM. Primary lung tumors in children: radiologic-pathologic correlation from the radiologic pathology archives. Radiographics 2018; 38(7): 2151-72.
[http://dx.doi.org/10.1148/rg.2018180192] [PMID: 30422774]

[50]　Bejiqi R, Retkoceri R, Bejiqi H. Prenatally diagnosis and outcome of fetuses with cardiac rhabdomyoma–single centre experience. Open Access Maced J Med Sci 2017; 5(2): 193-6.
[http://dx.doi.org/10.3889/oamjms.2017.040] [PMID: 28507627]

[51]  Wilk M, Zelger B. Mesenchymal and Neuronal Tumors. Braun-Falco's. Dermatology 2020; 1-35.

[52]  Isaacs H Jr. Fetal and neonatal cardiac tumors. Pediatr Cardiol 2004; 25(3): 252-73.
[http://dx.doi.org/10.1007/s00246-003-0590-4] [PMID: 15360117]

[53]  Holley DG, Martin GR, Brenner JI, *et al.* Diagnosis and management of fetal cardiac tumors: a multicenter experience and review of published reports. J Am Coll Cardiol 1995; 26(2): 516-20.
[http://dx.doi.org/10.1016/0735-1097(95)80031-B] [PMID: 7608458]

[54]  Rychik J, Khalek N, Gaynor JW, *et al.* Fetal intrapericardial teratoma: Natural history and management including successful in utero surgery. Am J Obstet Gynecol 2016; 215(6): 780e1-7.
[http://dx.doi.org/10.1016/j.ajog.2016.08.010]

[55]  Sallam A, Paes B, Bourgeois J. Neonatal hepatoblastoma: two cases posing a diagnostic dilemma, with a review of the literature. Am J Perinatol 2005; 22(8): 413-9.
[http://dx.doi.org/10.1055/s-2005-872592] [PMID: 16283600]

[56]  Wang ZP, Li K, Dong KR, Xiao XM, Zheng S. Congenital mesoblastic nephroma: Clinical analysis of eight cases and a review of the literature. Oncol Lett 2014; 8(5): 2007-11.
[http://dx.doi.org/10.3892/ol.2014.2489] [PMID: 25295083]

[57]  Vadeyar S, Ramsay M, James D, O'Neill D. Prenatal diagnosis of congenital Wilms' tumor (nephroblastoma) presenting as fetal hydrops. Ultrasound Obstet Gynecol 2000; 16(1): 80-3.
[http://dx.doi.org/10.1046/j.1469-0705.2000.00169.x] [PMID: 11084972]

[58]  Hrabovsky EE, Othersen HB Jr, deLorimier A, Kelalis P, Beckwith JB, Takashima J. Wilms' tumor in the neonate: A report from the national Wilms' tumor study. J Pediatr Surg 1986; 21(5): 385-7.
[http://dx.doi.org/10.1016/S0022-3468(86)80502-4] [PMID: 3012057]

[59]  Kim CH, Kim YH, Cho MK, *et al.* A case of fetal congenital mesoblastic nephroma with oligohydramnios. J Korean Med Sci 2007; 22(2): 357-61.
[http://dx.doi.org/10.3346/jkms.2007.22.2.357] [PMID: 17449950]

[60]  Do AY, Kim JS, Choi SJ, Oh S, Roh CR, Kim JH. Prenatal diagnosis of congenital mesoblastic nephroma. Obstet Gynecol Sci 2015; 58(5): 405-8.
[http://dx.doi.org/10.5468/ogs.2015.58.5.405] [PMID: 26430667]

[61]  Isaacs H Jr. Fetal and neonatal hepatic tumors. J Pediatr Surg 2007; 42(11): 1797-803.
[http://dx.doi.org/10.1016/j.jpedsurg.2007.07.047] [PMID: 18022426]

[62]  Weinberg AG, Finegold MJ. Primary hepatic tumors of childhood. Hum Pathol 1983; 14(6): 512-37.
[http://dx.doi.org/10.1016/S0046-8177(83)80005-7] [PMID: 6303939]

[63]  Huang LC, Ho M, Chang WC, Chen HY, Hung YC, Chiu TH. Prenatal diagnosis of fetal hepatoblastoma with a good neonatal outcome: case report and narrative literature review. Pediatr Hematol Oncol 2011; 28(2): 150-4.
[http://dx.doi.org/10.3109/08880018.2010.536299] [PMID: 21299342]

[64]  Catanzarite V, Hilfiker M, Daneshmand S, Willert J. Prenatal diagnosis of fetal hepatoblastoma: Case report and review of the literature. Journal of ultrasound in medicine: Official journal of the American Institute of Ultrasound in Medicine 2008; 27(7): 1095-8.
[http://dx.doi.org/10.7863/jum.2008.27.7.1095]

[65]  Feusner J, Plaschkes J. Hepatoblastoma and low birth weight: A trend or chance observation? Med Pediatr Oncol 2002; 39(5): 508-9.
[http://dx.doi.org/10.1002/mpo.10176] [PMID: 12228908]

[66]  Litwińska M, Litwińska E, Janiak K, Piaseczna-Piotrowska A, Szaflik K. Percutaneous intratumor laser ablation for fetal sacrococcygeal teratoma. Fetal Diagn Ther 2020; 47(2): 138-44.
[http://dx.doi.org/10.1159/000500775] [PMID: 31291630]

[67]  Kremer MEB, Althof JF, Derikx JPM, *et al.* The incidence of associated abnormalities in patients with sacrococcygeal teratoma. J Pediatr Surg 2018; 53(10): 1918-22.

[http://dx.doi.org/10.1016/j.jpedsurg.2018.01.013] [PMID: 29453131]

[68] Kremer MEB, Wellens LM, Derikx JPM, *et al.* Hemorrhage is the most common cause of neonatal mortality in patients with sacrococcygeal teratoma. J Pediatr Surg 2016; 51(11): 1826-9.
[http://dx.doi.org/10.1016/j.jpedsurg.2016.07.005] [PMID: 27502009]

[69] Dalal SS, Berry T, Pimentel VM. Prenatal sacrococcygeal teratoma diagnosed in a fetus with partial trisomy 13q22. Case reports in obstetrics and gynecology 2019; 2019.

[70] Crombleholme TM, Craigo SD, Garmel S, D'Alton ME. Fetal ovarian cyst decompression to prevent torsion. J Pediatr Surg 1997; 32(10): 1447-9.
[http://dx.doi.org/10.1016/S0022-3468(97)90558-3] [PMID: 9349765]

[71] Kirkinen P, Jouppila P. Perinatal aspects of pregnancy complicated by fetal ovarian cyst. J Perinat Med 1985; 21(1): 90-117.
[http://dx.doi.org/10.1515/jpme.1985.13.5.245]

[72] Enríquez G, Durán C, Torán N, *et al.* Conservative versus surgical treatment for complex neonatal ovarian cysts: outcomes study. AJR Am J Roentgenol 2005; 185(2): 501-8.
[http://dx.doi.org/10.2214/ajr.185.2.01850501] [PMID: 16037528]

[73] Hasiakos D, Papakonstantinou K, Bacanu AM, Argeitis J, Botsis D, Vitoratos N. Clinical experience of five fetal ovarian cysts: diagnosis and follow-up. Arch Gynecol Obstet 2008; 277(6): 575-8.
[http://dx.doi.org/10.1007/s00404-007-0508-0] [PMID: 18034256]

[74] Jafri SZ, Bree RL, Silver TM, Ouimette M. Fetal ovarian cysts: sonographic detection and association with hypothyroidism. Radiology 1984; 150(3): 809-12.
[http://dx.doi.org/10.1148/radiology.150.3.6695083] [PMID: 6695083]

[75] Erol O, Buyukkinaci Erol M, İsenlik BS, Özkiraz S, Karaca M. Prenatal diagnosis of fetal ovarian cyst: case report and review of the literature. J Turk Ger Gynecol Assoc 2013; 14(2): 119-22.
[http://dx.doi.org/10.5152/jtgga.2013.58855] [PMID: 24592088]

[76] Davis S, Rogers MAM, Pendergrass TW. The incidence and epidemiologic characteristics of neuroblastoma in the United States. Am J Epidemiol 1987; 126(6): 1063-74.
[http://dx.doi.org/10.1093/oxfordjournals.aje.a114745] [PMID: 3687918]

[77] Kang SY, Lee YJ, Park KH, *et al.* Congenital leukemia of fetus with acquired *AML1* gene duplication. Obstet Gynecol Sci 2014; 57(4): 325-9.
[http://dx.doi.org/10.5468/ogs.2014.57.4.325] [PMID: 25105108]

[78] Isaacs H Jr. Fetal and neonatal leukemia. J Pediatr Hematol Oncol 2003; 25(5): 348-61.
[http://dx.doi.org/10.1097/00043426-200305000-00002] [PMID: 12759620]

[79] Feygin T, Khalek N, Moldenhauer JS. Fetal brain, head, and neck tumors: Prenatal imaging and management. Prenat Diagn 2020; 40(10): 1203-19.
[http://dx.doi.org/10.1002/pd.5722] [PMID: 32350893]

[80] Hyett J. Intra-abdominal masses: prenatal differential diagnosis and management. Prenat Diagn 2008; 28(7): 645-55.
[http://dx.doi.org/10.1002/pd.2028] [PMID: 18567068]

[81] Debost-Legrand A, Laurichesse-Delmas H, Francannet C, *et al.* False positive morphologic diagnoses at the anomaly scan: marginal or real problem, a population-based cohort study. BMC Pregnancy Childbirth 2014; 14(1): 112.
[http://dx.doi.org/10.1186/1471-2393-14-112] [PMID: 24655605]

[82] Cavalheiro S, Moron AF, Hisaba W, Dastoli P, Silva NS. Fetal brain tumors. Childs Nerv Syst 2003; 19(7-8): 529-36.
[http://dx.doi.org/10.1007/s00381-003-0770-9] [PMID: 12908112]

[83] Victoria T, Johnson AM, Moldenhauer JS, Hedrick HL, Flake AW, Adzick NS. Imaging of fetal tumors and other dysplastic lesions: A review with emphasis on MR imaging. Prenat Diagn 2020;

40(1): 84-99.
[http://dx.doi.org/10.1002/pd.5630] [PMID: 31925807]

[84]   Suresh S, Indrani S, Vijayalakshmi S, Nirmala J, Meera G. Prenatal diagnosis of cerebral neuroblastoma by fetal brain biopsy. J Ultrasound Med 1993; 12(5): 303-6.
[http://dx.doi.org/10.7863/jum.1993.12.5.303] [PMID: 8345560]

[85]   Wapner RJ, Jenkins TM, Silverman N, Kaufmann M, Hannau C, McCue P. Prenatal diagnosis of congenital nephrosis byin utero kidney biopsy. Prenat Diagn 2001; 21(4): 256-61.
[http://dx.doi.org/10.1002/pd.38] [PMID: 11288113]

[86]   Waller EK, Huang S, Terstappen L. Changes in the growth properties of CD34+, CD38-bone marrow progenitors during human fetal development. Blood 1995; 86(2): 710-8.

[87]   Kontopoulos EV, Gualtieri M, Quintero RA. Successful in utero treatment of an oral teratoma *via* operative fetoscopy: case report and review of the literature. Am J Obstet Gynecol 2012; 207(1): e12-5.
[http://dx.doi.org/10.1016/j.ajog.2012.04.008] [PMID: 22541612]

[88]   Van den Veyver IB. Recent advances in prenatal genetic screening and testing. F1000 Res 2016; 5: 2591.
[http://dx.doi.org/10.12688/f1000research.9215.1] [PMID: 27853526]

[89]   Lancaster J, Wiseman R, Berchuck A. An inevitable dilemma: Prenatal testing for mutations in the brca1 breast-ovarian cancer susceptibility gene. Obstet Gynecol 1996; 87(2): 306-9.
[http://dx.doi.org/10.1016/0029-7844(95)00405-X] [PMID: 8559544]

[90]   Chasen ST, Chervenak FA, McCullough LB. The role of cephalocentesis in modern obstetrics. Am J Obstet Gynecol 2001; 185(3): 734-6.
[http://dx.doi.org/10.1067/mob.2001.117487] [PMID: 11568806]

[91]   Howse E, Teoh T, Kelly E, Chitayat D, McParland P, Ryan G. P21.04: The role of cephalocentesis in the management of the severely hydrocephalic fetus. Ultrasound Obstet Gynecol 2011; 38(S1): 237-8.
[http://dx.doi.org/10.1002/uog.9863]

[92]   Borsellino A, Zaccara A, Nahom A, *et al.* False-positive rate in prenatal diagnosis of surgical anomalies. J Pediatr Surg 2006; 41(4): 826-9.
[http://dx.doi.org/10.1016/j.jpedsurg.2005.12.024] [PMID: 16567202]

[93]   McEwing R, Hayward C, Furness M. Foetal cystic abdominal masses. Australas Radiol 2003; 47(2): 101-10.
[http://dx.doi.org/10.1046/j.0004-8461.2003.01136.x] [PMID: 12780436]

[94]   Thilaganathan B, Sairam S, Papageorghiou AT, Bhide A. Problem based obstetric ultrasound. CRC Press 2007.
[http://dx.doi.org/10.3109/9780203089996]

[95]   Cubas RF, Longshore S, Rodriguez S, Tagge E, Baerg J, Moores D. Atropine: a cure for persistent post laparoscopic pyloromyotomy emesis? J Neonatal Surg 2016; 6(1): 2.
[http://dx.doi.org/10.21699/jns.v6i1.485] [PMID: 28083488]

[96]   Yong R, Wu T, Mihatov N, Shen M, Brown M, Zaghloul K, *et al.* ST-035. Re-operation for recurrent glioblastoma multiforme. Neuro-oncology 2013; 15 (suppl_3).

[97]   Van Poppel M, Klimo P Jr, Dewire M, *et al.* Resection of infantile brain tumors after neoadjuvant chemotherapy: the St. Jude experience. J Neurosurg Pediatr 2011; 8(3): 251-6.
[http://dx.doi.org/10.3171/2011.6.PEDS11158] [PMID: 21882915]

[98]   Ryan G, Somme S, Crombleholme TM, Eds. Airway compromise in the fetus and neonate: Prenatal assessment and perinatal management. Seminars in Fetal and Neonatal Medicine 2016.

[99]   Laje P, Johnson MP, Howell LJ, *et al.* Ex utero intrapartum treatment in the management of giant

cervical teratomas. J Pediatr Surg 2012; 47(6): 1208-16.
[http://dx.doi.org/10.1016/j.jpedsurg.2012.03.027] [PMID: 22703795]

[100] Cavoretto P, Molina F, Poggi S, Davenport M, Nicolaides KH. Prenatal diagnosis and outcome of echogenic fetal lung lesions. Ultrasound Obstet Gynecol 2008; 32(6): 769-83.
[http://dx.doi.org/10.1002/uog.6218] [PMID: 18956429]

[101] Shamshirsaz AA, Nassr AA, Erfani H, *et al.* Fetoscopic laryngotracheoscopy: novel diagnostic modality to avoid unnecessary *ex-utero* intrapartum treatment (EXIT) in cases with suspected fetal airway compromise. Ultrasound Obstet Gynecol 2019; 53(3): 421-3.
[http://dx.doi.org/10.1002/uog.19033] [PMID: 29479755]

[102] Sheikh F, Akinkuotu A, Olutoye OO, *et al.* Prenatally diagnosed neck masses: long-term outcomes and quality of life. J Pediatr Surg 2015; 50(7): 1210-3.
[http://dx.doi.org/10.1016/j.jpedsurg.2015.02.035] [PMID: 25863543]

[103] Cruz-Martinez R, Moreno-Alvarez O, Garcia M, *et al.* Fetal endoscopic tracheal intubation: a new fetoscopic procedure to ensure extrauterine tracheal permeability in a case with congenital cervical teratoma. Fetal Diagn Ther 2015; 38(2): 154-8.
[http://dx.doi.org/10.1159/000362387] [PMID: 25228387]

[104] Curran PF, Jelin EB, Rand L, *et al.* Prenatal steroids for microcystic congenital cystic adenomatoid malformations. J Pediatr Surg 2010; 45(1): 145-50.
[http://dx.doi.org/10.1016/j.jpedsurg.2009.10.025] [PMID: 20105595]

[105] Pierce JM, LaCroix P, Heym K, *et al.* Pleuropulmonary blastoma: a single-center case series of 6 patients. J Pediatr Hematol Oncol 2017; 39(8): e419-22.
[http://dx.doi.org/10.1097/MPH.0000000000000972] [PMID: 28991133]

[106] Salomon LJ, Audibert F, Dommergues M, Vial M, Frydman R. Fetal thoracoamniotic shunting as the only treatment for pulmonary sequestration with hydrops: favorable long-term outcome without postnatal surgery. Ultrasound Obstet Gynecol 2003; 21(3): 299-301.
[http://dx.doi.org/10.1002/uog.76] [PMID: 12666228]

[107] Nicolini U, Cerri V, Groli C, Poblete A, Mauro F. A new approach to prenatal treatment of extralobar pulmonary sequestration. Prenat Diagn 2000; 20(9): 758-60.
[http://dx.doi.org/10.1002/1097-0223(200009)20:9<758::AID-PD899>3.0.CO;2-A] [PMID: 11015708]

[108] Adzick NS, Flake AW, Crombleholme TM. Management of congenital lung lesions. Semin Pediatr Surg 2003; 12(1): 10-6.

[109] Sepulveda W, Gómez E, Gutiérrez J. Intrapericardial teratoma. Ultrasound Obstet Gynecol 2000; 15(6): 547-8.
[http://dx.doi.org/10.1046/j.1469-0705.2000.00144.x] [PMID: 11005130]

[110] Grebille AG, Mitanchez D, Benachi A, *et al.* Pericardial teratoma complicated by hydrops: successful fetal therapy by thoracoamniotic shunting. Prenat Diagn 2003; 23(9): 735-9.
[http://dx.doi.org/10.1002/pd.698] [PMID: 12975784]

[111] Yuan SM. Fetal cardiac tumors: clinical features, management and prognosis. J Perinat Med 2018; 46(2): 115-21.
[http://dx.doi.org/10.1515/jpm-2016-0311] [PMID: 28343178]

[112] Leithiser RE Jr, Fyfe D, Weatherby E III, Sade R, Garvin AJ. Prenatal sonographic diagnosis of atrial hemangioma. AJR Am J Roentgenol 1986; 147(6): 1207-8.
[http://dx.doi.org/10.2214/ajr.147.6.1207] [PMID: 3535456]

[113] Kitagawa N, Ohhama Y, Fukuzato Y, *et al.* Pericardial hemangioma presenting fetal cardiac tamponade and postnatal bronchostenosis. Pediatr Surg Int 2004; 20(5): 376-7.
[http://dx.doi.org/10.1007/s00383-004-1202-y] [PMID: 15221363]

[114] Puligandla PS, Kay S, Morin L, *et al.* Pericardial hemangioma presenting as thoracic mass in utero. Fetal Diagn Ther 2004; 19(2): 178-81.
[http://dx.doi.org/10.1159/000075146] [PMID: 14764966]

[115] Ríos JC, Chávarri F, Morales G, *et al.* Cardiac myxoma with prenatal diagnosis. World J Pediatr Congenit Heart Surg 2013; 4(2): 210-2.
[http://dx.doi.org/10.1177/2150135112472210] [PMID: 23799738]

[116] Jabbari P, Hanaei S, Rezaei N. State of the art in immunotherapy of neuroblastoma. Immunotherapy 2019; 11(9): 831-50.
[http://dx.doi.org/10.2217/imt-2019-0018] [PMID: 31094257]

[117] Swamy R, Embleton N, Hale J. Sacrococcygeal teratoma over two decades: Birth prevalence, prenatal diagnosis and clinical outcomes. Prenat Diagn 2008; 28(11): 1048-51.
[http://dx.doi.org/10.1002/pd.2122] [PMID: 18973151]

[118] Samuel M, Spitz L. Infantile hepatic hemangioendothelioma: The role of surgery. J Pediatr Surg 1995; 30(10): 1425-9.
[http://dx.doi.org/10.1016/0022-3468(95)90397-6] [PMID: 8786479]

[119] Makin E, Davenport M. Fetal and neonatal liver tumours. Early Hum Dev 2010; 86(10): 637-42.
[http://dx.doi.org/10.1016/j.earlhumdev.2010.08.023] [PMID: 20956063]

[120] Tiao GM, Bobey N, Allen S, *et al.* The current management of hepatoblastoma: A combination of chemotherapy, conventional resection, and liver transplantation. J Pediatr 2005; 146(2): 204-11.
[http://dx.doi.org/10.1016/j.jpeds.2004.09.011] [PMID: 15689909]

[121] Sarin YK, Rahul SK, Sinha S, Khurana N, Ramji S. Antenatally diagnosed wilms' tumour. J Neonatal Surg 2014; 3(1): 8.
[http://dx.doi.org/10.47338/jns.v3.72] [PMID: 26023479]

[122] Van Mieghem T, Al-Ibrahim A, Deprest J, *et al.* Minimally invasive therapy for fetal sacrococcygeal teratoma: case series and systematic review of the literature. Ultrasound Obstet Gynecol 2014; 43(6): 611-9.
[http://dx.doi.org/10.1002/uog.13315] [PMID: 24488859]

[123] Benachi A, Durin L, Vasseur Maurer S, *et al.* Prenatally diagnosed sacrococcygeal teratoma: a prognostic classification. J Pediatr Surg 2006; 41(9): 1517-21.
[http://dx.doi.org/10.1016/j.jpedsurg.2006.05.009] [PMID: 16952584]

[124] Al-Refai A, Ryan G, Van Mieghem T. Maternal risks of fetal therapy. Curr Opin Obstet Gynecol 2017; 29(2): 80-4.
[http://dx.doi.org/10.1097/GCO.0000000000000346] [PMID: 28151754]

[125] Akin MA, Akin L, Özbek S, *et al.* Fetal-neonatal ovarian cysts--their monitoring and management: retrospective evaluation of 20 cases and review of the literature. J Clin Res Pediatr Endocrinol 2010; 2(1): 28-33.
[http://dx.doi.org/10.4274/jcrpe.v2i1.28] [PMID: 21274333]

[126] Mühler MR, Rake A, Schwabe M, *et al.* Value of fetal cerebral MRI in sonographically proven cardiac rhabdomyoma. Pediatr Radiol 2007; 37(5): 467-74.
[http://dx.doi.org/10.1007/s00247-007-0436-y] [PMID: 17357805]

[127] Mansouri HE, Zourair A, Hammaoui H, *et al.* Desmoid Tumor of the Pelvis in Children: One Case Report. OALib 2019; 6(1): 1-5.
[http://dx.doi.org/10.4236/oalib.1105122]

[128] Masmejan S, Baud D, Ryan G, Van Mieghem T. Management of fetal tumors. Best Pract Res Clin Obstet Gynaecol 2019; 58: 107-20.
[http://dx.doi.org/10.1016/j.bpobgyn.2019.01.006] [PMID: 30770283]

[129] Rudie JD, Rauschecker AM, Bryan RN, Davatzikos C, Mohan S. Emerging applications of artificial

intelligence in neuro-oncology. Radiology 2019; 290(3): 607-18.
[http://dx.doi.org/10.1148/radiol.2018181928] [PMID: 30667332]

[130] Palmeira P, Quinello C, Silveira-Lessa AL, Zago CA, Carneiro-Sampaio M. IgG placental transfer in healthy and pathological pregnancies. Clinical and Developmental Immunology 2012; 2012.
[http://dx.doi.org/10.1155/2012/985646]

[131] Kinder JM, Stelzer IA, Arck PC, Way SS. Immunological implications of pregnancy-induced microchimerism. Nat Rev Immunol 2017; 17(8): 483-94.
[http://dx.doi.org/10.1038/nri.2017.38] [PMID: 28480895]

[132] Peyce DM. Lower accessory pulmonary artery with intralobar sequestration of lung: A Report of seven cases. J Pathol Bacteriol 1946; 58(3): 457-67.
[http://dx.doi.org/10.1002/path.1700580316] [PMID: 20283082]

# CHAPTER 10

# Autism Spectrum Disorder during Infancy: Implications for Diagnosis, Prognosis, and Therapeutic Approaches

**Kimia Kazemzadeh[1,2], Parnian Shobeiri[2,3,4], Serge Brand[2,3,4] and Nima Rezaei[2,5,6,*]**

[1] *Students' Scientific Research Center, Tehran University of Medical Sciences, Tehran, Iran*

[2] *Network of Immunity in Infection, Malignancy and Autoimmunity (NIIMA), Universal Scientific Education and Research Network (USERN), Tehran, Iran*

[3] *School of Medicine, Tehran University of Medical Sciences, Tehran, Iran*

[4] *Center for Affective, Stress and Sleep Disorders, Psychiatric Clinics of the University of Basel, Basel, Switzerland*

[5] *Research Center for Immunodeficiencies, Pediatrics Center of Excellence, Children's Medical Center, Tehran University of Medical Sciences, Tehran, Iran*

[6] *Department of Immunology, School of Medicine, Tehran University of Medical Sciences, Tehran, Iran*

**Abstract:** Autism spectrum disorder (ASD) is a complex psychiatric and neurodevelopmental issue related to delays in the acquisition of behavioral and social skills. The main symptoms of ASD are impairments in communication, limited interest and skills in social interactions, and repetitive behavior. In the present chapter about ASD during infancy, we reviewed the behavioral indicators of ASD, different ways of diagnosis, and the significance of an early and correct diagnosis. While children with ASD are usually diagnosed between ages 2-4, many pediatricians and psychiatrists are interested in understanding the developmental course of ASD in early infancy and infancy. Such an understanding would help both infants with ASD and their family members to identify useful interventions to cope more favorably with difficulties related to the infants' symptoms of ASD. We highlighted that ASD traits unfavorably impact a child's and their family's social, behavioral, and the family's economic status and conditions. Given this, an early diagnosis and timely and appropriate interventions should mitigate ASD-related issues in everyday life. To this end, assessing a child's behavior is the gold standard for ASD diagnosis. Most of the symptoms appear in the second year of life; often language acquisition is impaired. Considering the signs of ASD in infancy, promising perspectives on ASD diagnosis will be introduced in the future.

---

* **Corresponding author Nima Rezaei:** Research Center for Immunodeficiencies, Children's Medical Center Hospital, Dr. Qarib St, Keshavarz Blvd, Tehran 14194, Iran; Tel: +9821-6692-9234; Fax: +9821-6692-9235; E-mail: rezaei_nima@yahoo.com

**Keywords:** ASD, Autism spectrum disorder, Behavioral skills, Brain development, Childhood, Children, Clinical approach, Communicational skill, Diagnosis, DSM-5, Early diagnosis, Early intervention, ICD-11, Infancy, Infant, Intervention, Neurodevelopmental disorder, Quality of life, Signs, Symptoms, Treatment.

## INTRODUCTION

Autism spectrum disorder (ASD) is a complex and lifelong neurodevelopmental disorder. The main etiology is unknown yet, but both environmental and genetic risk factors are associated with the onset of this disorder [1]. The prevalence of ASD significantly increased in early decades [2]: A comprehensive systematic review and meta-analysis including a total of 74 studies comprising 30,212,757 participants reported a worldwide prevalence rate of 0.6%. Importantly, prevalence rates varied among continents: Asia: 0.4%, Europe: 0.5%; America: 1%; Australia: 1.7%, and Africa 1% [3].

Children with ASD suffer from impairments in communication, limited interest and skills in social interactions, and repetitive behavior. Symptom severity may individually vary. Generally, in younger children with ASD, the following signs are observed: 1) avoiding eye contact with others, 2) repetitive movements, 3) not smiling when others are smiling at them, and 4) not talking as much as other same-aged children. In older children with ASD, the following additional behaviors are observed: 1) problems in making friends or preferring to stay alone, 2) showing great and increased interest in certain objects or very specific topics, 3) taking the content of a sentence completely literally (for example they may not perceive idioms, irony, sarcasm, verbal hints, word games, word ambiguities), 4) problems in understanding other people's feeling (*i.e.*, lack of empathy), 5) problems in expressing how they feel (*i.e.*, lack of emotional competencies), and 6) usually following a strict daily routine [4].

ASD imposes challenges on children with ASD and their parents. However, early detection and intervention can reduce this burden and lead to better developmental and cognitive improvement in the future. While ASD is usually diagnosed between the ages of 2 to 4 years, it is required to identify ASD in early infancy and infancy, thus, among infants and toddlers age up to 36 months. Typical behavioral signs are: Motor delays, lack of response to name, lack of proper eye contact, or a decreased variety of gesture types; further signs which will be elucidated in this chapter in more details are discussed below [5 - 7].

The aims of the present chapter are three-fold: a) To thoroughly show typical behavioral indicators of ASD, along with their impact on everyday life; b) To showcase the importance of the early diagnosis and detection of ASD to improve a favorable outcome of children with ASD; c) To streamline future directions of early diagnosis based on most recent publications in the field.

## WHAT IS AUTISM SPECTRUM DISORDER?

In 1943, Leo Kanner, an Austrian-American child psychiatrist, described three girls and eight boys, including a five-year-old boy called Donald. Unlike the general behavior of five-years-old children, Donald was the happiest when he was alone; he didn't cry to stay with his mother; he was indifferent to his father's homecoming and uninterested in visiting his relatives; in a room, he ignored people and was solely interested in objects; words' meanings were strict and unchangeable to him. He also didn't understand the meaning of facial expressions such as smiling. In 1944, Hans Asperger, an Austrian pediatrician, described four boys. A 6-year-old boy called Fritz was one of them who had some considerable behaviors such as: Quickly learned to talk and express himself in words, couldn't get involved in a group of playing kids, was indifferent to the respect to adults, talked to strangers without shyness, and also stereotypic habits and movements were observed. Both Kanner and Asperger portrayed a set of behavior not matching behaviors of typically developing children and of the general child population; their descriptions paved the ground for the today's autism spectrum disorder [8]. ASD is a psychiatric and neurological disorder characterized by significant delays in social and behavioral skills, communication, and language development. The etiology is unclear, but different immunological, biological, psychological [9], and genetic [10] models may explain the occurrence and development of ASD. In other words, ASD is a complex disorder with a relatively homogeneous pattern of symptoms and different possible etiologies. Further, pharmacological treatments target on mitigating symptoms and ASD-behavioral issues such as aggression, self-mutilation, sleep disorders, and repetitive behaviors [11].

Further, psychiatric, medical, or developmental co-occurring conditions are observed in almost 70% of individuals with ASD. Co-occurring conditions in childhood might cross into adolescence, while some of these conditions may develop in adulthood for the first time *(e.g.*, depression and epilepsy). A higher amount of co-occurring conditions is associated with more disabilities [8].

## MAIN TYPES OF AUTISM SPECTRUM DISORDER

Asperger syndrome is commonly used informally in ASD communities, but it has been used as the first level of autism spectrum disorder through medical professions. A child with Asperger syndrome may have problems with social communication but will have strong verbal skills and above-average intelligence. Other signs and symptoms are inflexibility in behavior, problems in executive functioning and switching between activities, interacting difficultly with others at school, and having flat and monotone speech.

Rett Syndrome is known as a considerable neurodevelopmental disorder in infancy. It happens rarely and mostly affects girls. The child can have a fulfilling life with the appropriate care, but s/he will experience different challenges affecting all aspects of their life. Loss of coordination and standard movements, speech and communication issues, and sometimes difficulty breathing are some of its signs and symptoms.

Childhood Disintegrative Disorder (CDD) is also known as Heller's syndrome. It is a neurodevelopmental disorder with a delayed onset of developmental issues in social function, motor skills, and language. It means that at first, the child has normal development in these areas, but then between ages 3 to 10, s/he will exhibit developmental problems. The etiology is unknown and is more common in boys (almost 90%). At the onset of this disorder, the child loses more than two developmental aspects of their life, including motor skills, social skills, vocabulary or language, and toileting skills.

Kanner's syndrome was identified by Leo Kanner, a psychiatrist, in 1943, as an infantile autism spectrum disorder. In medicine, this condition is also known as classic autism disorder. These children are alert, intelligent, and attractive. The common symptoms are lack of emotional attachment, obsession with handling objects, uncontrolled speech, and high degrees of visuospatial skills and memory.

Pervasive Developmental Disorder-Not Otherwise Specified (PDD-NOS) is a term for a mild type of this disorder with language and social development issues. It is also known as subthreshold ASD since it describes a person with some symptoms of ASD but not all of them [12].

## IMPORTANCE OF AUTISM SPECTRUM DISORDER ON THEIR QUALITY OF LIFE

Regarding the parent-child relationship, in comparison to parents with Typically Developing Children (TDC), parents with children with ASD report a higher degree of stress. Such a higher degree of stress is observed especially before a child's diagnosis, as parents of children with ASD might be unaware of their children's unpredictable behaviors and lack of interest in affection and interaction (known as typical markers of ASD). These parents might be unfamiliar with how to deal with these challenges or how to get help from others [9, 13]. Further, when treatment and care costs are high, this condition may lead to a considerable financial burden. In addition, the full-time care required for a child with ASD may impair parents' working schedules, including career plans and financial remunerations [14]. Also, children with ASD may develop other further different mental health disorders as co-existence conditions, such as depression, bipolar disorder, seizures (which occur in one out of four children with ASD), anxiety disorder, attention deficit hyperactivity disorder (ADHD), and eating disorders [15]. However, beyond all these issues for these children and their families, early diagnosis can be considered a helpful approach to reduce their challenges and to improve children's developmental and social outcomes in the future [14].

## NEONATAL RISK FACTORS FOR AUTISM SPECTRUM DISORDER

The etiology of ASD is not clear yet, and distinguishing whether the risk factors should be regarded as strictly genetic or environmental is neither possible nor helpful and necessary for the treatment. Guinchat *et al.* synthesized the following pre-, peri, and neonatal risk factors: Family-related factors are: Higher parental age and mother born abroad; maternal pregnancy factors are: bleeding and pre-eclampsia; delivery factors are: breech presentation, being small for gestational age (intrauterine growth restriction (IUGR)), and scheduled cesarean secetion. Regarding the neonatal risk factors, the most noticeable is a new-born with adverse conditions such as low Apgar score, prematurity, hyperbilirubinemia, encephalopathy, low birth weight, and birth defects [16].

In a meta-analysis by *Gardener et al.*, umbilical cord complications, birth trauma or injury, summer birth, abnormal presentation, fetal distress, multiple births, difficulties in feeding, neonatal anemia, Rh or ABO incompatibility, maternal hemorrhage, and congenital malformation were mentioned as associated factors. High birth weight, anesthesia, post-term birth, head circumference, and assisted vaginal delivery were known as not-associated factors of autism development [17].

Further risk factors for ASD were: Consanguineous marriage, passive smoking exposure during pregnancy, history of diabetes, family history of ASD, previous abortion, assisted fertility, and neonatal convulsion. In contrast, C-section and vitamin intake during pregnancy appeared to decrease the rate of ASD development [18].

## BRAIN DEVELOPMENT IN AUTISM SPECTRUM DISORDER

One of the most important findings in diverse studies on brain development in ASD was brain enlargement, which was not observed at birth but appeared one or two years later [19 - 21]. In other words, normal head size was observed at birth, but the head circumference enlarged obviously in about two years [19].

Total brain volume growth rate increased significantly in high familial risk for ASD (HR-ASD) infants compared to other infants in 12 to 24 months. Still, no differences in cortical thickness were detected between groups during the 6-24 months period. Further, higher severity scores of autism in the social domain at 24 months of age are related to greater brain volume growth rates across the 12-24 months period [22]. Next, infants who showed autism later, an excessive amount of cerebrospinal fluid (CSF) surrounded the brain's cortical surface in subarachnoid space in the first 6-9 months of life [23]. In this line, the amount of EA-CSF (extra-axial cerebrospinal fluid) in infants whose autism was diagnosed later was 18% more than in control groups (at six months of age). This excessive amount is correlated to motor deficits in the first year of their life [24].

In some other studies, some abnormalities were observed in white matter organizational structures among multiple fiber tracts *(e.g.,* increase in radial diffusivity and Fractional Anisotropy (FA) reduction for the left superior longitudinal fasciculus (LSLF)) at six months of age. Also, reductions in white matter organization were related to an abnormality of sensory responsiveness at 24 months of age [25 - 27].

Next, functional brain imaging (like fMRI Acquisition and IQ measuring) showed hypoactivity in response to language in temporal and frontal regions [28].

An fMRI study showed that many cortical regions, such as the left superior temporal gyrus, left fusiform gyrus, and left middle temporal gyrus had a reduction of activation. Also, greater activities in the right frontal lobe were shown in children with autism compared to typical same-aged children. In the group of children with ASD, in comparison to the control group, a trend towards greater recruitment of both the right temporal and right frontal regions was observed. Also, it was shown that in children with ASD right hemisphere plays a substantial role in language processing.

Bashat *et al.* reported an abnormal response of the right-lateralized temporal cortex to language in infants whose autism was diagnosed later at 14 months of age. This finding may be related to the failure of normal language development in these children [29]. Examining the autistic brain shows that brain overgrowth in the early years of life could result from an increased number of neurons, dendritic arbors, and synapses. With these possibilities, it is imaginable that resting state network development may be considered as evidence of over-connectivity, which was also reported in DTI (Diffusion Tensor Imaging) studies that showed increased FA in this period of time [30]. Check out Table **1** for more information on imaging studies.

**Table 1. Summary of Selected Neuroimaging Studies in Infants with ASD.**

| Author | Year | Country | ASD Patients [n] | Controls [n] | Main Findings |
|---|---|---|---|---|---|
| Courchesne *et al.* [66] | 2001 | USA | 60 | 52 | Abnormal regulation of brain growth, early overgrowth, and hyperplasia in cerebral gray matter and cerebellar white matter in ASD. |
| Hazlett *et al.* [67] | 2005 | USA | 51 | 25 | Generalized enlargement of white and gray matter cerebral volumes, but not cerebellar volume in autistic children at the age of two. |
| Hazlett *et al.* [68] | 2011 | USA | 59 | 38 | Generalized cerebral cortical enlargement and disproportionate enlargement in temporal lobe white matter in ASD. |
| Shen *et al.* [24] | 2017 | USA | 47 | 296 | Increased extra-axial CSF at 6 months in ASD. |
| Wolff *et al.* [25] | 2012 | USA | 28 | 64 | Abnormal development of white matter pathways might predict the manifestation of ASD in the first year of life. |
| Aylward *et al.* [69] | 2002 | USA | 67 | 83 | Larger brain volume in autistic children. |
| Kim *et al.* [70] | 2010 | South Korea | 31 | 20 | Bilateral enlargement of laterobasal subregions of the amygdala in autistic children. |
| Nordahl *et al.* [71] | 2012 | USA | 85 | 47 | Elevated amygdala volumes and total cerebral volumes in ASD at 37 months of age. |
| Maximo *et al.* [72] | 2019 | USA | 138 | 168 | Overconnectivity in unimodal networks and underconnectivity in supramodal networks in ASD. |
| Courchesne *et al.* [73] | 1993 | USA | 12 | 23 | Parietal lobes are reduced in volume in a portion of the autistic population. |

## BEHAVIORAL NEUROSCIENCE OF AUTISM SPECTRUM DISORDER

Network and synaptic dysregulation can cause behavioral problems in autistic children, such as abnormalities of circadian, serotonin, and sleep rhythm [31]. Regarding the irregularity of sleep rhythm, insomnia is highly prevalent among children with ASD [32]. By definition, insomnia is sleep latency of more than 30 minutes each night [33]. Problems in daytime functioning are the result of this prolonged night awakening. All cognitive levels of autistic children suffer from this disorder, and it has a high prevalence of 60-86% among them (two or three times more than healthy children) [32, 33]. It can cause their parents additional stress and change their sleep patterns [34]. Small and measurable variations among their sleep parameters were reported in studying children with ASD by actigraphy (ACT), a microcomputer like a wristwatch that generates a signal when it moves each time and senses physical motion [35].

Regarding the neurobiological hypothesis as the reason for this disorder, abnormal production of melatonin, circadian-relevant genes, maturational and organizational variations of brain waves, and also sensory and arousal dysregulation are the most significant ones. During Rapid Eye Movement (REM), there is an association between REM burst activity and slow wave activity in healthy children. However, this association was not reported in children with ASD; it may suggest the pattern of immature organization. In 1976, a study reported that in autistic children, mean Eye Movement (EM) burst length and the ratio of EMs within bursts to EMs outside of bursts are noticeably less than typical same-aged children. It showed that eye movement organization is immature in autistic children. Another finding in this study is that spindle EEG activity is found in autistic children but not found in the control group. It showed that sleep stages in children with ASD are not well differentiated [36]. Wakefulness and sleep in humankind, are regulated by the suprachiasmatic nucleus known as the circadian clock. This clock organizes the circadian rhythm, system of positive and negative feedback loops, which change the expression of the clock gene [37]. In 2002, the anomalies of clock genes or clock-related genes were suggested to have an association with core deficits of ASD, such as social timing and temporary synchrony deficits. Also, Wimpory *et al.* reported that the interaction of clock genes (such as hPER1, hPER2, and hPER3) and clock gene-gene might have a dual role in sleep and oscillator control related to social communication and concurrent development of the brain [38].

Another hypothesis for a reason for insomnia in autistic children is abnormal levels of melatonin. Pineal glands synthesize melatonin, which is then sent to the suprachiasmatic nucleus, which is the master clock in the brain, by MTNR1B and MTNR1A receptors, involved in various functions such as sleep induction, immune function, and regulation of seasonal and circadian rhythm. A delayed melatonin rhythm may be related to prolonged sleep latency, and a low melatonin amplitude may be related to night wakening in autistic children [37, 39]. Also, it has been reported in several studies that the level of melatonin and its primary metabolite (urinary 6 sulfatoxymelatonin) in plasma, serum, and urine of children with ASD is lower than in others [39, 40].

Recent studies focused on increased physiological and somatic arousal and cognitive arousal as the reason for insomnia in children with ASD. The hypothesis of cognitive arousal claims that increasing the rate of cognitive activity (worrying and thinking while trying to sleep) can prevent the start of the sleep process. The physiological arousal hypothesis claims that in individuals with insomnia, compared to good sleepers, sympathetic nervous system activation is greater [41 - 43]. Since children with ASD are described as hyper- or hypo-aroused to external and internal stimuli, they may have problems with their sleep rhythm [44].

Regarding the role of serotonin in behavior, Endocrine-Disrupting Chemicals (EDCs) were considered. EDCs are a large number of compounds, such as polycyclic aromatic hydrocarbons, pharmaceuticals, herbicides, industrial by-products, surface protectors, solvents, and flame retardants. During the early stages of development, exposure to many of these EDCs can cause problems for the endocrine system, and adverse reproductive, neurological, immune, and metabolic effects may be observed in the human body. For example, EDCs can cause problems with the synthesis and release of serotonin, glutamate, and dopamine. These neurotransmitters have a significant role in regulating behavior, learning, and cognition. As a hypothesis, exposure to EDCs which leads to endocrine disorders, can increase the risk of ASD as a neurodevelopmental disorder [45]. Also, another study shows that living near pesticide application sites during pregnancy can increase the risk of ASD by six times [46].

In a prospective longitudinal study by Bradshaw *et al.*, the neurobehavior of sixty neonates with a low and high familial likelihood of ASD was examined every month from 1 to 3 months old. In two years of the following duration, 18 participants were diagnosed with ASD and 36 participants developed typically. Consequently, the neurobehavioral development of the two groups of infants was largely similar to each other in the first three months of life. The only expectation was that object-focused attention development attenuated for autistic infants started at 2 to 3 months. This result significantly shows the importance of attention to objects as an early key sign of autism diagnosis [47].

## CLINICAL APPROACH TO AUTISM SPECTRUM DISORDER (CONSIDERING DIFFERENT WAYS OF DIAGNOSIS)

Some features with different degrees are used in diagnosis most of the time. In a study by Wing *et al.* [48], four different items were named as follows: social interaction, imagination, communication, and repetitive pattern of activities. Various degrees of social interactions are as follows: indifferent, only for physical needs, passive, and making odd one-sided approaches. Regarding social communication, no communication, for needs only, reply, and spontaneous (repetitive, unusual, one-sided) are the proposed degrees. Social imagination is classified into no imagination, copying others, using toys properly but repetitive and limited, and acting repetitively. There are also four degrees for repetitive patterns of activities: bodily-directed ad simple, object-directed and simple, complex routines, and verbal [49].

Developmental monitoring is known as a simple way for ASD diagnosis. It is an active and continuous process of observing child growth and developmental skills (based on developmental milestones) by parents, grandparents, and also education providers in early childhood [50]. Developmental screening is a more formal and detailed way than developmental monitoring, which takes a closer look at the child's development. The American Academy of Pediatrics (AAP) suggests developmental screening at 9, 18, and 30 months of age, especially for ASD, at 18 and 24 months. This screening is based on checklists and questions which compare the child to other same-aged children [51]. Additional screening should be done for children at high risk for ASD (for example, for children with a family history of this disorder). If the area of concern was identified in this screening, formal evaluation and an in-dept look at the developmental skills are needed for the final diagnosis by pediatricians and psychiatrists [52].

The DSM-5, which was released in 2013 by American Psychiatric Association [53], is currently used as a standard reference for ASD diagnosis: A) deficits in social interaction and communication (deficits in social-emotional interactions such as reduction of sharing interests and emotion, deficits in nonverbal behaviors such as body language and eye contact, deficits in understanding relationships such as being uninterested in making friends); B) repetitive and restricted patterns of behaviors(repetitive speech or motor movement, inflexible routines and persistent on sameness, abnormal and fixated interests, strange interest in environmental sensory inputs); C) onset of the symptoms must be in early developmental duration; D) symptoms cause important and clinical problems in social functioning; E) autism spectrum disorder and intellectual disability often co-occur [54].

## THE AMERICAN PSYCHIATRIC ASSOCIATION'S DIAGNOSTC AND STATISTIC MANUAL, FIFTH EDITION (DSM-5)

According to DSM-5, a child must show significant deficits in all aspects of social communication and interaction in addition to at least two types of repetitive behaviors. Three aspects of social interaction are as follows: 1) deficits in sharing interests and emotions, 2) deficits in nonverbal communicative behaviors, and 3) deficits in the development and understanding of the relationship. Four aspects of restricted and repetitive behaviors are as follows: 1) repetitive motor movements, 2) inflexible adherence to routines, 3) highly fixated and abnormal interest in unusual subjects/objects, and 4) hypo/hyperreactivity to sensory input from the environment [55].

## AUTISM SPECTRUM DISORDER IN THE INTERNATIONAL CLASSIFICATION OF DISEASE [ICD-11]

ICD-11 is offered by the World Health Organization (WHO) and included ASD in its category as a mental, behavioral and neurodevelopmental disorder besides other disorders such as Attention Deficit Hyperactivity Disorder (ADHD), developmental learning disorders, and developmental motor coordination disorder. In order to diagnose ASD, ICD-11 noted that: "Autism spectrum disorder is characterized by persistent deficits in the ability to initiate and to sustain reciprocal social interaction and social communication, and by a range of restricted, repetitive, and inflexible patterns of behavior and interests" [56].

## DIFFERENCES IN SIGNS AND PRESENTATIONS OF AUTISM SPECTRUM DISORDER AMONG TWO GENDERS

Comparing girls and boys diagnosed with ASD, girls are more likely to have better cognitive development and decreased symptoms over time than boys. Girls are less described as struggling socially than boys since they are more likely to stay close to others than boys. Also, girls less tend to show repetitive interest or behavior than boys. Girls' motivation for making friends and social attention is observed better than in boys. However, difficulties in social challenges and adaptive functioning may happen more for girls than boys when they become adults [57].

## SIGNS OF AUTISM SPECTRUM DISORDER IN INFANTS

Although ASD diagnosis in infancy is not common today, some articles reported different studies on the signs of ASD in infants, which draw a promising way for the future to diagnose children with autism spectrum disorder as soon as possible. We summarize some of them herein.

A lack of response to name might be observed in developmental abnormalities, but it can be considered a general identification in these disorders. However, a prospective worked on this feature as a sign of ASD. Home videos of the behavior of children later diagnosed with autism and normally developed children were compared to each other. As a result, significantly fewer children whose ASD was diagnosed later tend to respond to their names in the first days of birth. It claims that the co-occurrence of this behavior with other signs, such as lack of attention to faces, can be a reliable marker for early ASD diagnosis [58].

Another study claims that motor delays in infancy, such as head lag, can identify the high risks of ASD. In other words, the effect of the visual and vestibular system on the head righting longitudinally can be related to high and low risks of

ASD, respectively, because of the association between the association of quantity and quality of sensorimotor skills and communication and social behavior. In summary, head lag can be known as identification for autism diagnosis in early development [6].

Some other studies reported the Autism Observation Scale for Infants (AOSI) as an index for detecting signs of autism in infants (age 6-18 months), especially with older autistic siblings [59]. There are 19 different target behaviors in AOSI: 1) eye contact: the ability to have proper eye contact with the examiner, 2) imitation: the ability to repeat a particular action by the examiner, 3) orientation to name: the ability to have proper response such as moving eyes or head toward the examiner when calling his name, 4) behavioral reactivity: general response to examiner's activities, 5) sharing interest: in an event or object with others, 6) engagement of attention: the ability to focus attention on events or objects, 7) abnormal motor behavior: such as repetitive motor movements and abnormal gait or motor posture, 8) abnormal sensory behavior: such as abnormal staring on objects, 9) transition: easily relinquish activity or toy and move to another, 10) visual tracking: disengagement of attention: easily disengage attention from environmental stimuli, 11) visual tracking: ability to follow the movement of objects with his eyes, 12) anticipatory social response: the ability to enjoy social cause-effect relationships, 13) coordination of actions and eye gaze on objects, 14) motor control: degree to modulation, goal direction and organization of motor behavior, 15) reciprocal social smile: ability to smile as a response to examiner's smile, 16) differential response to different facial emotion of examiner, 17) insistence on a special activity: showing repetitive behavior or interest, 18) social babbling: ability to have engagement with examiner in back and forth vocalization, 19) social interest and shared affect: easily being interested in activities and sharing their good affects with others [5].

Another study with a retrospective video analysis design considered social interaction gestures among infants aged 9-12 months. As a result, they claimed that there is an association between decreased variety in gesture types (not the total number of gestures or onset of gestures) and later ASD diagnosis [7]. See Table **2** to find out the presentations of ASD in infants reported in case series.

**Table 2. Summary of Presentations of ASD in Infants Reported in Case Series.**

| Author | Year | Country | Sex | Age | Follow-up Duration | Presentation |
|---|---|---|---|---|---|---|
| Miniscalco *et al.* [74] | 2021 | Sweden | Boy | 3.1 years | 5.2 years | Family history of ASD, speaking in sentences, a high score on RDSL receptive, average or above average performance IQ and language test result, age-appropriate speech, interested in reading, average result in non-verbal skills. |
| | | | Boy | 2.3 years | 5.5 years | Family history of ASD, not using more than a handful of words, low score on RDSL receptive, difficulties in social interaction and understanding others, avoiding eye contact, rarely answering questions, non-fluent speech, above average non-verbal skills. |
| | | | Boy | 2.7 years | 4.6 years | No family history of ASD, used a few single words, difficulties in social interaction, used very few gestures or mimics, overtime facial expressions such as smile while happiness improved, echolalia in speech, below average non-verbal functioning, recalling sentences, and receptive vocabulary. |
| | | | Girl | 29 months | 4.5 years | Older brother with ASD, no difficulties with language development, frequent tantrums and behavioral difficulties, multi-world utterance, epilepsy, no problems with receptive or expressive speech and language. |
| | | | Girl | 3 years | 4.4 years | No family history of ASD, a typical development during the first year of life, used single words as expected and then lost her early words, severe problems with language comprehension, performance IQ=86, age-appropriate speech, below average on recalling sentences, receptive vocabulary and language, difficulties in remembering the story content. |
| | | | Girl | 3.8 years | 3.5 years | No family history of ASD, not interested in sharing or showing her interests, satisfied to be by herself, playing with small toy animals lining them up in long lines and sorting them depending on their color, not understanding any world in a receptive language test, using echolalia, average vocabulary receptive test, severe difficulties with story retelling, repeat sentences below average. |
| Dawson *et al.* [75] | 2000 | USA | Boy | birth | 2 years | Difficulties in oral motor coordination and muscle tone, hypersensitive to touch, responding socially to others by smiling and cooing in the first six months of life, difficulties in social interaction, poor eye contact, no evidence of significant impairment in working memory, response inhibition, and speech perception. |

*(Table 2) cont.....*

| Bryson et al. [76] | 2007 | Canada | Boy | 6 months | 30 months | Oriented to his mom talking and events in his environment but not oriented to name calling, delayed motor development, being upset by changes, not walking independently, striking sensory interests, has very poor self-regulation, very poor sleeper, absence of smiling and facial expressiveness generally. |
|---|---|---|---|---|---|---|
| | | | Girl | 6 months | 30 months | Limited motor control, little social smiling, imitated action on an object, atypical motor behavior, approaching new toys slowly, over-reactive to certain sounds, limited food preferences, shivering spells, grass on feet, upset if the door on toy house is open, a poor sleeper, sensitive to touch. |
| | | | Girl | 6 months | 30 months | Prolonged distress with frequent crying, fleeting eye contact, clinging to mom and touching mom's hair and face when distressed, watching TV for a prolonged period, attentive to details, distressed by fluorescent lights and sound of running water and noise in stores. |
| | | | Boy | 6 months | 30 months | Difficult to engage in face-to-face interaction, not oriented to name calls or people talking, difficulty engaging his attention in activities/toys, generally under-reactive to toys and people and people talking, atypical motor behavior. |
| | | | Boy | 6 months | 30 months | Upset when not held, not sleeping through the night, ripping paper and holding remote control even at bedtime, resistance to giving up particular toys, wanting to hug it for the vibration, several repetitive behaviors. |
| | | | Girl | 6 months | 30 months | Reportedly had three words [mama, dada, baby], reacted negatively to being held, poorly modulated eye contact, no sharing of interest in an object/event with others, atypical sensory behaviors and gait, very active, running around with toy in hand, dislike any dirt on her, light sleeper. |
| | | | Boy | 6 months | 30 months | Equivocal imitation, no social smiling, atypical motor behavior, no social-communicative initiations, atypical sensory behavior, repetitive banging of toy, inconsistent orienting to name called. |
| | | | Boy | 6 months | 30 months | Fleeting eye contact, with lots of vocalizations and some social babbling, equivocal imitation, occasional hand flapping, very difficult to get his attention and move it elsewhere, very slow to warm up. |
| | | | Girl | 6 months | 30 months | Limited interest in and responsiveness to others, eye gaze at her parent, few vocalizations, no social babbling, atypical sensory behaviors, motor mannerisms, watching TV for long periods, difficulty falling asleep, has only three single words. |

RDLS: reynell developmental language scale

## IMPORTANCE OF AUTISM SPECTRUM DISORDER DIAGNOSIS AS SOON AS POSSIBLE

Research shows that when ASD is diagnosed early in a child, the probability of developmental, adaptive functional, cognitive, and social skill improvement is higher than in later diagnosed children [60]. Another reason is that parents of undiagnosed autistic children experience much more stress because of their unawareness. Also, early diagnosis can help these children better understand themselves in the future, such as when they may not attain their best at school. Gradually knowing more about their disease, they better know they are not alone in how they feel. When the parents are more trained and aware in this field, they can better help their children and manage their difficult conditions. With early diagnosis, parents have more time to accept that although their child is similar to other children in many aspects, there are some limitations for them, and they should revise their future plans and expectations. Undeniably, some of the most successful people were diagnosed with ASD. Proper care as the result of early diagnosis had an essential role for these individuals [61]. Dawson *et al.* reported that in children with ASD, the best time for consequent intervention is before age four [62] because early intervention in autism can improve their social behavior and daily living skills [63]. Intervention in preschool age is common today, but the intervention's development in infants is needed for a better outcome [64].

## INTERVENTIONS TO TREAT AUTISM SPECTRUM DISORDERS [ASD] IN INFANCY AND CHILDHOOD

Applied Behavior Analysis (ABA) therapists try to use an evidence-based approach for early intervention and help autistic children to suffer less from the symptoms of ASD and live as much independent as possible. Their interventions include: 1) Early Intensive Behavioral Intervention (EIBI) which is a behavioral therapy used for children under five years and sometimes for children under three years old. Each child has his/her private therapist. They learn social behavior, manage their tantrum emotions or anger and reduce their self-injurious actions. Consequently, their language skills, IQ, and adaptive behaviors improve. 2) Early Start Denver Model (ESDM) is another way used for very young aged autistic children (12-48 months). Parents and therapists are involved in this therapy by playing fun games for the children. In this way, they try to support these children to learn social interactions and improve their language skills, cognition, and brain activity. 3) Speech therapy in which therapists try to help autistic children with their speech issues by strengthening their mouth muscles to form the words better. 4) Social skills therapy helps them interact with other people through conversation and problem-solving. 5) Prescribing medications decreases the risk of seizures, a common issue among autistic children. 6) Physical therapy helps them to strengthen their muscle and have healthier bodies since struggling with strength is a mutual problem among children with ASD. 7) Occupational therapy teaches these children how to prepare meals or clean the house and self-hygiene to experience a more independent life [65].

## CONCLUSION

Despite the fact that autism is a developmental disorder with a very early onset, research on the behavioral symptoms of ASD in early infancy and infancy is sparse. In contrast, the understanding of traits of ASD in newborns and infants has been dramatically expanded due to new research methodologies, in general, and recently performed prospective studies, in specific. In this view, it turned out that focusing on the early detection and identification of ASD-traits in early infancy and infancy leads to beneficial health outcomes both for the child with ASD and their family system.

## CONSENT FOR PUBLICATION

Not applicable.

## CONFLICT OF INTEREST

The authors declare no conflict of interest, financial or otherwise.

## ACKNOWLEDGEMENT

Declared none.

## REFERENCES

[1]     Newschaffer CJ, Croen LA, Daniels J, *et al.* The epidemiology of autism spectrum disorders. Annu Rev Public Health 2007; 28(1): 235-58.
[http://dx.doi.org/10.1146/annurev.publhealth.28.021406.144007] [PMID: 17367287]

[2]     Chiarotti F, Venerosi A. Epidemiology of autism spectrum disorders: a review of worldwide prevalence estimates since 2014. Brain Sci 2020; 10(5): 274.
[http://dx.doi.org/10.3390/brainsci10050274] [PMID: 32370097]

[3]     Salari N, Rasoulpoor S, Rasoulpoor S, *et al.* The global prevalence of autism spectrum disorder: a comprehensive systematic review and meta-analysis. Ital J Pediatr 2022; 48(1): 112.
[http://dx.doi.org/10.1186/s13052-022-01310-w] [PMID: 35804408]

[4]     Signs of autism in children. 2019. Available From: https://www.nhs.uk/conditions/autism/signs/

[5]     Bryson SE, Zwaigenbaum L, McDermott C, Rombough V, Brian J. The Autism Observation Scale for Infants: scale development and reliability data. J Autism Dev Disord 2008; 38(4): 731-8.
[http://dx.doi.org/10.1007/s10803-007-0440-y] [PMID: 17874180]

[6]     Flanagan JE, Landa R, Bhat A, Bauman M. Head lag in infants at risk for autism: a preliminary study. Am J Occup Ther 2012; 66(5): 577-85.
[http://dx.doi.org/10.5014/ajot.2012.004192] [PMID: 22917124]

[7]     Colgan SE, Lanter E, McComish C, Watson LR, Crais ER, Baranek GT. Analysis of social interaction gestures in infants with autism. Child Neuropsychol 2006; 12(4-5): 307-19.
[http://dx.doi.org/10.1080/09297040600701360] [PMID: 16911975]

[8]     Lai MC, Lombardo MV, Baron-Cohen S. Autism. Lancet 2014; 383(9920): 896-910.
[http://dx.doi.org/10.1016/S0140-6736(13)61539-1] [PMID: 24074734]

[9]     Sadeghi S, Pouretemad HR, Brand S. Cognitive control and cognitive flexibility predict severity of depressive symptoms in parents of toddlers with autism spectrum disorder. Curr Psychol 2022; 1-8.
[http://dx.doi.org/10.1007/s12144-022-03682-y]

[10]    Ghafouri-Fard S, Noroozi R, Brand S, *et al.* Emerging Role of Non-coding RNAs in Autism Spectrum Disorder. J Mol Neurosci 2022; 72(2): 201-16.
[http://dx.doi.org/10.1007/s12031-021-01934-3] [PMID: 34767189]

[11]    Bahmani M, Sarrafchi A, Shirzad H, Rafieian-Kopaei M. Autism: Pathophysiology and promising herbal remedies. Curr Pharm Des 2015; 22(3): 277-85.
[http://dx.doi.org/10.2174/1381612822666151112151529] [PMID: 26561063]

[12]    What are the 5 types of autism? 2021. Available From: https://www.integrityinc.org/what-are-th--5-types-of-autism/

[13]    Hayes SA, Watson SL. The impact of parenting stress: a meta-analysis of studies comparing the experience of parenting stress in parents of children with and without autism spectrum disorder. J Autism Dev Disord 2013; 43(3): 629-42.
[http://dx.doi.org/10.1007/s10803-012-1604-y] [PMID: 22790429]

[14]    Elder J, Kreider C, Brasher S, Ansell M. Clinical impact of early diagnosis of autism on the prognosis and parent-child relationships. Psychol Res Behav Manag 2017; 10: 283-92.
[http://dx.doi.org/10.2147/PRBM.S117499] [PMID: 28883746]

[15]    Coexisting Conditions Autism, Aspergers, ASD: SpectrumLife magazine/autism empowerment. 2022. Available From: https://www.autismempowerment.org/understanding-autism/co-existing-conditions/

[16]    Guinchat V, Thorsen P, Laurent C, Cans C, Bodeau N, Cohen D. Pre-, peri- and neonatal risk factors for autism. Acta Obstet Gynecol Scand 2012; 91(3): 287-300.
[http://dx.doi.org/10.1111/j.1600-0412.2011.01325.x] [PMID: 22085436]

[17]    Gardener H, Spiegelman D, Buka SL. Perinatal and neonatal risk factors for autism: a comprehensive meta-analysis. Pediatrics 2011; 128(2): 344-55.
[http://dx.doi.org/10.1542/peds.2010-1036] [PMID: 21746727]

[18]    Arafa A, Mahmoud O, Salah H, Abdelmonem AA, Senosy S. Maternal and neonatal risk factors for autism spectrum disorder: A case-control study from Egypt. PLoS One 2022; 17(6): e0269803.
[http://dx.doi.org/10.1371/journal.pone.0269803] [PMID: 35704613]

[19]    Hazlett HC, Poe MD, Gerig G, *et al.* Early brain overgrowth in autism associated with an increase in cortical surface area before age 2 years. Arch Gen Psychiatry 2011; 68(5): 467-76.
[http://dx.doi.org/10.1001/archgenpsychiatry.2011.39] [PMID: 21536976]

[20]    Hazlett HC, Poe M, Gerig G, *et al.* Magnetic resonance imaging and head circumference study of brain size in autism: birth through age 2 years. Arch Gen Psychiatry 2005; 62(12): 1366-76.
[http://dx.doi.org/10.1001/archpsyc.62.12.1366] [PMID: 16330725]

[21]    Schumann CM, Bloss CS, Barnes CC, *et al.* Longitudinal magnetic resonance imaging study of cortical development through early childhood in autism. J Neurosci 2010; 30(12): 4419-27.
[http://dx.doi.org/10.1523/JNEUROSCI.5714-09.2010] [PMID: 20335478]

[22]    Hazlett HC, Gu H, Munsell BC, *et al.* Early brain development in infants at high risk for autism spectrum disorder. Nature 2017; 542(7641): 348-51.
[http://dx.doi.org/10.1038/nature21369] [PMID: 28202961]

[23]    Shen MD, Nordahl CW, Young GS, *et al.* Early brain enlargement and elevated extra-axial fluid in

infants who develop autism spectrum disorder. Brain 2013; 136(9): 2825-35.
[http://dx.doi.org/10.1093/brain/awt166] [PMID: 23838695]

[24] Shen MD, Kim SH, McKinstry RC, *et al.* Increased extra-axial cerebrospinal fluid in high-risk infants who later develop autism. Biol Psychiatry 2017; 82(3): 186-93.
[http://dx.doi.org/10.1016/j.biopsych.2017.02.1095] [PMID: 28392081]

[25] Wolff JJ, Gu H, Gerig G, *et al.* Differences in white matter fiber tract development present from 6 to 24 months in infants with autism. Am J Psychiatry 2012; 169(6): 589-600.
[http://dx.doi.org/10.1176/appi.ajp.2011.11091447] [PMID: 22362397]

[26] Wolff JJ, Swanson MR, Elison JT, *et al.* Neural circuitry at age 6 months associated with later repetitive behavior and sensory responsiveness in autism. Mol Autism 2017; 8(1): 8.
[http://dx.doi.org/10.1186/s13229-017-0126-z] [PMID: 28316772]

[27] Libero LE, Burge WK, Deshpande HD, Pestilli F, Kana RK. White matter diffusion of major fiber tracts implicated in autism spectrum disorder. Brain Connect 2016; 6(9): 691-9.
[http://dx.doi.org/10.1089/brain.2016.0442] [PMID: 27555361]

[28] Anderson JS, Lange N, Froehlich A, *et al.* Decreased left posterior insular activity during auditory language in autism. AJNR Am J Neuroradiol 2010; 31(1): 131-9.
[http://dx.doi.org/10.3174/ajnr.A1789] [PMID: 19749222]

[29] Redcay E, Courchesne E. Deviant functional magnetic resonance imaging patterns of brain activity to speech in 2-3-year-old children with autism spectrum disorder. Biol Psychiatry 2008; 64(7): 589-98.
[http://dx.doi.org/10.1016/j.biopsych.2008.05.020] [PMID: 18672231]

[30] Ben Bashat D, Kronfeld-Duenias V, Zachor DA, *et al.* Accelerated maturation of white matter in young children with autism: A high b value DWI study. Neuroimage 2007; 37(1): 40-7.
[http://dx.doi.org/10.1016/j.neuroimage.2007.04.060] [PMID: 17566764]

[31] Takumi T, Tamada K, Hatanaka F, Nakai N, Bolton PF. Behavioral neuroscience of autism. Neurosci Biobehav Rev 2020; 110: 60-76.
[http://dx.doi.org/10.1016/j.neubiorev.2019.04.012] [PMID: 31059731]

[32] Goodlin-Jones BL, Tang K, Liu J, Anders TF. Sleep patterns in preschool-age children with autism, developmental delay, and typical development. J Am Acad Child Adolesc Psychiatry 2008; 47(8): 930-8.
[http://dx.doi.org/10.1097/CHI.0b013e3181799f7c] [PMID: 18596550]

[33] Owens JA, Mindell JA. Pediatric Insomnia. Pediatr Clin North Am 2011; 58(3): 555-69.
[http://dx.doi.org/10.1016/j.pcl.2011.03.011] [PMID: 21600342]

[34] Meltzer LJ. Brief report: sleep in parents of children with autism spectrum disorders. J Pediatr Psychol 2007; 33(4): 380-6.
[http://dx.doi.org/10.1093/jpepsy/jsn005] [PMID: 18250091]

[35] Elrod MG, Hood BS. Sleep differences among children with autism spectrum disorders and typically developing peers: a meta-analysis. J Dev Behav Pediatr 2015; 36(3): 166-77.
[http://dx.doi.org/10.1097/DBP.0000000000000140] [PMID: 25741949]

[36] Tanguay PE, Ornitz EM, Forsythe AB, Ritvo ER. Rapid eye movement (REM) activity in normal and autistic children during REM sleep. J Autism Child Schizophr 1976; 6(3): 275-88.
[http://dx.doi.org/10.1007/BF01543468] [PMID: 186448]

[37] Yang Z, Matsumoto A, Nakayama K, *et al.* Circadian-relevant genes are highly polymorphic in autism spectrum disorder patients. Brain Dev 2016; 38(1): 91-9.
[http://dx.doi.org/10.1016/j.braindev.2015.04.006] [PMID: 25957987]

[38] Wimpory D, Nicholas B, Nash S. Social timing, clock genes and autism: a new hypothesis. J Intellect Disabil Res 2002; 46(4): 352-8.
[http://dx.doi.org/10.1046/j.1365-2788.2002.00423.x] [PMID: 12000587]

[39]   Bourgeron T, Ed. The possible interplay of synaptic and clock genes in autism spectrum disorders Cold Spring harbor symposia on quantitative biology. Cold Spring Harbor Laboratory Press 2007.

[40]   Tordjman S, Anderson GM, Pichard N, Charbuy H, Touitou Y. Nocturnal excretion of 6-sulphatoxymelatonin in children and adolescents with autistic disorder. Biol Psychiatry 2005; 57(2): 134-8.
[http://dx.doi.org/10.1016/j.biopsych.2004.11.003] [PMID: 15652871]

[41]   Levenson JC, Kay DB, Buysse DJ. The pathophysiology of insomnia. Chest 2015; 147(4): 1179-92.
[http://dx.doi.org/10.1378/chest.14-1617] [PMID: 25846534]

[42]   Bonnet MH, Arand DL. Hyperarousal and insomnia: State of the science. Sleep Med Rev 2010; 14(1): 9-15.
[http://dx.doi.org/10.1016/j.smrv.2009.05.002] [PMID: 19640748]

[43]   Feige B, Baglioni C, Spiegelhalder K, Hirscher V, Nissen C, Riemann D. The microstructure of sleep in primary insomnia: An overview and extension. Int J Psychophysiol 2013; 89(2): 171-80.
[http://dx.doi.org/10.1016/j.ijpsycho.2013.04.002] [PMID: 23583625]

[44]   Hutt C, Hutt SJ, Lee D, Ounsted C. Arousal and childhood autism. Nature 1964; 204(4961): 908-9.
[http://dx.doi.org/10.1038/204908a0] [PMID: 14235732]

[45]   De Luca F, Ed. Endocrinological abnormalities in autism. Seminars in Pediatric Neurology. Elsevier 2020.

[46]   Roberts EM, English PB, Grether JK, Windham GC, Somberg L, Wolff C. Maternal residence near agricultural pesticide applications and autism spectrum disorders among children in the California Central Valley. Environ Health Perspect 2007; 115(10): 1482-9.
[http://dx.doi.org/10.1289/ehp.10168] [PMID: 17938740]

[47]   Bradshaw J, Shi D, Hendrix CL, Saulnier C, Klaiman C. Neonatal neurobehavior in infants with autism spectrum disorder. Dev Med Child Neurol 2022; 64(5): 600-7.
[http://dx.doi.org/10.1111/dmcn.15096] [PMID: 34713902]

[48]   Wing L. Autism: Possible clues to the underlying pathology: Clinical facts Aspects of autism-biological research. London: Gaskell. 1988.

[49]   Baird G, Cass H, Slonims V. Diagnosis of autism. BMJ 2003; 327(7413): 488-93.
[http://dx.doi.org/10.1136/bmj.327.7413.488] [PMID: 12946972]

[50]   Screening and Diagnosis of Autism Spectrum Disorder. 2022. Available From: https://www.cdc.gov/ncbddd/autism/screening.html

[51]   Lord C, Risi S, DiLavore PS, Shulman C, Thurm A, Pickles A. Autism from 2 to 9 years of age. Arch Gen Psychiatry 2006; 63(6): 694-701.
[http://dx.doi.org/10.1001/archpsyc.63.6.694] [PMID: 16754843]

[52]   Hyman SL, Levy SE, Myers SM, *et al.* Council on Children with Disabilities, Section on Developmental and Behavioral Pediatrics. Identification, evaluation, and management of children with autism spectrum disorder. Pediatrics 2020; 145(1): e20193447.
[http://dx.doi.org/10.1542/peds.2019-3447] [PMID: 31843864]

[53]   Association AP. Diagnostic and Statistical Manual of Mental Disorders (DSM-5-TR). Available From: https://psychiatry.org/psychiatrists/practice/dsm (cited: 9th April 2023).

[54]   Autism diagnosis criteria autism speaks. Available From: https://www.autismspeaks.org/autism-diagnosis-criteria-dsm-5

[55]   Diagnostic criteria/ autism spectrum disorder. 2022. Available From: https://www.cdc.gov/ncbddd/autism/hcp-dsm.html

[56]   International classification of diseases for mortality and morbidity statistics (11th Revision). 2018. Available From: https://icd.who.int/browse11/l-m/en

[57]   Lai MC, Szatmari P. Sex and gender impacts on the behavioural presentation and recognition of autism. Curr Opin Psychiatry 2020; 33(2): 117-23.
[http://dx.doi.org/10.1097/YCO.0000000000000575] [PMID: 31815760]

[58]   Nadig AS, Ozonoff S, Young GS, Rozga A, Sigman M, Rogers SJ. A prospective study of response to name in infants at risk for autism. Arch Pediatr Adolesc Med 2007; 161(4): 378-83.
[http://dx.doi.org/10.1001/archpedi.161.4.378] [PMID: 17404135]

[59]   Bryson SE, Zwaigenbaum L. Autism observation scale for infants Comprehensive guide to autism New York. Springer 2014; pp. 299-310.
[http://dx.doi.org/10.1007/978-1-4614-4788-7_12]

[60]   The impact of an early diagnosis. Available From: https://www.autismspectrum.org.au/blog/the-impact-of-an-early-diagnosis

[61]   Autism-the importance of early diagnosis. Available From: https://www.priorygroup.com/blog/autism-the-importance-of-early-diagnosis

[62]   Dawson G, Rogers S, Munson J, *et al.* Randomized, controlled trial of an intervention for toddlers with autism: the Early Start Denver Model. Pediatrics 2010; 125(1): e17-23.
[http://dx.doi.org/10.1542/peds.2009-0958] [PMID: 19948568]

[63]   Remington B, Hastings RP, Kovshoff H, *et al.* Early intensive behavioral intervention: outcomes for children with autism and their parents after two years. Am J Ment Retard 2007; 112(6): 418-38.
[http://dx.doi.org/10.1352/0895-8017(2007)112[418:EIBIOF]2.0.CO;2] [PMID: 17963434]

[64]   Bradshaw J, Steiner AM, Gengoux G, Koegel LK. Feasibility and effectiveness of very early intervention for infants at-risk for autism spectrum disorder: a systematic review. J Autism Dev Disord 2015; 45(3): 778-94.
[http://dx.doi.org/10.1007/s10803-014-2235-2] [PMID: 25218848]

[65]   Early Autistic Interventions: The Best Methods. 2021. Available From: https://www.elemy.com/studio/autism-treatment/early-interventions/

[66]   Courchesne E, Karns CM, Davis HR, *et al.* Unusual brain growth patterns in early life in patients with autistic disorder: An MRI study. Neurology 2001; 57(2): 245-54.
[http://dx.doi.org/10.1212/WNL.57.2.245] [PMID: 11468308]

[67]   Hazlett HC, Poe M, Gerig G, *et al.* Magnetic resonance imaging and head circumference study of brain size in autism: birth through age 2 years. Arch Gen Psychiatry 2005; 62(12): 1366-76.
[http://dx.doi.org/10.1001/archpsyc.62.12.1366] [PMID: 16330725]

[68]   Hazlett HC, Poe MD, Gerig G, *et al.* Early brain overgrowth in autism associated with an increase in cortical surface area before age 2 years. Arch Gen Psychiatry 2011; 68(5): 467-76.
[http://dx.doi.org/10.1001/archgenpsychiatry.2011.39] [PMID: 21536976]

[69]   Aylward EH, Minshew NJ, Field K, Sparks BF, Singh N. Effects of age on brain volume and head circumference in autism. Neurology 2002; 59(2): 175-83.
[http://dx.doi.org/10.1212/WNL.59.2.175] [PMID: 12136053]

[70]   Kim JE, Lyoo IK, Estes AM, *et al.* Laterobasal amygdalar enlargement in 6- to 7-year-old children with autism spectrum disorder. Arch Gen Psychiatry 2010; 67(11): 1187-97.
[http://dx.doi.org/10.1001/archgenpsychiatry.2010.148] [PMID: 21041620]

[71]   Nordahl CW, Scholz R, Yang X, *et al.* Increased rate of amygdala growth in children aged 2 to 4 years with autism spectrum disorders: a longitudinal study. Arch Gen Psychiatry 2012; 69(1): 53-61.
[http://dx.doi.org/10.1001/archgenpsychiatry.2011.145] [PMID: 22213789]

[72]   Maximo JO, Kana RK. Aberrant "deep connectivity" in autism: A cortico-subcortical functional connectivity magnetic resonance imaging study. Autism Res 2019; 12(3): 384-400.
[http://dx.doi.org/10.1002/aur.2058] [PMID: 30624021]

[73]   Courchesne E, Press GA, Yeung-Courchesne R. Parietal lobe abnormalities detected with MR in

patients with infantile autism. AJR Am J Roentgenol 1993; 160(2): 387-93.
[http://dx.doi.org/10.2214/ajr.160.2.8424359] [PMID: 8424359]

[74]   Miniscalco C, Carlsson E. A longitudinal case study of six children with autism and specified language and non-verbal profiles. Clin Linguist Phon 2022; 36(4-5): 398-416.
[http://dx.doi.org/10.1080/02699206.2021.1874536] [PMID: 33554685]

[75]   Dawson G, Osterling J, Meltzoff AN, Kuhl P. Case Study of the Development of an Infant with Autism from Birth to Two Years of Age. J Appl Dev Psychol 2000; 21(3): 299-313.
[http://dx.doi.org/10.1016/S0193-3973(99)00042-8] [PMID: 23667283]

[76]   Bryson SE, Zwaigenbaum L, Brian J, *et al.* A prospective case series of high-risk infants who developed autism. J Autism Dev Disord 2007; 37(1): 12-24.
[http://dx.doi.org/10.1007/s10803-006-0328-2] [PMID: 17211728]

**CHAPTER 11**

# Medical Futility in Pediatrics: Challenges, Hopes, and New Perspectives



**Ardeshir Khorsand**[1,2,3], **Zahra Mohajer**[2,3], **Soroush Khojasteh-Kaffash**[2,3,4], **Zahra Hosseini Bajestani**[3,5,6], **Azar Ghasemi**[2,7], **Farbod Ghobadinezhad**[2,3,7] and **Noosha Samieefar**[2,3,8,*]

[1] *Department of Oral and Maxillofacial Surgery, School of Dentistry, Shahid Beheshti University of Medical Sciences, Tehran, Iran*

[2] *USERN Office, Shahid Beheshti University of Medical Sciences, Tehran, Iran*

[3] *School of Medicine, Shahid Beheshti University of Medical Sciences, Tehran, Iran*

[4] *Student Research Committee, School of Medicine, Birjand University of Medical Sciences, Birjand, Iran*

[5] *Student Research Committee, Mazandaran University of Medical Sciences, Sari, Iran*

[6] *USERN Office, Mazandaran University of Medical Sciences, Sari, Iran*

[7] *USERN Office, Kermanshah University of Medical Sciences, Kermanshah, Iran*

[8] *Network of Interdisciplinarity in Neonates and Infants (NINI), Universal Scientific Education and Research Network (USERN), Tehran, Iran*





**Abstract:** The concept of medical futility is explored, particularly in relation to the challenge of defining futile treatments, and the difficulties in identifying patient subgroups that strictly match the criteria for treatment futility. The issue of categorizing perinatal disorders as fatal is an important topic, with a focus on the moral and legal repercussions of identifying lethal malformation. The identification of a lethal malformation often has moral and legal repercussions, and the phrase "lethal" should be avoided unless it is precisely defined, used consistently, and covered in transparency in perinatal counseling following prenatal diagnosis.

We argue that a nuanced and carefully considered approach is required, one that takes into account the complex medical and ethical issues involved, and that focuses on the best interests of the patient and their family.

Overall, we highlight the importance of ethical considerations and effective communication in the provision of perinatal palliative care for fetuses with genetic disorders and congenital defects. Also, while there is much that remains uncertain and



---



***** **Corresponding author Noosha Samieefar:** Shahid Beheshti University of Medical Sciences, Tehran, Iran; Tel: +982123871; Fax:+9821-2243-9907; E-mail: nooshasamieefar@gmail.com

controversial in this field, continued research and discussions are necessary to ensure that the best possible care is provided for all patients and their families.

**Keywords:** Futility, Medical Futility, Medicine, Pediatrics.

## INTRODUCTION

Medical futility has always remained a controversial issue in all fields of medicine, and pediatrics is no exception. Medical futility is defined as treatment or interventions that patients might not benefit from them. Some argue that patients should be autonomous regarding choosing whether they want to be over-treated or to be left untreated. To put it another way, withdrawing or withholding medical treatment must be optional for patients. However, the matter is far more complicated. The dilemma is even much more complex when you are facing an infant or a child [1, 2].

In recent decades, patients' autonomy has claimed considerable credit due to the emphasis on it as a major patient right, at least partly by social forces and philosophical contributions [3]. As a result, the patient-physician relationship has transformed from a paternalistic model to a partnership model [4]. The principle of autonomy states that the patient has the capacity to choose and the right to decide what is done with her body.

Pediatric ethics is challenging, as the pediatrician might behave according to the child's best interest and put a high priority on the child's rather than the parents' preferences. These facts might result in conflict among the child, parents, and pediatrician. Cultural, social, and religious differences might add complexity. Therefore, the physician must balance respecting the parents' responsibility and following the child's autonomy [5].

Far-reaching advances in medical technology have led to many realistic and unrealistic expectations, and doctors are sometimes faced with demands that are professionally futile, with no effect or benefit [4]. This study aims to review nuanced aspects of medical futility in pediatrics and shed light on the most controversial issues by highlighting future perspectives.

## A BRIEF INTRODUCTION TO THE HISTORY AND DEFINITION OF MEDICAL FUTILITY IN PEDIATRICS

It is difficult to define medical futility, but as a working definition, one may call a preventive, diagnostic, or therapeutic medical intervention futile on the condition that it has no benefit for the patient [6]. Although the idea has surfaced since the 1960s, there's an aeonic background [7]. Hippocrates advises his students that whenever the extent of a patient's illness is far beyond available treatments, they should not expect to overcome it [8]. At that time, physicians were free to decide, and patients' preferences had a minute role in medical decision-making [9].

The word futilis is from Greek mythology, in which trying to draw water in leaky sieves is condemned to failure [10]. Webster's definition of futility is "a useless act or gesture" [4].

There is not an all-inclusive definition of futility in medicine, but one of the best-known conceptions is due to Schneiderman. According to him, a futile medical intervention is one with an unacceptable probability of achieving a therapeutic benefit for the patient. For Schneiderman, medical futility has both quantitative and qualitative aspects. Quantitative futility is established when a treatment doesn't result in the desired outcome in recent 100 cases. He considers this aspect of medical futility as an adaptation of famous Hippocrates' instruction to his pupils that providing futile treatments in such conditions is evidence of co-occurring ignorance and insanity [11].

Qualitative futility is a treatment that falls short of supplying a satisfactory quality of life for the patient [12], or a treatment that preserves the patient in the unconscious state or is incapable of freeing her from intensive medical care [3]. This concept is adapted from Plato's dialogue The Republic, in which Asclepius, the deity of medicine, is mentioned as not treating and prolonging the miserable life of people with very severe diseases. Furthermore, some experts place qualitative futility into two categories: first, when the disadvantages of treatment outweigh its benefits, and second, when the treatment is of little value for the patient's quality of life, so remaining alive doesn't worth it [13]. It must be noted here that providing care and relief for a patient's pain and suffering is never futile and should continue at all costs.

Besides these common conceptions, other definitions of medical futility have also been proposed. For instance, Youngner, in 1988, distinguished between two other types of medical futility:

Physiologic futility: a treatment that is unable to meet the physiological goals of the physician. Here, the physician and the patient are in mutual agreement about the goal of treatment, but they argue about whether treatment can achieve that goal.

Normative futility: a treatment that can fulfill the goals of the patient or her surrogates, but these goals are worthless from the physician's point of view. Here, the dispute is on the value of the goals of the patient or her surrogates. Many commentators consider these two types of futility equivalent to quantitative and qualitative futility, respectively [14].

Scofield in 1994 and Susan Rubin in 1998 held that the introduction of the concept of medical futility is an effort by doctors to increase their power against patients [15, 16]. Also, earlier in 1988, Wulff stated that the concept of futility had been proposed in reaction to the enhancement of patient autonomy and that doctors are trying to return to their previous control over patients [17]. In response, Schneiderman rejects the supposition of there being a battlefield between patients and doctors over decision-making, but the problem is opponents' failure to appreciate the central place of the principle of beneficence in medicine. It is the physician who knows which treatment is beneficial to the patient, so she should decide which treatment to offer and which one to lay aside [18]. One must also act according to the principle of beneficence in pediatrics. If a physician realizes that treatment is futile, she should refuse it.

## FROM THE PATERNALISTIC PARADIGM TO THE SHARED DECISION-MAKING MODEL

Long before, pediatricians used to seek innovative therapies for prematurity, administration of antenatal corticosteroids, pulmonary surfactants in neonates, and advancing ventilators for Neonatal Intensive Care Units (NICUs) [19]. With the rise of bioethics, previous models of decision-making in healthcare which were paternalist and authorized physicians, were questioned. Medical decision-making shifted towards patient autonomy, so patients and parents claimed to choose whether to proceed with or decline treatment in the moment of choice [20].

The shared decision-making method was now born, an intermediary approach on the spectrum of decision-making. One extreme of this spectrum is physician paternalism, and the other is patient autonomy [19]. In this model, the main focus is to consider patients' or their surrogates' values and preferences. So, to facilitate medical decisions that align with this, by emphasizing concepts of autonomy and informed consent, a reciprocal exchange of knowledge occurs between so-called parties. In shared decision-making, medical practitioners carry a decisional responsibility, and to do so, they give recommendations to the parents as the infant's surrogate based on their values and moral frameworks [20]. However, physicians are not assumed to be mere knowledge suppliers, and they are not supposed to leave parents to decide on their own; instead, the surrogate decision-makers have a limitation on authority, as well. That is why physicians have to confirm that surrogates are given adequate info to make a decision, although possessing adequate information and data is not the only prominent qualification they must have [21]. These surrogate decision-makers also need to be powerful enough to make reasonable judgments and be emotionally stable, which is very difficult considering the major emotional burden they carry [22].

## Dependency on Parents

Guidelines state that, like other fields of medicine, neonatologists are expected to adopt a shared decision-making approach when they come across an end-of-life decision and area [23 - 25]. As mentioned before, in this approach, both parties agree on a joint decision that considers their knowledge, values, and preferences. Parents might prefer different roles when facing these situations [26 - 28].

All physicians might face decisions concerning whether or not to continue life-sustaining treatments, but in ICUs, these situations happen nearly daily [29]. This situation is primarily challenging because of moral dilemmas. What makes it even more difficult in intensive care units is the absence of a previous connection and relationship between the physicians and the patients, who are now not able to communicate their values and wishes [30, 31]. In NICUs, there is a point that makes this situation significantly challenging, family members are the patient's surrogate decision-makers, and they might not have an equal preference about their amount of involvement in the decision-making process [32, 33].

## Autonomy

Till the uprising of modern bioethics, calling a practice futile was exclusively based on the physicians' decisions and their prognostic skills. It all started when more and more emphasis was put on the concept of autonomy [34]. The right of autonomy was first assumed to be a negative legal right to refuse treatment. Then it metamorphosized into a presumptive moral right to demand treatment. The principle of autonomy is commonly defined as a patient's legal and moral right to refuse treatment, even if it is life-saving.

Step by step, a shift from the traditional doctor-centered definitions occurred, and the physician's role became more restricted. Patients' interests are now the ultimate answer for these decisions. Futility is a criterion that has to be applied to the decisions about withholding or withdrawing a medical intervention which can be a continued life-sustaining treatment. Many believe that this decision needs to be made by committees and institutional policies and not at the bedside. We know this decision must arise between physicians and their patients, and subjective and psychological components with objective clinical features should interlink [35].

Exploring the rich literature on relative aspects of subjectivity, autonomous individuals are conceptualized as agents situated within and dependent on specific social contexts, while the role of the body and embodiment in perception and choice is seldom addressed [36 - 39]. Embodiment is about the necessity to elaborate on what could also be tagged as the autos of autonomous decision making, and phenomenologically, it is one's own reflected decisions that have characterized most of the autonomy discussion in bioethics [40].

Phenomenological accounts of an embodiment generally begin from a radical departure from mind versus body and subject versus object dichotomies, usually along the lines of Maurice Merleau Ponty's works. Subjectivity is known as embodied and embedded in the world, the bodily subject exists neither solely as consciousness nor as a thing, and also the concept of the lived body is introduced to refer to the "intertwining" of body and world [41]. My lived body, "to the extent that it's indivisible from a view of the world and is that view itself realized, is the condition of possibility" for me and an area of the world, oriented in and conditioned by it [42]. By the lived body, I have a lived relation to a world plunged in meaning, unfolded to me through my bodily senses, and a place for self-becoming, "in which the interface with others—both objects and living beings—constructs a dynamic self in which abstract singularity plays no part [43]."

**Family Interaction**

Family-centered care paradigm has caused many policy statements in pediatric medicine to establish shared decision-making as a component of care for critically ill infants. In the NICU, there is a significant level of uncertainty in most decisions, and this brings along moral dilemmas and keeps applying shared decision-making in the NICU an everlasting challenge [44]. In neonatal palliative care, families and parents are involved in decision-making as their infant's surrogates; as mentioned above, it is one of the foremost priorities in pediatrics. Involving parents does not mean leaving families unsupported to make a decision; instead, it involves cultivating trust, informing them with accurate and realistic data, embracing and empowering them, and last but not least, creating general accordance with their values and wishes [45]. Thereby to deliver palliative care, a whole community of healthcare suppliers is needed who are compassionate with parents and support them in the decisions they make, therein they are being provided guidance by the healthcare team as a supportive whole to confirm that choices are in the best interest of the infant [46]. By this means, a truly multidisciplinary approach is demanded to do so [47, 48].

The concept of neonatal palliative care entails a family-centered and multidisciplinary approach. The main objective of this approach is to attain sensitive and empathetic care, treat the infant with dignity, and provide empathetic support toward the family's experience [47, 49]. In practice, there are repeatedly multiple challenges which might be physical, psychological, and social. To be able to alleviate all these issues requires an integrated approach to care. This integration needs a strategic connection between multiple disciplines across the spectrum of caring, which includes the physical, emotional, social, and spiritual needs of the infant and the surrogates [50]. Healthcare as a whole should provide care to the infant and advocate for avoiding unnecessary or invasive procedures and the ones that can be potentially painful or obtrusive [51]. At the same time, relieving the suffering of a dying infant must be taken into consideration [47].

## The Concept of Suffering in Pediatric Decision-Making

In modern medicine, human suffering is more recognized and, therefore, raises a crucial question for pediatrics practice: What specifically does it mean to mention that a child suffers? The lives of sick children depend on how clinicians evaluate their suffering. A recent literature review indicated that over the past years, the term "suffering" was repeated 651 times in articles on pediatric ethics. And a particular finding of this review was that the concept of a child suffering was three times more likely to refer to a life-ending decision than a life-extending one [52]. Reflective on these findings, Salter believes that a label of suffering could imply the very fact that, in practice, physicians find a severely ill or disabled child's life not worth living [53].

To shed light on these ethical and linguistic challenges and ambiguities, the sphere of pediatric medicine desires an in-depth understanding and exhaustive definition of child suffering. What is even more unsettling is that the presiding theory on the concept of human suffering in today's medicine, which is based on Eric Cassell's ideas, does not acknowledge that children can suffer meaningfully and is built merely around the experiences of adults [54]. Cassell explicitly states that children cannot suffer because they are equipped with language and cannot assign meaning to their experiences. In his opinion, there is a distinction between suffering and pain, so if a being cannot reflect on and articulate its suffering, it's not suffering; instead, it's experiencing pain which is a basic emotional response to its surroundings [55]. This understanding of suffering dismisses the suffering of a large population of pediatric patients who are nonverbal because of young age or even maybe due to cognitive impairment.

In pediatric medicine, the opposite of Cassell's claim is supported philosophically, and there is a broad acknowledgment that children can suffer, even if they are not able to articulate their suffering and attach meaning to their experience [56 - 59]. The notice that children can suffer despite their inability to acknowledge and mention that they are suffering makes a new challenge arise: who has the right to decide when and to what extent nonverbal children are suffering? Does validation of suffering dwell in the judgment of clinicians or children's parents? Does the confirmation of suffering need objective information, for example, vital signs and physical examination findings?

In pediatrics, suffering is mostly treated as a subjective phenomenon, and for children who can represent themselves, the presence or absence of suffering is decided subjectively by surrogates. Unlike Cassell's focus on personal experience and the capability for a self-report, which confines suffering to the first-person distressing experience. For a 6-month-old infant at the NICU, who is sedated by fentanyl and midazolam and is attached to an extracorporeal ventilator, there can be no subjective experience. In this case, the subjective experience of the infant's caretakers is projected onto the child; therefore, the subjective distress or subjective hope experienced by this caretaker becomes the presence or absence of suffering for the child [60].

Phenomenologists have offered elaborate examinations of experiences of pain and illness. Previous such work has explored how intense and moderate pain could lead to a "Spatio-temporal constriction", where the subject in pain cannot but attend to his or her hurting bodily here and now, and the way this transforms the experience of time and space [61]. Additionally, examining how others' ways of encountering the subject in pain will facilitate forming his or her experience of pain [62, 63]. The subject-in pain might experience his or her pain differently depending on how others encounter and acknowledge him or her as somebody in distress. The suffering child and, therefore, the parent are dynamically shaped in relation to one another within a shared space, and therefore the child's way of curling up in bed will form others' ways of seeing him or her as suffering, even as their method of responding to his or her pain can form the method he or she emerges as suffering [64].

Philosophically, no logical reason exists that a clinician or a court of law, or even a parent, can ever thoroughly comprehend the lived experience of a child, and none of these parties can guarantee whether a nonverbal child is suffering or not. There exists one phenomenon other than pure subjectivity that ceases this incomprehensibility of pediatric suffering, and that phenomenon is the child's body. Some things should not be done to a human body, and this is accountable regardless of the parents' opinions because parents are sometimes wrong. That being said, a shift towards a more objective theory of pediatric suffering is needed to know when and where to draw this line. The complicated physical, biological, linguistic, psychological, theological, social, historical, and spiritual realities that make the interconnection between children and their parents have to be taken into account and explained by this theory to place all parties meaning doctor, patient, and parent in their dynamic relationship [60].

## MEDICAL FUTILITY IN THE NEONATAL INTENSIVE CARE UNIT

### Unconventional Medicine

It has been said that we live in a time when medical practice is akin to performing a miracle. In the world of NICU, this is plain to see. While modern neonatology has undoubtedly helped many babies, it has also had unfortunate consequences. However, it is only sometimes evident to the neonatologist or the patient's family whether or not life-sustaining treatment should be continued or discontinued. When making decisions for critically ill newborns, the American Academy of Pediatrics (AAP) Committee on Bioethics endorses a "best-interests-of-the-child" ethical standard and the idea of shared decision-making between the treatment team and the family [65].

It presents a moral conundrum to provide treatment to newborns with lesions incompatible with life or conditions that will not permit meaningful survival. Providing "futile care", which is sometimes very expensive, to infants who are not likely to improve despite extensive medical intervention is problematic [66].

### Medical, Lethal, and Ethical Aspects

Infant intensive care has faced a perception of futility for the previous 35 years. Attempts to ascertain which care procedures are warranted by neonatologists predate the Baby Doe restrictions and the establishment of ethical committees. Given the prevalence of severe abnormalities, birth asphyxia, and extreme preterm, the responsible physician is frequently faced with whether or not the proposed therapy would be helpful. The therapeutic armament has grown more potent and intricate, making it harder to pick the proper intervention among the many available. Parents' rights to make their own choices were progressively recognized. Limits on medical autonomy were established in the 1980s by the federal government, the courts, and several accident judgments. In the 1990s, third-party payors were more forceful in their efforts to curb costs. There is often tension between these legal and social requirements. Therefore, the question of medical futility concerning newborns in the United States is still open [67, 68].

The American Academy of Pediatrics emphasizes that parents may withdraw their child from life-sustaining care, notwithstanding the treating physician's opinion. The parents typically justify this decision by asserting their kid's "right to die." The physician may "invoke existing child-protecting measures" if the parties fail to resolve their differences with the assistance of ethical committees or consultants. However, what if doctors recommend discontinuing life-sustaining therapy, but the child's parents disagree and want it to continue? Treatment beyond what is necessary for comfort has been deemed "futile" since it either does not enhance the patient's prognosis or only delays death. AAP has been largely mute on the topic of "futility", maybe because it is riddled with medical, ethical, and legal uncertainties [3].

## Imminent Demise Futility, Lethal Condition Futility, Qualitative Futility, Ethical Issues

Infants born with extremely low birth weights now have a better chance of surviving because of recent developments in medical research and the application of technology. Despite the impaired long-term fate of these infants, parental anticipation had grown dramatically. Similar difficulties have arisen in caring for newborns with lesions incompatible with life or situations that will not enable meaningful survival. It has become a moral conundrum to save these helpless newborns [69, 70]. Treatment of these infants at this point may be considered "futile care" because it is not helping the baby in the long run [71, 72]. There is consequently moral and financial stress on pediatricians who care for newborns. Parental counseling can help with some of the challenges of newborn management, but there are also financial and logistical considerations to bear in mind. Costs associated with 'futile care' are substantial and can make up a sizable amount of total hospital expenditures, as was previously demonstrated. Finding and eliminating unnecessary treatments have significantly saved costs in adult critical care units (ICUs) [73 - 75]. However, some contradictory findings have been made in Pediatric Intensive Care Units (PICUs) [76, 77]. Unfortunately, there is a dearth of literature documenting the prevalence of unnecessary interventions in the NICU [78].

## Uncertainty

However, there is much disagreement over what is truly in a child's best interest. There are situations in which even the most caring of families and most compassionate doctors cannot agree on whether or not life-sustaining therapy should be maintained.

## Resource Allocation

Because of the high expense of neonatal intensive care, doctors must weigh factors, including parental desire, medical urgency, and therapeutic need, when deciding whether or not to provide a specific course of treatment.

The public often argues that the healthcare system places too much emphasis on end-of-life care and not enough on treatment and prevention [79]. Because of these worries, discussions about resource allocation often center around the intensive care unit (ICU), where poor allocation choices are typically thought to occur [80]. Various alternatives are put up. Patients' wishes are the subject of criticism. Individuals claim that patients are coerced into receiving the care they do not want because physicians are pressured to keep up with technological advances [81]. Promotion of advance directives would facilitate refusal of therapy [82].

Babies born with low birth weight and the elderly often need expensive and scarce resources and have a poor prognosis if they need emergency medical attention. Because of this, rationing plans disproportionately affect specific demographics [83].

Respiratory failure deaths in adults in the ICU constitute a significant drain on hospital resources. It has been argued that preterm newborns should not be treated because their survival rate is so poor [84]. Deficient birth weight infants have a minimal chance of life, although their care is inexpensive if they do not make it. Resources should be redistributed to those patients still alive, as this is a matter of distributive justice. To put this in perspective, compared to the less than 50% spent on intensive care for patients 85 or older and the less than 20% spent on mechanically ventilated patients 85 or older, over 80% of the money spent on NICU care for babies as little as 750 g will be spent on infants who survive [85].

## MEDICAL FUTILITY IN THE PEDIATRIC CARE UNIT

### Unconventional Medicine

Unconventional medicine is being used more frequently now. The primary motivation for applying this type of treatment to children who are admitted to pediatric intensive care with serious diseases is to explore every therapeutic option [86 - 91]. Since treatment in these circumstances is tougher in some ways than that for adults, having a child with these conditions is emotionally draining for families [92]. This stress could be correlated with the increased usage of unconventional medicines. The most often expressed motivation for choosing alternative medicines isn't to cure the disease but rather to enhance the child's overall health. The parents in these situations frequently see what they were providing as just a part of their responsibility as parents: to give the child everything they would need to mature into adulthood in excellent shape. The overwhelming perception that these therapies are at the very least "slightly successful" provides reassurance to parents. The most popular particular methods employed by patients are dietary modifications, nutritional supplements, and herbal treatments [93]. Even dietary modifications and nutritional supplements may have an impact on tumor progression and the bioavailability of standard therapeutic medicines. The effects of antimetabolites may also be hindered by dietary supplements and herbal remedies [94]. The majority of people who use unconventional medicines use more than one method, which opens the door to potentially complicated interactions.

## Medical, Lethal, and Ethical Aspects

Healthcare professionals cannot interfere without the proper authorization unless the patient's life is in urgent danger, and they are unable to consult with the patient or a representative to decide what to do. The general consent papers used for hospital admission or for transportation of a patient to a tertiary care center do not grant medical professionals permission to do any actions of that sort. The patient or the patient's legitimate surrogate is at the center of the medical decision-making process, as has been the case since the judicial articulation of the law of informed consent [95]. A complicated interactive procedure is required for real legitimate consent for diagnosis and treatment, as opposed to a single action that is marked by a signature on paper [96]. As a result, there is now widespread agreement that healthcare professionals should ensure the person giving consent has the mental capacity (also known as competency in the law) to comprehend what they are being asked to authorize as well as that they have adequate and understandable knowledge about the advantages, risks, and available alternatives to the suggested intervention (including the suggestion of no intervention). The approval must also be freely provided, without any indication that the patient or surrogate is being coerced into accepting a treatment they do not desire [97, 98].

## Imminent Demise Futility, Lethal Condition Futility, Qualitative Futility, Ethical Issues

Observations indicate that a large number of medical professionals agree that intensive care that has no therapeutic effects should be stopped [99 - 103]. According to research, referrals for intensive care during a severe illness are not just made for children who were previously healthy. Many of the individuals who died recently had underlying diseases or deformities, some of which would be considered fatal disorders. One can only assume that in these situations, the choice to stop or reduce treatment will be impacted by the anticipated rise in the total burden of the disease if the patient lives. Acute critical illness in children is usually unanticipated, and the burden of loss for the parents is serious. Tragically, the futility of a particular treatment, like mechanical ventilation, may not become apparent until after it has built unrealistic expectations of long-term survival. Therefore, it should come as no surprise that patients who had been admitted for intensive care and had a fatal underlying disease also died after failing Cardio-Pulmonary Resuscitation (CPR). This implied that a "Do-Not-Resuscitate (DNR) order" had not obtained permission or parental approval. When the family has had enough time to process everything that has been stated, this is an unexpected conclusion. Even yet, there could be a lot of emotional pressure to keep through with the futile treatment rather than stop it. These problems must be identified early, and addressed in an honest and caring manner. Due to their education, professional experience, and interactions with the families involved, intensive care professionals are specially qualified to reconcile such ethical and clinical complexities. However, it may be challenging and perhaps arbitrary to determine whether continuing to live while severely ill or disabled is beneficial enough. Many clinical scenarios, according to critics, render it hard to make an objective medical determination about whether a treatment is futile since futility is not restricted to a single, measurable amount but rather spans a range of probabilities [103, 104].

## Uncertainty

Although medical professionals frequently expect that the parents of seriously ill children would provide their consent for recommended diagnoses and treatments, there are times when this assumption can be problematic. Potential conflicts of interest between the child and their parents, such as those involving child abuse or neglect, parental denial or insistence on treatment based on religious views, or unwarranted parental focus on matters related to the child's welfare, are a few examples of such situations. Another example is when parents and children differ on the best course of action to take or when parents are unable to make decisions for themselves. There are also times when giving parents access to pertinent information may jeopardize the minor child's valid privacy rights. In the United States, state law continues to play a role in determining who makes decisions for a minor child whose parents have been charged with abuse or neglect severe enough to need ICU treatment. In several states, unless a judge formally revokes that ability, even parents who have been found guilty of criminally assaulting their children have the right to make medical decisions for their children. The influence of a child's illness on the rest of the family may be so intense that in such situations, parental interests may collide with those of their children. Since the phenomenon of child abuse and neglect has come to light, "the best interests of the child" has been a central concept in legal and ethical theory [105].

Most people today believe that kids, including a large number of those with Down syndrome, who can experience life have genuine autonomous moral and legal claims to life-saving care, including intensive care, even if their parents would prefer the kid to die. There is an assumption in this extremely broad moral agreement that, notwithstanding the parents' objections, the quality of life for these patients is high enough to warrant complex and expensive care. Cases, when doctors are unable to provide solid prognostic information, and the planned actions might have a significant negative impact on the family are even more challenging. These circumstances include those where taking care of the child might force parents to quit their jobs, where continued reliance on technology and medical care necessitates 24-hour monitoring, or where the attention required by the child depletes the time and energy available to other family members, such as the elderly or young children [106, 107].

Parents and children can also have differing perspectives on medical care, especially intensive care. Patients with degenerative conditions like cystic fibrosis or muscular dystrophy who are growing reliant on hospital equipment are two examples of those who do not want to go back to the ICU for mechanical ventilation due to pneumonia or septic shock. Children who are knowledgeable about their underlying illness and have expertise with life support are typically involved in these circumstances. Although their parents or physicians may disagree, the youngsters may come to the conclusion that death is the best option. According to the few empirical data on how children acquire the ability to make mature medical decisions, it is commonly believed that by the age of 14, it is difficult to tell the difference between a minor's and an adult's decision-making abilities. The kid's maturity and decision-making abilities are influenced by factors such as intelligence, experience, the number of independent decision-making opportunities the child has previously been given, and the specifics of the connection between the child and parents. This means that PICU professionals have an ethical and occasionally legal obligation to take their young patients' feelings and wishes seriously, particularly when those views diverge from the parents' [108, 109]. Another important issue regarding PICU is that the consent to treat a patient is invalid if it was given by parents under the influence of drugs or alcohol, including those that were legally administered by medical professionals or who had a significant mental disability or were suffering from a medical condition themselves, such as when all members of a family had been injured in an accident. Naturally, immediate life-saving intervention is excluded from the standard consent procedures. Thus the professionals should provide emergency care as necessary [98].

## Resource Allocation

With the widespread concern about cost containment related to healthcare reform, the role and responsibility of doctors and healthcare institutions in situations of medical futility have gained increased attention. Well-known examples like Stephanie Keene (Baby K), who was born with anencephaly, show that there is a lot of interest in pediatric medical decision-making but no general agreement [110]. Knaus *et al.* [111] suggested evaluating the appropriateness of treatment for critically ill patients based on the severity of their disease. Measures of disease severity, including the Acute Physiology and Chronic Health Evaluation (APACHE), have been used to predict non-survivors in the adult population with excellent specificity and the ability to save significant amounts of resources. Although this problem has hardly been brought up in the PICU context, it is evident that there is still debate over it in the adult ICU situation [112 - 115]. Schneiderman *et al.* [3] have made a proposition to declare futility following unsuccessful treatment attempts in the previous 100 cases. In an effort to recognize patients who were expected to die as a result of their underlying diseases but were not essential during the current hospitalization, an operational definition of lethal disease futility was established. And the criteria for adults were modified for the children. This definition covered the most futile care patient days. However, the fact that these patients frequently live for considerable periods of time makes the definition controversial.

Several researchers have argued that it may be necessary to restrict such care, although this may not always result in less resource consumption [3]. When it is known upfront that the likelihood of a favorable outcome is low, resources might be seen from the perspective of society as having been wasted. Even if the children do not survive in these situations, significant resources must be spent on them because they have a real chance of having a positive outcome. And it should not be declared a waste of resources. Clinical decisions in the PICU should not be made with the intention of reducing costs by lowering the care given to high-risk patients. And efforts to minimize resource consumption by focusing on medical futility may fail [76].

## DO-NOT-RESUSCITATE ORDER IN INFANTS AND CHILDREN

DNR instructions were first discussed in a 2003 study published in Critical Care Medicine [116]. An order for DNR from a doctor means that CPR will not be attempted in the case of cardiac or respiratory arrest [117].

The report says that DNR orders "placed a proper constraint on the widespread administration of CPR for the dying patient," but it adds that "even today, many of the early concerns persist." There is much written about DNR orders but less about them precisely as they relate to newborn and older pediatric patients. Of course, the moral concerns involved in carrying out a DNR order for an old patient will differ from those involved with a newborn or a child [118].

## Medical, Lethal, and Ethical Aspects

Children are ethically unique regarding end-of-life issues, which is the first and arguably the most important factor in understanding the ethical challenges that follow pediatric and infant DNR orders [118].

"The last days, hours, and minutes of the kid's life will most likely remain eternally in the parents' memories, and how their child dies is of critical relevance to the parents' following lives". Postovsky *et al.* wrote in two separate studies. It seems that parents, in their capacity as surrogate decision-makers, would be more hesitant to consent to a DNR order on behalf of their children than would be the case with older patients' surrogates or even the patients themselves [119].

Moreover, "most of our patients do not want to discontinue intensive care if there is a potential of life, and most are prepared to sustain medical intervention even in the face of a high likelihood prognosis of morbidity," as stated by Singh *et al.* [120].

DNR orders are a sensitive topic, and parents and doctors may be hesitant to bring them up. In turn, the literature overwhelmingly observes that DNR orders are "addressed with parents all too seldom and too late in clinical practice," suggesting that doctors' reluctance to raise the topic with their patients' parents may constitute an ethical problem in and of itself. It is difficult for most doctors to have difficult conversations with patients' loved ones or surrogates concerning end-of-life care, as stated by Garros *et al.* [121]. Only 41% of patients in the study talked to their doctors about CPR, and in 80% of those situations, the doctors misunderstood the patients' wishes [122].

When discussing a child's health, Hilden *et al.* [123] note that "both physicians and parents desire to apply all available treatment possibilities".

Postovsky *et al.* argue that DNR orders enforced only a short time before the patient dies may diminish or even eliminate the benefits of DNR orders. If a DNR order is placed within the last 24 hours of a patient's life, it is not timely since it does not give parents and other relatives enough time to prepare for the child's death. It would be difficult to overstate the emotional and psychological support that DNR orders might give to parents dealing with the loss of a child. The considerable "discrepancy between parents' opinion of the child's final prognosis and that of his/her treating physician," as shown by Postovsky *et al.* [124], is another interesting finding. One study found that parents, on average, acknowledged the end of treatment hopes more than 100 days later than doctors [117].

There is a lack of comfort in issuing DNR orders among newborn and pediatric end-of-life decision-makers, as shown by the findings in citation [125].

A recent study sheds insight into the cultural perspective on children that shapes end-of-life decisions and the clinical and economic differences that make care for pediatric patients unique. The development of neonatal medicine has allowed for the survival of babies who might have otherwise not made it. Since survival can cause morbidity and neurological harm to infants, careers, and society, the morality of life-sustaining treatment (LST) has been questioned. Every neonatal team is responsible for determining when to issue DNR or LST orders [126].

Many moral concerns need to be addressed. First, if the DNR is not implemented correctly, it might lead to an unnecessary extension of suffering. According to Postovsky *et al.*, DNR orders are necessary for young people with cancer so that doctors can concentrate on pain relief and respect for the patient's wishes rather than euthanasia [119].

Unfortunately, as noted by Einav *et al.*, competent patients' wishes are often disregarded in favor of the medical staff's preferences. Patients' wishes are routinely disregarded in favor of medical necessity, leading to unnecessary procedures and tests up until death [127]. Newborn and pediatric DNR analyses are different because of a lack of competence. Postovsky *et al.* [119] and Singh *et al.* [120] indicate that the disparities between how doctors see babies and adults increase the likelihood that pediatric patients, including newborns, may be "subjected to medical operations until death" [127].

Parents may find it easier to consent to DNR orders for their children if they restrict treatment rather than actively end life support [122].

Many philosophers and ethicists have argued for years that refusing to begin life-sustaining treatment is no different from stopping it. This view has not been reflected in actual medical practice. Several studies have shown that there is more significant hesitance to end LST than to cease providing it [121].

## Opposing Families' Wishes

The possibility of clinicians disagreeing with a parent's DNR decision is perhaps the most significant ethical challenge for those caring for neonatal patients in end-of-life scenarios. In a study of babies born extremely early, doctors almost always followed parents' wishes when deciding whether or not to attempt resuscitation: "Whereas treatment was invariably withheld when parents desired comfort care only, resuscitation was provided in 50% of the cases in which physicians preferred comfort care only" [128]. Physicians who blindly follow the parents' wishes about euthanasia may act unethically against their newborn patients. As one author puts it, "The medical motive of avoiding any pointless suffering of the infant may occasionally collide with the principle of acting following the parents' opinion about which course of action is in the best interest of their child " [125].

DNR orders are used to instruct medical professionals not to do CPR in the event of cardiac arrest, but the treating medical professional's competence ultimately determines whether or not to do so [121].

It is not uncommon for doctors to avoid discussing DNR orders with their patients' families for fear of adverse reactions or the argument that "it is unfair to ask parents to be involved in the decision-making process involving life and death". Inappropriate intensive care being given for an inordinate amount of time has resulted in a dramatic rise in the number of disabled survivors and a lack of intensive care beds [129].

**Unilateral**

A doctor is not ethically or legally required to follow a surrogate's DNR order. This does not mean the doctor or care team will not follow the parent's wishes for prudential reasons. The criticism is reflexive compliance or following the parents' lead. The DNR statute in New York formalizes the notion that a doctor's clinical judgment, while guided by ethical norms, still governs a DNR order. When a patient is incompetent and has no known surrogates, doctors may issue a DNR order based on medical futility under New York's DNR law [130].

Doctors should be able to use their professional judgment when making recommendations and acting upon those recommendations when appropriate. This includes making decisions regarding DNR status conflicts with the healthcare provider's personal judgment regarding what actions are or are not necessary for a neonatal or pediatric patient. Denying this would mean renouncing the expert role that directs the patient's or surrogate's therapeutic decision. According to Kevin Gibson, choosing surgery over-medication is a pointless choice if no one else is on board and involved [131].

It is not always necessary to comply with the surrogate's DNR requests for pediatric or neonatal patients, even if the surrogate may disagree with the provider's decision.

This is not to argue for a doctor's absolute power or to deny the possibility of abuse. The provider's tone when communicating judgment and recommendations is also important. The argument that providers should share recommendations even when they differ with patients or surrogates should not imply support for abusive power.

"Active listening" may help reduce abusive behavior. Active listening "focuses on patients' hints, *i.e.,* utterances and actions that may have a unique meaning and imply unshared ideas, concerns, and expectations. To detect and examine these signs, attentive listening is needed [132].

Gregg Bloche argues that active listening skills may be necessary when patients can "no longer define preferences" [133]. He also advocates mediation approaches in end-of-life decision-making: "Good mediation technique can clarify misunderstandings, soften wrath, and reduce unjustified suspicion [134]."

The goal is to present advice that both the patient and surrogate find useful while emphasizing the moral significance of ethical communication.

Bloche notes that "large literature suggests that party-crafted solutions come with a sense of shared ownership that dampens discord" [133]. It is hard to imagine collaborative decision-making when the provider acquiesces to the surrogate's decisions. Sharing responsibilities may mean more than equal collaboration [135]. The clinician must exercise their judgment, discuss it with the patient and surrogate, and, in some situations, use it to disagree with the surrogate's decision about neonatal or pediatric DNR status.

## MEDICAL FUTILITY IN PEDIATRIC BRAIN DEATH

Death is defined as the complete and irreversible cessation of all body organs' function. According to the role of the brain in body function, brain death and lack of brain function are also known as a form of death [136]. Brain death is associated with dysfunction of the cortex and brain stem and vegetative life. Brain death occurs as a result of extensive brain damage, such as extensive brain ischemia, extensive brain hemorrhages, hypoxic-ischemic encephalopathy, *etc* [137 - 139]. The most common causes of brain death in children include trauma, anoxic encephalopathy, infections, and brain neoplasms [140]. The diagnostic criteria of brain death are mainly clinical, but to confirm the diagnosis legally, it is necessary to prove neurological dysfunction. Of course, the legal laws regarding brain death and its diagnostic tests are different in different parts of the world, and there is no single global protocol in this matter. In order to perform brain death diagnostic tests, there are some clinical characteristics as prerequisites, which are [141 - 143]:

1. Clinical or neuroimaging evidence of an acute central nervous system (CNS)

injury that is consistent with a clinical diagnosis of brain death and there is a definite cause for brain death.

2. Absence of evidence of drug intoxication or poisoning causing neurological symptoms.
3. Exclusion of other medical causes that mimic conditions and symptoms of brain death, such as severe electrolyte imbalance, acid-base defects, endocrine disorders, and shock.

Also, for the neurological evaluation, it is necessary to set the core temperature to be higher than 36 degrees Celsius and the systolic blood pressure to be set to more than 100 mmHg so that there is no disturbance in the results of the tests.

Neurological examination is performed in patients with clinical suspicion of brain death with the aim of proving dysfunction in the brain and brain stem. These neurological examinations include [141, 142]:

1. Absence of pupillary reflex to light, pupils in the middle position or dilated (4-9 mm).
2. Absence of corneal reflex.
3. Absence of oculovestibular reflex (caloric responses), of course, in infants from 30 days to one year, the use of oculocephalic reflex is recommended instead of oculovestibular reflex.
4. Absence of gag reflex.
5. Absence of jaw jerk.
6. Absence of cough with tracheal suction.
7. Coma.
8. Apnea during the apnea test.
9. Absence of movement responses with a nervous origin of the brain (such as seizures, decerebrate or decorticate condition) and lack of response to pain stimuli above the neck
10. Absence of sucking or rooting reflex.
11. Subtle and semi-rhythmic movements of the facial muscles that are innervated by the facial nerve or the 7th cranial nerve.
12. Finger flexor movements.
13. Neck tonic reflexes and Lazarus sign.
14. Triple flexion response in the form of flexion in the hip, knee, and ankle with stimulation of the soles of the feet (such as stimulation during the skin-plantar test).
15. Trunk movements such as the asymmetric opisthotonos position of the trunk and, at the same time, the presence of superficial and deep abdominal reflexes.
16. Presence of Babinski's sign.

17. Flexion, extension, and pronation in the upper limbs.
18. Extensive fasciculation in the trunk and upper and lower limbs.

## Confirmation of Brain Death in Pediatric

Diagnosis and confirmation of brain death in children are different in adults [144]. It is not possible to diagnose brain death in preterm neonates with a gestational age of fewer than 37 weeks. Also, hypothermia, metabolic disorders, hypotension, and all factors and medications treatments that cause disruption in neurological examinations should be investigated and solved. During the period when the patient is monitored for brain death, 2 apnea tests should be performed after each round of neurological examination for the patient. It is recommended that the neurological examination be evaluated by two different physicians and the apnea test done by one physician. The length of the observation period is 24 hours for term neonates until the 30$^{th}$ day and 12 hours for infants and children (30 days to 18 years old). Also, if there is still doubt about brain death after the observation period and neurological tests, the observation will continue for another 24 hours.

## Brain Death Confirmation, A Bioethical Challenge

In the years before the 1960s, complete cardio-respiratory arrest was known as a criterion to confirm death. With scientific progress and more understanding of brain functions, neurological criteria, including complete brain damage and interruption in its functions, are also used as criteria to confirm death [145]. In the United States, two standards are used to confirm death in patients: (1) irreversible cessation of the cardiorespiratory system or (2) irreversible cessation of all functions of the entire brain. Today, if any of these standards are definitively diagnosed, the patient's death is confirmed. The second standard is also known as Death by Neurological Criteria (DNC), which is examined in patients with suspected brain death and irreversible cessation of brain functions. Performing DNC to confirm the death of patients is always criticized. According to opponents, patients with DNC confirmation who are known as the deceased person still have fertility, immunity against infectious agents, wound healing, digestion and metabolism, and stress response to surgical incisions, etc., and these patients only depend on mechanical ventilation and have cerebral quadriplegia [146, 147]. Although the use of DNC to confirm death in patients is still discussed clinically and theoretically, according to the latest decisions, there is no problem in doing it ethically and legally, and it helps a lot in the diagnosis of brain death in patients [145, 148]. Despite criticizing DNC as a test to confirm death legally and not biologically, many critics still consider this test legally and morally correct [149, 150]. Investigations demonstrate that despite the legality of the DNC, legal cases have also been formed in this regard, and the most common reasons for the formation of these legal cases include the following [145]:

1. The need of the patient's family for physiological support after the DNC.
2. Pursuing patients' families to receive damages due to early DNC due to negligence.
3. Pursuing patients' families to receive damages due to intentional early DNC.
4. Pursuing patients' families to receive damages due to emotional trauma after DNC.
5. Pregnancy restrictions at the DNC.

## Futile Care in Brain-Dead

One of the common causes of futile care in patients who are diagnosed with brain death is organ transplantation [151]. In order to prepare the patient and transplant conditions, it is necessary for the patient to be hospitalized for some time in the ICU and be under mechanical support. All medical procedures at this stage are not for the treatment and recovery of the patient but for the preservation of the patient's organs for transplantation. Therefore, due to the fact that the patient does not benefit from the care provided at this time, this care process is called futile [151]. Care performed in the ICU during this stage is called Elective Intensive Care (EIC) or Elective Ventilation (EV), which has created many challenges in bioethics [152]. One of the important principles in EIC is to avoid malice towards the patient. Long-term futile care by creating a vegetative life for patients has caused various injuries to them so that sudden death will be easier [151]. Therefore, it is recommended to reduce as much as possible the duration of unnecessary care for any reason in order to reduce harm and damage to the patient [153, 154]. It is recommended to perform neurological and cardio-respiratory examinations in a short period of time after the onset of symptoms, and after these tests and the final diagnosis, the patient can be a candidate for life support [155, 156]. Another principle is to refrain from malice towards the patient's family. In the era of futile care and EIC, human care can give way to technology and reduce the metaphysical and spiritual relationship between the family and the patient [157]. The third principle in EIC is to avoid malice towards health care providers. Many caregivers and doctors working in ICU who are related to useless care, after a while, feel useless. This causes less acceptance, moral suffering, professional misunderstanding, and the resignation of some employees [158]. The last principle is to refrain from malice towards society. Spreading the idea of futile care can reduce public trust in doctors and healthcare systems. Also, creating the thought of death after performing useless care and simplifying death and its concept in society can cause the normalization of this bitter event and lead people to easy death and suicide [151].

Examining the futility of care performed on patients depends on the purpose of performing medical procedures. In brain death, due to the irreversible interruption of brain function, it seems futile to provide medical care, including mechanical ventilation, for the treatment and recovery of patients. But in such a situation, if the purpose of mechanical ventilation is to preserve the function of body organs for organ transplantation, this care will not be futile. It should be noted that some medical procedures performed on brain death patients, who are not candidates for transplantation, can also be useful and lead to the achievement of a medical goal. For example, intubation for a brain-dead patient is performed with the aim of establishing an advanced airway, and it is not considered futile care.

## Parental Refusal of DNC

The American Academy of Neurology does not consider it correct to receive informed consent from parents for the examination of brain death and considers physicians morally and professionally responsible for the examination of brain death in pediatric [159]. Of course, this is not agreed upon by everyone, and many physicians do not accept such evaluations [160, 161]. Legally, after the death of the child, the parents have no right to request further treatment. In patients suspected of brain death or patients who died based on cardiorespiratory criteria, due to the lack of proof of death by neurological criteria (DNC), legally the patient is still alive, and the parents have the legal right to make medical decisions [162]. In different states of the United States, the decision regarding the need to obtain consent from parents for the DNC examination is also different. It is necessary to obtain medical consent for all medical procedures. Consent is not required only in emergency cases due to the need for early procedures and diagnostic procedures such as blood sampling for routine tests. If the parents do not consent to DNC, the child is legally alive, and the medical decision rests with the child's parents. Therefore, how to oblige parents to perform DNC and the principle of necessity to obtain parental consent for DNC are discussed. Unlike many medical practices that are based on the benefit of the patient, DNC finally confirms brain death and provides the possibility of one-way mechanical ventilation disconnection from the patient. Therefore, based on the principle of the patient's benefit, the parents' refusal to perform DNC can be justified [163]. There are also justifications for performing DNC without parental consent. Continuing life using mechanical support is not beneficial for the patient in the long term and cannot create better conditions for the patient other than survival. Also, based on the principle of doctors' responsibility to provide the best possible treatment based on the final diagnosis, DNC can be performed without parental consent [164]. Of course, the refusal of parents to perform diagnostic tests is significant if it is clear, preventive, and without the possibility of harming the child, and the physician cannot reject them at all [165]. Also, due to the limitation of special care facilities and mechanical support, if long-term mechanical support in a patient with an initial diagnosis of brain death makes it impossible to care for other patients, a physician can perform DNC to confirm the diagnosis without obtaining the consent of the parents [166]. Finally, studies have demonstrated that performing DNC against the consent and wishes of the parents is not morally justifiable. Unilateral DNC is different in different countries and can be done legally in many parts of the world, but it is not acceptable from an ethical point of view. Regarding the parent's reasons for not consenting to the DNC, there are some issues. First, due to the condition of the child and the deterioration of his clinical condition, the relationship between the parents and the medical staff has weakened, and the parent's trust in the physician has decreased [167]. In different parts of the world, according to different beliefs, religions, and customs, parents' decisions regarding DNC, brain death, and death are different [168, 169].

Also, in some cases, the parents can't accept the condition psychologically, and hoping for the improvement of the child's clinical condition causes them to refrain from performing DNC. Nowadays, it is recommended that in order to satisfy the parents to perform DNC, the doctors should put the child under cardio-respiratory and neurological monitoring for a while and inform the family about the daily conditions of the child. It is expected that after some time, due to the lack of improvement in the child's condition and by proving the clinical condition to the parents, their consent to perform DNC will be obtained. It is also recommended that physicians refrain from expressions that convey the feeling of the child's aliveness to the parents when talking to the patient's family. Also, considering the improvement of some body organs in children after hypoxia, it is necessary to explain the importance of the brain and its irreversibility after enduring hypoxia to parents [170]. Also, at the time of mentoring, it is necessary to get help from services such as bio-ethical consent and palliative care teams in order to obtain parental consent. The presence of psychological counseling teams alongside parents can also be effective.

## Genetic Disorders and Congenital Defects

The categorization of a perinatal disorder as fatal can be regarded theoretically in a variety of ways, including the following. A disorder causing fetal death in the uterus without exceptions, a disorder undoubtedly causing death in the fetus or the newborn despite medical treatment [47, 171 - 173], a disorder usually resulting in death in the fetus or the newborn [174 - 177], and a disorder correlated with death in the fetus or the newborn [178 - 180]. Many type-specified disorders do not categorize with the first description mentioned above. The second definition seems to be the most realistic, a disorder that makes it impossible to survive past the neonatal stage. Nevertheless, the second definition does not adequately represent a large number of congenital defects that are frequently referred to as fatal [181]. The identification of a lethal malformation often has moral and legal repercussions. According to some researchers, congenital anomalies serve as a platform for the need for perinatal palliative care [47, 182, 183].

As we know, medical futility has evolved in response to an increase in patient-physician disagreements, and notable disagreements about life-sustaining treatments [184]. The theory suggested that doctors would be ethically justified in declining to administer ineffective treatments if they could properly identify them [3]. Although the idea of futility has drawn a lot of attention over the past decades, there are a number of well-explained issues with it [12, 185]. The primary issue is the challenge of defining futile treatments. Futility is occasionally categorized into qualitative and quantitative forms. A treatment method with an extremely slim possibility of being successful is regarded as quantitatively futile. Nevertheless, there is disagreement over the precise threshold at which treatment is quantitatively futile. When a treatment method may theoretically be effective in maintaining life, but it is believed that the patient would not profit from it, it is regarded as qualitative futility. Giving intensive care to a patient who is in a prolonged vegetative state is one illustration that comes to mind. However, the amount of cognitive function required to benefit the patient is still under debate, which is the challenge for identifying qualitative futility [3]. Lethal deformities are similarly subject to these definitional issues. There is currently no consensus on the likelihood of death that would allow a condition to be classified as fatal. Similar to qualitative futility, some definitions of lethal malformations include diseases that result in a chronic vegetative state or lack of cognitive development; however, there is disagreement over the precise amount of function that would support this title [186 - 188]. It has been observed that patients with trisomy 13 and 18, hydranencephaly, and holoprosencephaly can be aware of their surroundings, perceive and respond to sounds, and learn and recall things [189, 190]. The challenge of identifying whether a specific treatment conforms to a given criterion is the second significant issue with futility. It is challenging to predict how frequently survival would be feasible if all treatments were given. Studies of prognosis that claim to be able to identify patient populations for which treatment is unsuccessful frequently rely on too little data to be confidently statistically inferred [191]. The next issue with futility is that, even while it is feasible to identify patient subgroups that strictly match the criteria for treatment futility, this only ends up being true in a limited number of circumstances. One definition employs the term "physiological futility," which refers to a treatment that fails to accomplish its physiological goal [184]. Similarly, lethality may be limited to diseases that always result in perinatal mortality, regardless of therapy (definition 2). However, this description appears to apply primarily to renal agenesis among the illnesses that are usually referred to be fatal. In perinatal counseling following prenatal diagnosis, the phrase lethal should be avoided unless it is precisely defined, used consistently, and covered in transparency. As a result, parents may be misled regarding the prognosis of serious defects. If treatment is offered, counselors should be clear about the prognosis and the effects of that treatment on the fetus or child. In many instances, this will call for acknowledging uncertainty.

## CONCLUSION

The ethical issues surrounding perinatal care are complex and multifaceted. It is essential to consider not only the medical aspects of perinatal care but also the moral, social, and legal implications that arise. The decision to provide or withhold medical treatment to a fetus or newborn with a life-limiting condition requires careful consideration of the patient's best interests, the parent's wishes, and the healthcare provider's duty to do no harm. Additionally, it is important to consider the impact of these decisions on the wider society and healthcare system [192]. One philosophical framework that has been proposed to guide decision-making in perinatal care is the principle of beneficence. According to this principle, healthcare providers have an obligation to act in the best interests of the patient, taking into account their medical condition and personal preferences. However, the principle of beneficence must be balanced against the principle of non-maleficence, which requires healthcare providers to avoid causing harm to the patient. In some cases, providing medical treatment to a fetus or newborn may cause more harm than good, and withholding treatment may be the most compassionate option [193]. Another important philosophical consideration in perinatal care is the concept of autonomy. The principle of autonomy acknowledges the patient's right to make decisions about their own healthcare, based on their values and beliefs. In perinatal care, this principle must be applied in a nuanced way, taking into account the patient's age, cognitive ability, and level of maturity. In cases where the patient is unable to make their own decisions, the parents or legal guardians may be called upon to make decisions on their behalf [194, 195]. However, healthcare providers must ensure that these decisions are made in the best interests of the patient and are not unduly influenced by societal pressures or personal biases. In conclusion, perinatal care is a complex area of healthcare that requires careful consideration of medical, ethical, social, and legal factors. Healthcare providers must strive to balance the principles of beneficence and non-maleficence, while respecting the autonomy of the patient and their caregivers. Ultimately, the goal of perinatal care should be to provide compassionate and respectful care to all patients, regardless of their medical condition or prognosis.

## CONSENT FOR PUBLICATION

Not applicable.

## CONFLICT OF INTEREST

The authors declare no conflict of interest, financial or otherwise.

## ACKNOWLEDGMENT

This article is wholeheartedly dedicated to the memory of our beloved friend, Mahdi Azadi, who recently departed. The one who has been our source of inspiration and gave us strength when we thought of giving up.

## REFERENCES


[1]     Clark PA. Medical futility in pediatrics: is it time for a public policy? J Public Health Policy 2002; 23(1): 66-89.
        [http://dx.doi.org/10.2307/3343119] [PMID: 12013717]

[2]     Bernat JL. Medical futility: definition, determination, and disputes in critical care. Neurocrit Care 2005; 2(2): 198-205.
        [http://dx.doi.org/10.1385/NCC:2:2:198] [PMID: 16159066]

[3]     Schneiderman LJ, Jecker NS, Jonsen AR. Medical futility: its meaning and ethical implications. Ann Intern Med 1990; 112(12): 949-54.
        [http://dx.doi.org/10.7326/0003-4819-112-12-949] [PMID: 2187394]

[4]     Aghabarary M, Dehghan Nayeri N. Medical futility and its challenges: a review study. J Med Ethics Hist Med 2016; 9: 11.
        [PMID: 28050241]

[5]     Orioles A, Morrison WE. Medical ethics in pediatric critical care. Crit Care Clin 2013; 29(2): 359-75.
        [http://dx.doi.org/10.1016/j.ccc.2012.12.002] [PMID: 23537680]

[6]     Aramesh, k., Medical futility. Iranian Journal of Medical Ethics and History of Medicine 2008; 1(4): 47-52.

[7]     Callahan D. Medical futility, medical necessity. The-problem-without-a-name. Hastings Cent Rep 1991; 21(4): 30-5.
        [http://dx.doi.org/10.2307/3562999] [PMID: 1938349]

[8]     Youngner SJ, Arnold RM. The Oxford handbook of ethics at the end of life. Oxford University Press 2016.

[9]     Sigerist HE. A history of medicine. Oxford University Press 1987; Vol. 2.

[10]    Vergano M, Gristina GR. Futility in medicine. Trends in Anaesthesia and Critical Care 2014; 4(6): 167-9.
        [http://dx.doi.org/10.1016/j.tacc.2014.10.004]

[11]    Schneiderman LJ. The futility debate: effective versus beneficial intervention. J Am Geriatr Soc 1994; 42(8): 883-6.
        [http://dx.doi.org/10.1111/j.1532-5415.1994.tb06564.x] [PMID: 8046201]

[12]    Brody BA, Halevy A. Is futility a futile concept? J Med Philos 1995; 20(2): 123-44.
        [http://dx.doi.org/10.1093/jmp/20.2.123] [PMID: 7636419]

[13]    Geppert CMA. Futility in chronic anorexia nervosa: a concept whose time has not yet come. Am J

Bioeth 2015; 15(7): 34-43.
[http://dx.doi.org/10.1080/15265161.2015.1039720] [PMID: 26147264]

[14]	Bagheri A. Medical Futility: A cross-national study. World Scientific 2013; p. 312.
[http://dx.doi.org/10.1142/p881]

[15]	Rubin SB. When doctors say no: The battleground of medical futility. Indiana University Press 1998.

[16]	Scofield GR. Medical futility: can we talk? Generations 1994; 18(4): 66-70.
[PMID: 11657021]

[17]	Wolf SM. Conflict between doctor and patient. Law Med Health Care 1988; 16(3-4): 197-203.
[http://dx.doi.org/10.1111/j.1748-720X.1988.tb01946.x] [PMID: 3205050]

[18]	Schneiderman LJ, Jecker NS, Jonsen AR. Medical futility: response to critiques. Ann Intern Med 1996; 125(8): 669-74.
[http://dx.doi.org/10.7326/0003-4819-125-8-199610150-00007] [PMID: 8849152]

[19]	Kon AA, Morrison W. Shared decision-making in pediatric practice: a broad view. Pediatrics 2018; 142 (Suppl. 3): S129-32.
[http://dx.doi.org/10.1542/peds.2018-0516B] [PMID: 30385618]

[20]	Haward MF, Kirshenbaum NW, Campbell DE. Care at the edge of viability: medical and ethical issues. Clin Perinatol 2011; 38(3): 471-92.
[http://dx.doi.org/10.1016/j.clp.2011.06.004] [PMID: 21890020]

[21]	Tl B, Childress J. Principles of biomedical ethics. New York: Oxford University Press 2009.

[22]	Sullivan A, Cummings C. Historical Perspectives: Shared Decision Making in the NICU. Neoreviews 2020; 21(4): e217-25.
[http://dx.doi.org/10.1542/neo.21-4-e217] [PMID: 32238484]

[23]	Franck L. Critical care decisions in fetal and neonatal medicene: Ethical issues. 2006.

[24]	Lemyre B, Moore G. Counselling and management for anticipated extremely preterm birth. Paediatr Child Health 2017; 22(6): 334-41.
[http://dx.doi.org/10.1093/pch/pxx058] [PMID: 29485138]

[25]	Dageville C, Bétrémieux P, Gold F, Simeoni U. The French Society of Neonatology's proposals for neonatal end-of-life decision-making. Neonatology 2011; 100(2): 206-14.
[http://dx.doi.org/10.1159/000324119] [PMID: 21471705]

[26]	Charles C, Gafni A, Whelan T. Shared decision-making in the medical encounter: What does it mean? (or it takes at least two to tango). Soc Sci Med 1997; 44(5): 681-92.
[http://dx.doi.org/10.1016/S0277-9536(96)00221-3] [PMID: 9032835]

[27]	Opel DJ. A 4-step framework for shared decision-making in pediatrics. Pediatrics 2018; 142 (Suppl. 3): S149-56.
[http://dx.doi.org/10.1542/peds.2018-0516E] [PMID: 30385621]

[28]	Schouten ES, Beyer MF, Flemmer AW, de Vos MA, Kuehlmeyer K. Conversations About End-o--Life Decisions in Neonatology: Do Doctors and Parents Implement Shared Decision-Making? Front Pediatr 2022; 10: 897014.
[http://dx.doi.org/10.3389/fped.2022.897014] [PMID: 35676897]

[29]	Davidson JE, Aslakson RA, Long AC, *et al.* Guidelines for family-centered care in the neonatal, pediatric, and adult ICU. Crit Care Med 2017; 45(1): 103-28.
[http://dx.doi.org/10.1097/CCM.0000000000002169] [PMID: 27984278]

[30]	Kon AA, Davidson JE, Morrison W, Danis M, White DB. Shared decision making in ICUs: an American College of critical care medicine and American thoracic Society policy statement. Crit Care Med 2016; 44(1): 188-201.
[http://dx.doi.org/10.1097/CCM.0000000000001396] [PMID: 26509317]

[31] Cohen S, Sprung C, Sjokvist P, *et al.* Communication of end-of-life decisions in European intensive care units. Intensive Care Med 2005; 31(9): 1215-21.
[http://dx.doi.org/10.1007/s00134-005-2742-x] [PMID: 16041519]

[32] Curtis JR, Tonelli MR. Shared decision-making in the ICU: value, challenges, and limitations. American Thoracic Society 2011; pp. 840-1.

[33] Akkermans AA, Lamerichs JMWJJ, Schultz MJM, *et al.* How doctors actually (do not) involve families in decisions to continue or discontinue life-sustaining treatment in neonatal, pediatric, and adult intensive care: A qualitative study. Palliat Med 2021; 35(10): 1865-77.
[http://dx.doi.org/10.1177/02692163211028079] [PMID: 34176357]

[34] Schloendorff V. Society of New York hospital. 211 NY 125, 105 NE 92 1914. Court of appeals of New York, 14th April 1914.

[35] Pellegrino ED. Futility in medical decisions: the word and the concept. HEC Forum 2005; 17(4): 308-18.
[http://dx.doi.org/10.1007/s10730-005-5156-9] [PMID: 16637443]

[36] Freeman L. Reconsidering relational autonomy: A feminist approach to selfhood and the other in the thinking of Martin Heidegger. Inquiry (Oslo) 2011; 54(4): 361-83.
[http://dx.doi.org/10.1080/0020174X.2011.592342]

[37] Donchin A. Understanding autonomy relationally: toward a reconfiguration of bioethical principles. J Med Philos 2001; 26(4): 365-86.
[http://dx.doi.org/10.1076/jmep.26.4.365.3012] [PMID: 11484130]

[38] Christman J. Relational autonomy, liberal individualism, and the social constitution of selves. Philos Stud 2004; 117(1/2): 143-64.
[http://dx.doi.org/10.1023/B:PHIL.0000014532.56866.5c]

[39] Mackenzie C, Stoljar N. Relational autonomy: Feminist perspectives on autonomy, agency, and the social self. Oxford University Press 2000.

[40] Zeiler K. On the autós of autonomous decision making: Intercorporeality, temporality, and enacted normativities in transplantation medicine. 2018.

[41] Merleau-Ponty M. The visible and the invisible Evanston. IL: North 1968.

[42] Merleau-Ponty M, Smith C. Phenomenology of perception. 1979.

[43] Shildrick M. Embodying the monster. Embodying the Monster 2001; pp. 1-154.

[44] Weise KL, Okun AL, Carter BS, *et al.* Guidance on forgoing life-sustaining medical treatment. Pediatrics 2017; 140(3): e20171905.
[http://dx.doi.org/10.1542/peds.2017-1905] [PMID: 28847979]

[45] Behrman RE, Field MJ. When children die: Improving palliative and end-of-life care for children and their families. Washington (DC): National Academies Press (US); 2003.

[46] MacDonald H, Fetus C. Perinatal care at the threshold of viability. Pediatrics 2002; 110(5): 1024-7.
[http://dx.doi.org/10.1542/peds.110.5.1024] [PMID: 12415047]

[47] Catlin A, Carter B. Creation of a neonatal end-of-life palliative care protocol. J Perinatol 2002; 22(3): 184-95.
[http://dx.doi.org/10.1038/sj.jp.7210687] [PMID: 11948380]

[48] Gilmour D, Davies MW, Herbert AR. Adequacy of palliative care in a single tertiary neonatal unit. J Paediatr Child Health 2017; 53(2): 136-44.
[http://dx.doi.org/10.1111/jpc.13353] [PMID: 27701795]

[49] Reid S, Bredemeyer S, Berg CVD, Cresp T, Martin T, Miara N. Palliative care in the neonatal nursery: Guidelines for neonatal nurses in Australia. Neonatal Paediatr Child Health Nurs 2011; 14(2): 2-8.

[50]  Mendel TR. The use of neonatal palliative care: Reducing moral distress in NICU nurses. J Neonatal Nurs 2014; 20(6): 290-3.
[http://dx.doi.org/10.1016/j.jnn.2014.03.004]

[51]  Kain VJ, Chin SD. Conceptually Redefining Neonatal Palliative Care. Adv Neonatal Care 2020; 20(3): 187-95.
[http://dx.doi.org/10.1097/ANC.0000000000000731] [PMID: 32384328]

[52]  Friedrich AB, Dempsey KM, Salter EK. The use of suffering in pediatric bioethics and clinical literature: A qualitative content analysis. Pediatric Ethicscope 2019; 32: 2.

[53]  Salter EK. The new futility? The rhetoric and role of "suffering" in pediatric decision-making. Nurs Ethics 2020; 27(1): 16-27.
[http://dx.doi.org/10.1177/0969733019840745] [PMID: 31032704]

[54]  Cassell EJ. The nature of suffering.The Oxford handbook of ethics at the end of life. 2016; pp. 216-26.

[55]  Cassell EJ. The nature of healing: The modern practice of medicine. Oxford University Press 2012.
[http://dx.doi.org/10.1093/acprof:oso/9780195369052.001.0001]

[56]  Tate T, Pearlman R. What we mean when we talk about Suffering—and why ERIC Cassell should not have the last word. Perspect Biol Med 2019; 62(1): 95-110.
[http://dx.doi.org/10.1353/pbm.2019.0005] [PMID: 31031299]

[57]  Brady MS. Suffering and virtue. Oxford University Press 2018.
[http://dx.doi.org/10.1093/oso/9780198812807.001.0001]

[58]  Waldman E. Children, fatal illness and the nature of suffering. Sci Am 2018.

[59]  Clément de Cléty S, Friedel M, Verhagen AAE, Lantos JD, Carter BS. Please do whatever it takes to end our daughter's suffering! Pediatrics 2016; 137(1): e20153812.
[http://dx.doi.org/10.1542/peds.2015-3812] [PMID: 26644491]

[60]  Tate T. Pediatric Suffering and the Burden of Proof. Pediatrics 2020; 146 (Suppl. 1): S70-4.
[http://dx.doi.org/10.1542/peds.2020-0818N] [PMID: 32737236]

[61]  Leder D. The absent body. University of Chicago Press 1990.

[62]  Zeiler K. A phenomenological analysis of bodily self-awareness in the experience of pain and pleasure: on dys-appearance and eu-appearance. Med Health Care Philos 2010; 13(4): 333-42.
[http://dx.doi.org/10.1007/s11019-010-9237-4] [PMID: 20162369]

[63]  Carel H. Illness: The Cry of the Flesh. Routledge 2008: p. 226.

[64]  Käll LF. Intercorporeality and the sharability of pain. Dimensions of pain. Routledge 2012; pp. 27-40.
[http://dx.doi.org/10.4324/9780203087381-13]

[65]  Bioethics AAPC. Ethics and the care of critically ill infants and children. Pediatrics 1996; 98(1): 149-52.
[http://dx.doi.org/10.1542/peds.98.1.149] [PMID: 8668392]

[66]  Chadwick J, Mann WN. The medical works of Hippocrates. Oxford Blackwell Scientific Publications 1950.

[67]  Jecker NS. Knowing when to stop: the limits of medicine. Hastings Cent Rep 1991; 21(3): 5-8.
[http://dx.doi.org/10.2307/3563315] [PMID: 1885297]

[68]  Lundberg GD. American health care system management objectives. The aura of inevitability becomes incarnate. JAMA 1993; 269(19): 2554-5.
[http://dx.doi.org/10.1001/jama.1993.03500190098045] [PMID: 8487424]

[69]  Dunn PM. Appropriate care of the newborn: ethical dilemmas. J Med Ethics 1993; 19(2): 82-4.
[http://dx.doi.org/10.1136/jme.19.2.82] [PMID: 8331642]

[70]  Lantos JD. Ethical Problems in Decision Making in the Neonatal ICU. N Engl J Med 2018; 379(19):

1851-60.
[http://dx.doi.org/10.1056/NEJMra1801063] [PMID: 30403936]

[71]　Bernat JL. Medical futility: definition, determination, and disputes in critical care. Neurocrit Care 2005; 2(2): 198-205.
[http://dx.doi.org/10.1385/NCC:2:2:198] [PMID: 16159066]

[72]　Chervenak FA, McCullough LB. Ethics in perinatal medicine: A global perspective.Seminars in Fetal and Neonatal Medicine. Elsevier 2015.
[http://dx.doi.org/10.1016/j.siny.2015.05.003]

[73]　Esserman L, Belkora J, Lenert L. Potentially ineffective care. A new outcome to assess the limits of critical care. JAMA 1995; 274(19): 1544-51.
[http://dx.doi.org/10.1001/jama.1995.03530190058034] [PMID: 7474223]

[74]　Atkinson S, Mason R, McColl LI, Bihari D, Smithies M, Daly K. Identification of futility in intensive care. Lancet 1994; 344(8931): 1203-6.
[http://dx.doi.org/10.1016/S0140-6736(94)90514-2] [PMID: 7934546]

[75]　Engelmann C, Thomsen KL, Zakeri N, *et al.* Validation of CLIF-C ACLF score to define a threshold for futility of intensive care support for patients with acute-on-chronic liver failure. Crit Care 2018; 22(1): 254.
[http://dx.doi.org/10.1186/s13054-018-2156-0] [PMID: 30305132]

[76]　Sachdeva RC, Jefferson LS, Coss-Bu J, Brody BA. Resource consumption and the extent of futile care among patients in a pediatric intensive care unit setting. J Pediatr 1996; 128(6): 742-7.
[http://dx.doi.org/10.1016/S0022-3476(96)70323-2] [PMID: 8648530]

[77]　Goh AY, Mok Q. Identifying futility in a paediatric critical care setting: a prospective observational study. Arch Dis Child 2001; 84(3): 265-8.
[http://dx.doi.org/10.1136/adc.84.3.265] [PMID: 11207181]

[78]　Graham S. Futile care in the neonatal intensive care unit: Is aggressive care always justifiable? J Neonatal Nurs 1999; 5: 23-6.

[79]　Lubitz JD, Riley GF. Trends in Medicare payments in the last year of life. N Engl J Med 1993; 328(15): 1092-6.
[http://dx.doi.org/10.1056/NEJM199304153281506] [PMID: 8455667]

[80]　Birnbaum M, Walleck CA. Rationing health care. Impact on critical care. Crit Care Clin 1993; 9(3): 585-602.
[http://dx.doi.org/10.1016/S0749-0704(18)30187-8] [PMID: 8353793]

[81]　Veatch RM. The ethics of resource allocation in critical care. Crit Care Clin 1986; 2(1): 73-89.
[http://dx.doi.org/10.1016/S0749-0704(18)30626-2] [PMID: 3135928]

[82]　Wolf SM, Boyle P, Callahan D, *et al.* Sources of concern about the patient self-determination act. N Engl J Med 1991; 325(23): 1666-71.
[http://dx.doi.org/10.1056/NEJM199112053252334] [PMID: 1944466]

[83]　Warrell DA, *et al.* Oxford textbook of medicine. Oxford University Press 2003.

[84]　Zarfin J, Aerde JV, Perlman M, Pape K, Chipman M. Predicting survival of infants of birth weight less than 801 grams. Crit Care Med 1986; 14(9): 768-72.
[http://dx.doi.org/10.1097/00003246-198609000-00002] [PMID: 3743094]

[85]　Lantos JD, Meadow W, Miles SH, *et al.* Providing and forgoing resuscitative therapy for babies of very low birth weight. J Clin Ethics 1992; 3(4): 283-7.
[http://dx.doi.org/10.1086/JCE199203406] [PMID: 1463880]

[86]　Eisenberg DM, Davis RB, Ettner SL, *et al.* Trends in alternative medicine use in the United States, 1990-1997: results of a follow-up national survey. JAMA 1998; 280(18): 1569-75.
[http://dx.doi.org/10.1001/jama.280.18.1569] [PMID: 9820257]

[87]     Ernst E. Prevalence of use of complementary/alternative medicine: a systematic review. Bull World Health Organ 2000; 78(2): 252-7.
[PMID: 10743298]

[88]     Ernst E, Willoughby M, Weihmayr T. Nine possible reasons for choosing complementary medicine. Perfusion 1995; 8(11): 356-9.

[89]     Cleary PD. Chiropractic use: a test of several hypotheses. Am J Public Health 1982; 72(7): 727-30.
[http://dx.doi.org/10.2105/AJPH.72.7.727] [PMID: 7091466]

[90]     Cook C, Baisden D. Ancillary use of folk medicine by patients in primary care clinics in southwestern West Virginia. South Med J 1986; 79(9): 1098-101.
[http://dx.doi.org/10.1097/00007611-198609000-00014] [PMID: 3749993]

[91]     McGuire MB, Kantor D. Ritual healing in suburban America. Rutgers University Press 1988.

[92]     Barakat LP, Kazak AE, Meadows AT, Casey R, Meeske K, Stuber ML. Families surviving childhood cancer: a comparison of posttraumatic stress symptoms with families of healthy children. J Pediatr Psychol 1997; 22(6): 843-59.
[http://dx.doi.org/10.1093/jpepsy/22.6.843] [PMID: 9494321]

[93]     Brigden ML. Unproven (questionable) cancer therapies. West J Med 1995; 163(5): 463-9.
[PMID: 8533410]

[94]     Borsi JD, Wesenberg F, Stokland T, Moe PJ. How much is too much? Folinic acid rescue dose in children with acute lymphoblastic leukaemia. Eur J Cancer Clin Oncol 1991; 27(8): 1006-9.
[http://dx.doi.org/10.1016/0277-5379(91)90269-J] [PMID: 1832883]

[95]     Faden RR, Beauchamp TL. A history and theory of informed consent. Oxford University Press 1986.

[96]     Lidz CW, Appelbaum PS, Meisel A. Two models of implementing informed consent. Arch Intern Med 1988; 148(6): 1385-9.
[http://dx.doi.org/10.1001/archinte.1988.00380060149027] [PMID: 3377623]

[97]     Making health care decisions. President's Commission for the Study of Ethical Problems in Medicine and Biomedical and Behavioral Research 1982; Vol. 1.

[98]     Frader J, Thompson A. Ethical issues in the pediatric intensive care unit. Pediatr Clin North Am 1994; 41(6): 1405-21.
[http://dx.doi.org/10.1016/S0031-3955(16)38879-4] [PMID: 7984392]

[99]     Vernon DD, Dean JM, Timmons OD, Banner W Jr, Allen-Webb EM. Modes of death in the pediatric intensive care unit. Crit Care Med 1993; 21(11): 1798-802.
[http://dx.doi.org/10.1097/00003246-199311000-00035] [PMID: 7802736]

[100]    Mink RB, Pollack MM. Resuscitation and withdrawal of therapy in pediatric intensive care. Pediatrics 1992; 89(5): 961-3.
[http://dx.doi.org/10.1542/peds.89.5.961] [PMID: 11654011]

[101]    Lantos JD, Berger AC, Zucker AR. Do-not-resuscitate orders in a children's hospital. Crit Care Med 1993; 21(1): 52-5.
[http://dx.doi.org/10.1097/00003246-199301000-00012] [PMID: 8420730]

[102]    Ryan CA, Byrne P, Kuhn S, Tyebkhan J. No resuscitation and withdrawal of therapy in a neonatal and a pediatric intensive care unit in Canada. J Pediatr 1993; 123(4): 534-8.
[http://dx.doi.org/10.1016/S0022-3476(05)80946-1] [PMID: 8410503]

[103]    Balfour-Lynn IM, Tasker RC. At the coalface--medical ethics in practice. Futility and death in paediatric medical intensive care. J Med Ethics 1996; 22(5): 279-81.
[http://dx.doi.org/10.1136/jme.22.5.279] [PMID: 8910779]

[104]    Tomlinson T, Brody H. Futility and the ethics of resuscitation. JAMA 1990; 264(10): 1276-80.
[http://dx.doi.org/10.1001/jama.1990.03450100066027] [PMID: 2388379]

[105]   Caplan AL, Blank RH, Merrick JC. Compelled compassion: Government intervention in the treatment of critically ill newborns. Springer Science & Business Media 2012.

[106]   Hardwig J. What about the Family? Hastings Cent Rep 1990; 20(2): 5-10.
[http://dx.doi.org/10.2307/3562603] [PMID: 2318632]

[107]   Strong C. The neonatologist's duty to patient and parents. Hastings Cent Rep 1984; 14(4): 10-6.
[http://dx.doi.org/10.2307/3561159] [PMID: 6237074]

[108]   Melton GB. Children's competence to consent.Children's competence to consent. Springer 1983; pp. 1-18.
[http://dx.doi.org/10.1007/978-1-4684-4289-2_1]

[109]   Weithorn LA, Campbell SB. The competency of children and adolescents to make informed treatment decisions. Child Dev 1982; 53(6): 1589-98.
[http://dx.doi.org/10.2307/1130087] [PMID: 7172783]

[110]   Annas GJ. Asking the courts to set the standard of emergency care--the case of Baby K. Mass Medical Soc. 1994; pp. 1542-5.

[111]   Knaus WA, Wagner DP, Lynn J. Short-term mortality predictions for critically ill hospitalized adults: science and ethics. Science 1991; 254(5030): 389-94.
[http://dx.doi.org/10.1126/science.1925596] [PMID: 1925596]

[112]   Chang RWS, Jacobs S, Lee B, Pace N. Predicting deaths among intensive care unit patients. Crit Care Med 1988; 16(1): 34-42.
[http://dx.doi.org/10.1097/00003246-198801000-00007] [PMID: 3123138]

[113]   Knaus WA, Draper EA, Wagner DP. The use of intensive care: new research initiatives and their implications for national health policy. Milbank Mem Fund Q Health Soc 1983; 61(4): 561-83.
[http://dx.doi.org/10.2307/3349873] [PMID: 6557371]

[114]   Rogers J, Fuller HD. Use of daily Acute Physiology and Chronic Health Evaluation (APACHE) II scores to predict individual patient survival rate. Crit Care Med 1994; 22(9): 1402-5.
[http://dx.doi.org/10.1097/00003246-199409000-00008] [PMID: 8062561]

[115]   Luce JM, Wachter RM. The ethical appropriateness of using prognostic scoring systems in clinical management. Crit Care Clin 1994; 10(1): 229-41.
[http://dx.doi.org/10.1016/S0749-0704(18)30158-1] [PMID: 8118731]

[116]   Burns JP, Edwards J, Johnson J, Cassem NH, Truog RD. Do-not-resuscitate order after 25 years. Crit Care Med 2003; 31(5): 1543-50.
[http://dx.doi.org/10.1097/01.CCM.0000064743.44696.49] [PMID: 12771631]

[117]   Fallat ME, Deshpande JK. Do-not-resuscitate orders for pediatric patients who require anesthesia and surgery. Pediatrics 2004; 114(6): 1686-92.
[http://dx.doi.org/10.1542/peds.2004-2119] [PMID: 15574636]

[118]   Sabouneh R, Lakissian Z, Hilal N, Sharara-Chami R. The State of the Do-Not-Resuscitate Order in a Pediatric Intensive Care Unit in the Middle East: A Retrospective Study. J Palliat Care 2022; 37(2): 99-106.
[http://dx.doi.org/10.1177/08258597211073228] [PMID: 35014894]

[119]   Postovsky S, Arush MWB. Care of a child dying of cancer: the role of the palliative care team in pediatric oncology. Pediatr Hematol Oncol 2004; 21(1): 67-76.
[http://dx.doi.org/10.1080/pho.21.1.67.76] [PMID: 14660308]

[120]   Singh J, Lantos J, Meadow W. End-of-life after birth: death and dying in a neonatal intensive care unit. Pediatrics 2004; 114(6): 1620-6.
[http://dx.doi.org/10.1542/peds.2004-0447] [PMID: 15574624]

[121]   Goldberg DS. The Ethics of DNR Orders as to Neonatal & (and) Pediatric Patients: The Ethical Dimension of Communication. Hous J Health L & Pol'y 2007; 7: 57.

[122] Garros D, Rosychuk RJ, Cox PN. Circumstances surrounding end of life in a pediatric intensive care unit. Pediatrics 2003; 112(5): e371-1.
[http://dx.doi.org/10.1542/peds.112.5.e371] [PMID: 14595079]

[123] Kisska-Schulze K, Holden JT. Betting on Education. Ohio St LJ 2020; 81: 465.

[124] Postovsky S, Levenzon A, Ofir R, Arush MWB. "Do not resuscitate" orders among children with solid tumors at the end of life. Pediatr Hematol Oncol 2004; 21(7): 661-8.
[http://dx.doi.org/10.1080/08880010490501088] [PMID: 15626022]

[125] van der Heide A, van der Maas PJ, van der Wal G, Kollée LAA, de Leeuw R, Holl RA. The role of parents in end-of-life decisions in neonatology: physicians' views and practices. Pediatrics 1998; 101(3): 413-8.
[http://dx.doi.org/10.1542/peds.101.3.413] [PMID: 9481006]

[126] Roy R, Aladangady N, Costeloe K, Larcher V. Decision making and modes of death in a tertiary neonatal unit. Arch Dis Child Fetal Neonatal Ed 2004; 89(6): F527-30.
[http://dx.doi.org/10.1136/adc.2003.032912] [PMID: 15499147]

[127] Einav S, Avidan A, Brezis M, Rubinow A. Attitudes of medical practitioners towards "Do Not Resuscitate" orders. Med Law 2006; 25(1): 219-28.
[PMID: 16681124]

[128] Doron MW, Veness-Meehan KA, Margolis LH, Holoman EM, Stiles AD. Delivery room resuscitation decisions for extremely premature infants. Pediatrics 1998; 102(3): 574-82.
[http://dx.doi.org/10.1542/peds.102.3.574] [PMID: 9738179]

[129] Fine RL, Whitfield JM, Carr BL, Mayo TW. Medical futility in the neonatal intensive care unit: hope for a resolution. Pediatrics 2005; 116(5): 1219-22.
[http://dx.doi.org/10.1542/peds.2004-2790] [PMID: 16264011]

[130] Hassan FM. "Do Not Resuscitate Order" By Competent Adults: The Legal Position in the United States and Canada Perspectives. Int J Humanit Soc Sci 2018; 8: 9.
[http://dx.doi.org/10.30845/ijhss.v8n9p6]

[131] Gibson K. Mediation in the medical field. Is neutral intervention possible? Hastings Cent Rep 1999; 29(5): 6-13.
[http://dx.doi.org/10.2307/3527730] [PMID: 10587804]

[132] Lang F, Floyd MR, Beine KL. Clues to patients' explanations and concerns about their illnesses. A call for active listening. Arch Fam Med 2000; 9(3): 222-7.
[http://dx.doi.org/10.1001/archfami.9.3.222] [PMID: 10728107]

[133] Bloche MG. Managing conflict at the end of life. N Engl J Med 2005; 352(23): 2371-3.
[http://dx.doi.org/10.1056/NEJMp058104] [PMID: 15944420]

[134] Dubler NN, Liebman CB. Bioethics mediation: A guide to shaping shared solutions. Vanderbilt University Press 2011.
[http://dx.doi.org/10.2307/j.ctv17z84h3]

[135] Levine C, Zuckerman C. The trouble with families: Toward an ethic of accommodation. American College of Physicians 1999; pp. 148-52.

[136] Bernat JL. Ethical issues in the perioperative management of neurologic patients. Neurol Clin 2004; 22(2): 457-471, 457-471.
[http://dx.doi.org/10.1016/j.ncl.2003.12.004] [PMID: 15062523]

[137] Goudreau JL, Wijdicks EFM, Emery SF. Complications during apnea testing in the determination of brain death: Predisposing factors. Neurology 2000; 55(7): 1045-8.
[http://dx.doi.org/10.1212/WNL.55.7.1045] [PMID: 11061269]

[138] Saposnik G, Bueri JA, Mauriño J, Saizar R, Garretto NS. Spontaneous and reflex movements in brain death. Neurology 2000; 54(1): 221-3.

[http://dx.doi.org/10.1212/WNL.54.1.221] [PMID: 10636153]

[139]  Wijdicks EFM, Rabinstein AA, Manno EM, Atkinson JD. Pronouncing brain death: Contemporary practice and safety of the apnea test. Neurology 2008; 71(16): 1240-4.
[http://dx.doi.org/10.1212/01.wnl.0000327612.69106.4c] [PMID: 18852438]

[140]  Goh AY-T, Mok Q. Clinical course and determination of brainstem death in a children's hospital. Acta Paediatr 2004; 93(1): 47-52.
[http://dx.doi.org/10.1111/j.1651-2227.2004.tb00673.x] [PMID: 14989439]

[141]  Gardiner D, Shemie S, Manara A, Opdam H. International perspective on the diagnosis of death. Br J Anaesth 2012; 108 (Suppl. 1): i14-28.
[http://dx.doi.org/10.1093/bja/aer397] [PMID: 22194427]

[142]  Neurology QSSAA. Practice parameters for determining brain death in adults. Neurology 1995; 45(5): 1012-4.
[http://dx.doi.org/10.1212/WNL.45.5.1012] [PMID: 7746374]

[143]  Wijdicks EFM, Varelas PN, Gronseth GS, Greer DM. Evidence-based guideline update: Determining brain death in adults: Report of the Quality Standards Subcommittee of the American Academy of Neurology. Neurology 2010; 74(23): 1911-8.
[http://dx.doi.org/10.1212/WNL.0b013e3181e242a8] [PMID: 20530327]

[144]  Nakagawa TA, Ashwal S, Mathur M, Mysore M. Clinical report—Guidelines for the determination of brain death in infants and children: an update of the 1987 task force recommendations. Pediatrics 2011; 128(3): e720-40.
[http://dx.doi.org/10.1542/peds.2011-1511] [PMID: 21873704]

[145]  Pope TM. Legal briefing: Brain death and total brain failure. J Clin Ethics 2014; 25(3): 245-7.
[http://dx.doi.org/10.1086/JCE201425309] [PMID: 25192349]

[146]  Shewmon DA. Constructing the death elephant: a synthetic paradigm shift for the definition, criteria, and tests for death. J Med Philos 2010; 35(3): 256-98.
[http://dx.doi.org/10.1093/jmp/jhq022] [PMID: 20439358]

[147]  Truog RD, Miller FG. Defining death: the importance of scientific candor and transparency. Intensive Care Med 2014; 40(6): 885-7.
[http://dx.doi.org/10.1007/s00134-014-3301-0] [PMID: 24807081]

[148]  Kirkpatrick JN, Beasley KD, Caplan A. Death is just not what it used to be. Camb Q Healthc Ethics 2010; 19(1): 7-16.
[http://dx.doi.org/10.1017/S096318010999020X] [PMID: 20025798]

[149]  Shah SK, Truog RD, Miller FG. Death and legal fictions. J Med Ethics 2011; 37(12): 719-22.
[http://dx.doi.org/10.1136/jme.2011.045385] [PMID: 21810923]

[150]  Truog RD, Miller FG. Changing the conversation about brain death. Am J Bioeth 2014; 14(8): 9-14.
[http://dx.doi.org/10.1080/15265161.2014.925154] [PMID: 25046286]

[151]  Baumann A, Audibert G, Guibet Lafaye C, Puybasset L, Mertes PM, Claudot F. Elective non-therapeutic intensive care and the four principles of medical ethics. J Med Ethics 2013; 39(3): 139-42.
[http://dx.doi.org/10.1136/medethics-2012-100990] [PMID: 23355225]

[152]  Salih MA, Harvey I, Frankel S, Coupe DJ, Webb M, Cripps HA. Potential availability of cadaver organs for transplantation. BMJ 1991; 302(6784): 1053-5.
[http://dx.doi.org/10.1136/bmj.302.6784.1053] [PMID: 2036502]

[153]  Browne A, Gillett G, Tweeddale M. Elective ventilation: reply to Kluge. Bioethics 2000; 14(3): 248-53.
[http://dx.doi.org/10.1111/1467-8519.00194] [PMID: 11658136]

[154]  Settergren G, MacHado C. Allow elective ventilation to recruit more organ donors. Acta Anaesthesiol Scand 2011; 55(3): 340-3.

[http://dx.doi.org/10.1111/j.1399-6576.2010.02386.x] [PMID: 21288217]

[155] DeVita MA, Brooks MM, Zawistowski C, Rudich S, Daly B, Chaitin E. Donors after cardiac death: validation of identification criteria (DVIC) study for predictors of rapid death. Am J Transplant 2008; 8(2): 432-41.
[http://dx.doi.org/10.1111/j.1600-6143.2007.02087.x] [PMID: 18190657]

[156] Puybasset L, Bazin JE, Beloucif S, *et al.* [Critical appraisal of organ procurement under Maastricht 3 condition]. Ann Fr Anesth Reanim 2012; 31(5): 454-61.
[http://dx.doi.org/10.1016/j.annfar.2012.02.009] [PMID: 22465653]

[157] Rady MY, Verheijde JL, McGregor JL. Scientific, legal, and ethical challenges of end-of-life organ procurement in emergency medicine. Resuscitation 2010; 81(9): 1069-78.
[http://dx.doi.org/10.1016/j.resuscitation.2010.05.007] [PMID: 20678461]

[158] Joris J, Kaba A, Lauwick S, *et al.* End of life care in the operating room for non-heart-beating donors: organization at the University Hospital of Liège. Transplant Proc 2011; 43(9): 3441-4.
[http://dx.doi.org/10.1016/j.transproceed.2011.09.034] [PMID: 22099816]

[159] Russell JA, Epstein LG, Greer DM, Kirschen M, Rubin MA, Lewis A. Brain death, the determination of brain death, and member guidance for brain death accommodation requests. Neurology 2019; 92(5): 228-32.
[http://dx.doi.org/10.1212/WNL.0000000000006750] [PMID: 31358673]

[160] Wahlster S, Wijdicks EFM, Patel PV, *et al.* Brain death declaration: Practices and perceptions worldwide. Neurology 2015; 84(18): 1870-9.
[http://dx.doi.org/10.1212/WNL.0000000000001540] [PMID: 25854866]

[161] Truog RD, Tasker RC. Counterpoint: should informed consent be required for apnea testing in patients with suspected brain death? Chest 2017; 152(4): 702-4.
[http://dx.doi.org/10.1016/j.chest.2017.05.032] [PMID: 28625580]

[162] Pope T. Brain death and the law: hard cases and legal challenges. Hastings Cent Rep 2018; 48 (Suppl. 4): S46-8.
[http://dx.doi.org/10.1002/hast.954] [PMID: 30584858]

[163] Robertson JA. Involuntary euthanasia of defective newborns: a legal analysis. Stanford Law Rev 1975; 27(2): 213-69.
[http://dx.doi.org/10.2307/1228265] [PMID: 1235925]

[164] Lewis A, Adams N, Chopra A, Kirschen MP. Organ support after death by neurologic criteria in pediatric patients. Crit Care Med 2017; 45(9): e916-24.
[http://dx.doi.org/10.1097/CCM.0000000000002452] [PMID: 28471816]

[165] Diekema D. Parental refusals of medical treatment: the harm principle as threshold for state intervention. Theor Med Bioeth 2004; 25(4): 243-64.
[http://dx.doi.org/10.1007/s11017-004-3146-6] [PMID: 15637945]

[166] Wilkinson D, Savulescu J. Ethics, conflict and medical treatment for children: From disagreement to dissensus. Elsevier 2018.

[167] Lee BM, Trowbridge A, McEvoy M, Wightman A, Kraft SA, Clark JD. Can a Parent Refuse the Brain Death Examination? Pediatrics 2020; 145(4): e20192340.
[http://dx.doi.org/10.1542/peds.2019-2340] [PMID: 32220905]

[168] Flamm AL, Smith ML, Mayer PA. Family members' requests to extend physiologic support after declaration of brain death: a case series analysis and proposed guidelines for clinical management. J Clin Ethics 2014; 25(3): 222-37.
[http://dx.doi.org/10.1086/JCE201425307] [PMID: 25192347]

[169] Morioka M. Reconsidering brain death: a lesson from Japan's fifteen years of experience. Hastings Cent Rep 2001; 31(4): 41-6.
[http://dx.doi.org/10.2307/3527955] [PMID: 12945466]

[170]   Tawil I, Brown LH, Comfort D, *et al.* Family presence during brain death evaluation: a randomized controlled trial. Crit Care Med 2014; 42(4): 934-42.
[http://dx.doi.org/10.1097/CCM.0000000000000102] [PMID: 24335446]

[171]   Hunfeld JAM, Wladimiroff JW, Passchier J, Uden MUV-V, Frets PG, Verhage F. Emotional reactions in women in late pregnancy (24 weeks or longer) following the ultrasound diagnosis of a severe or lethal fetal malformation. Prenat Diagn 1993; 13(7): 603-12.
[http://dx.doi.org/10.1002/pd.1970130711] [PMID: 8415426]

[172]   Schechtman KB, Gray DL, Baty JD, Rothman SM. Decision-making for termination of pregnancies with fetal anomalies: analysis of 53,000 pregnancies. Obstet Gynecol 2002; 99(2): 216-22.
[http://dx.doi.org/10.1097/00006250-200202000-00010] [PMID: 11814500]

[173]   Munson D, Leuthner SR. Palliative care for the family carrying a fetus with a life-limiting diagnosis. Pediatr Clin North Am 2007; 54(5): 787-798, xii.
[http://dx.doi.org/10.1016/j.pcl.2007.06.006] [PMID: 17933623]

[174]   Courtwright AM, Laughon MM, Doron MW. Length of life and treatment intensity in infants diagnosed prenatally or postnatally with congenital anomalies considered to be lethal. J Perinatol 2011; 31(6): 387-91.
[http://dx.doi.org/10.1038/jp.2010.124] [PMID: 21164425]

[175]   Czeizel AE. First 25 years of the Hungarian congenital abnormality registry. Teratology 1997; 55(5): 299-305.
[http://dx.doi.org/10.1002/(SICI)1096-9926(199705)55:5<299::AID-TERA1>3.0.CO;2-V]   [PMID: 9261923]

[176]   Dommergues M, Mandelbrot L, Mahieu-Caputo D, Boudjema N, Durand-Zaleski I. Termination of pregnancy following prenatal diagnosis in France: how severe are the foetal anomalies? Prenat Diagn 2010; 30(6): 531-9.
[http://dx.doi.org/10.1002/pd.2510] [PMID: 20509152]

[177]   Lewis S, McGillivray G, Rowlands S, Halliday J. Perinatal outcome following suspected fetal abnormality when managed through a fetal management unit. Prenat Diagn 2010; 30(2): 149-55.
[http://dx.doi.org/10.1002/pd.2431] [PMID: 20063325]

[178]   Goldenberg RL, Humphrey JL, Hale CB, Wayne JB. Lethal congenital anomalies as a cause of birth-weight-specific neonatal mortality. JAMA 1983; 250(4): 513-5.
[http://dx.doi.org/10.1001/jama.1983.03340040053032] [PMID: 6864951]

[179]   Milunsky A. Lethal congenital anomalies. JAMA 1983; 250(4): 517-8.
[http://dx.doi.org/10.1001/jama.1983.03340040057034] [PMID: 6864953]

[180]   Young ID, Clarke M. Lethal malformations and perinatal mortality: a 10 year review with comparison of ethnic differences. BMJ 1987; 295(6590): 89-91.
[http://dx.doi.org/10.1136/bmj.295.6590.89] [PMID: 3113647]

[181]   Wilkinson DJC, Thiele P, Watkins A, De Crespigny L. Fatally flawed? A review and ethical analysis of lethal congenital malformations. BJOG 2012; 119(11): 1302-8.
[http://dx.doi.org/10.1111/j.1471-0528.2012.03450.x] [PMID: 22827258]

[182]   Bhatia J. Palliative care in the fetus and newborn. J Perinatol 2006; 26(S1) (Suppl. 1): S24-6.
[http://dx.doi.org/10.1038/sj.jp.7211468] [PMID: 16625220]

[183]   Breeze ACG, Lees CC, Kumar A, Missfelder-Lobos HH, Murdoch EM. Palliative care for prenatally diagnosed lethal fetal abnormality. Arch Dis Child Fetal Neonatal Ed 2007; 92(1): F56-8.
[http://dx.doi.org/10.1136/adc.2005.092122] [PMID: 16705007]

[184]   Wilkinson DJC, Savulescu J. Knowing when to stop: futility in the ICU. Curr Opin Anaesthesiol 2011; 24(2): 160-5.
[http://dx.doi.org/10.1097/ACO.0b013e328343c5af] [PMID: 21293267]

[185]  Helft PR, Siegler M, Lantos J. The rise and fall of the futility movement. Mass Medical Soc. 2000; pp. 293-6.

[186]  Chervenak FA, McCullough LB. An ethically justified, clinically comprehensive management strategy for third-trimester pregnancies complicated by fetal anomalies. Obstet Gynecol 1990; 75(3 Pt 1): 311-6.
[PMID: 2304702]

[187]  Babnik J. Ethical decisions in the delivery room. Textbook of Perinatal Medicine. The Parthenon publishing group Ltd.: London 1998.

[188]  Chervenak FA, McCullough LB. The fetus as a patient: An essential ethical concept for maternal-fetal medicine. J Matern Fetal Med 1996; 5(3): 115-9.
[http://dx.doi.org/10.1002/(SICI)1520-6661(199605/06)5:3<115::AID-MFM3>3.0.CO;2-P]  [PMID: 8796779]

[189]  Barr M Jr, Cohen MM Jr. Holoprosencephaly survival and performance. Am J Med Genet 1999; 89(2): 116-20.
[http://dx.doi.org/10.1002/(SICI)1096-8628(19990625)89:2<116::AID-AJMG10>3.0.CO;2-4] [PMID: 10559767]

[190]  Fenton LJ. Trisomy 13 and 18 and quality of life: Treading "softly". Am J Med Genet A 2011; 155(7): 1527-8.
[http://dx.doi.org/10.1002/ajmg.a.34084] [PMID: 21671397]

[191]  Gabbay E, Calvo-Broce J, Meyer KB, Trikalinos TA, Cohen J, Kent DM. The empirical basis for determinations of medical futility. J Gen Intern Med 2010; 25(10): 1083-9.
[http://dx.doi.org/10.1007/s11606-010-1445-3] [PMID: 20645019]

[192]  Bell EF. Noninitiation or withdrawal of intensive care for high-risk newborns. Pediatrics 2007; 119(2): 401-3.
[http://dx.doi.org/10.1542/peds.2006-3180] [PMID: 17272630]

[193]  Brock DW. Life and Death: Philosophical Essays in Biomedical Ethics. Cambridge University Press 1993; 24: pp. 43-4.

[194]  Cassel EJ. The nature of suffering and the goals of medicine. N Engl J Med 1982; 306(11): 639-45.
[http://dx.doi.org/10.1056/NEJM198203183061104] [PMID: 7057823]

[195]  Wool C, Northam S. The Perinatal Palliative Care Perceptions and Barriers Scale Instrument©. Adv Neonatal Care 2011; 11(6): 397-403.
[http://dx.doi.org/10.1097/ANC.0b013e318233809a] [PMID: 22123471]

# SUBJECT INDEX

## A

Abnormalities 14, 15, 81, 108, 110, 111, 112, 118, 121, 122, 135, 184, 191, 193, 194, 195, 196, 215, 216
  central nervous system 135
  chromosomal 110, 194
  congenital 14, 15
  epileptiform 121
  genetic 191, 195
  metabolic 112
  neuroendocrine 196
  thyroid 81
Acidosis 120, 146, 147, 148, 149, 150, 152, 153, 157, 158, 162, 174, 176, 177
  lactic 153
  metabolic 120, 147, 148, 149, 150, 162, 174, 176, 177
  respiratory 158
Activation, sympathetic nervous system 218
Additional MH 39, 40
  problems 40
  risks 39
Additional neurologic symptoms 122
Agents 157, 160, 235, 251
  cardiotonic 157
  infectious 251
Airway malformations 187
Alcohol consumption 9, 12
Alkalosis, respiratory 149, 157
Amino acids 117
Aminoglycoside 160
Amniocentesis 13
Amniotic fluid 145, 146, 148, 149, 150, 153, 162, 170, 171, 173, 177
Applied behavior analysis (ABA) 224
Arrest 245, 248
  cardiac 248
  respiratory 245
Arrhythmias, fetal cardiac 149
Arrhythmogenic right ventricular dysplasia (ARVD) 132

Asthma, severe 7
Astrocytoma 185
Asymmetric opisthotonos position 250
Atelectasis 151, 154, 158, 162
Attention deficit 37, 38, 39, 41, 42, 45, 51, 60, 62, 85, 86, 214, 220
  and hyperactive disorder (ADHD) 37, 38, 39, 41, 42, 45, 51, 60, 62, 85, 86, 214, 220
  hyperactivity disorder 85, 214, 220
Autism 37, 38, 124, 210, 211, 212, 213, 214, 216, 218, 219, 220, 221, 224
  observation scale for infants (AOSI) 221
  spectrum disorder 37, 38, 124, 210, 211, 212, 213, 214, 216, 218, 219, 220, 224
Autistic spectrum disorders 6, 117
Autoimmune 81, 109
  encephalitis 109
  thyroiditis 81

## B

Bipolar disorder 214
Blood 160, 161
  deoxygenated 160
  oxygenated 161
Brain magnetic resonance spectroscopy 112

## C

Cancers 7, 14, 62, 82, 84, 87, 182, 183, 195, 200, 247
  breast 87, 195
  thyroid 14
Cardiac diseases in children 135
Cardiomyopathies 132, 135, 138
Cardio-pulmonary resuscitation (CPR) 243, 245, 246, 248
Cardiotocography 155
Cardiovascular diseases 12, 84, 85, 130, 131, 133, 134, 137, 138, 139, 140